Orthopedic Biomaterials in Research and Practice

Orthopedic Biomaterials in Research and Practice

Editor: Griffin Haynes

AMERICAN
MEDICAL PUBLISHERS
www.americanmedicalpublishers.com

AMERICAN
MEDICAL PUBLISHERS
www.americanmedicalpublishers.com

Cataloging-in-Publication Data

Orthopedic biomaterials in research and practice / edited by Griffin Haynes.
p. cm.
Includes bibliographical references and index.
ISBN 978-1-63927-775-9
1. Orthopedic implants--Materials. 2. Biomedical materials. 3. Orthopedic apparatus. 4. Orthopedics.
5. Biomedical engineering. I. Haynes, Griffin.
RD755.5 .O78 2023
617.95--dc23

American Medical Publishers,
41 Flatbush Avenue,
1st Floor, New York,
NY 11217, USA

ISBN 978-1-63927-775-9 (Hardback)

Contents

Preface

Every book is initially just a concept; it takes months of research and hard work to give it the final shape in which the readers receive it. In its early stages, this book also went through rigorous reviewing. The notable contributions made by experts from across the globe were first molded into patterned chapters and then arranged in a sensibly sequential manner to bring out the best results.

A biomaterial is a substance that has been created to take on a shape that can be employed either alone or as a component of a complex system. The biomaterials in orthopedics have progressed from temporary bone-fixing implants to durable implant materials and bioabsorbable implants. They are typically used in one of three surgical specialty categories, which include upper extremity, lower extremity or spine. Furthermore, each of these specialties is subdivided into three main categories, namely, reconstruction, pediatric and trauma. Technological and scientific advances in orthopedic surgery have led to the development of more sophisticated and advanced orthopedic biomaterials that have contributed in improving the quality of life for patients. This book elucidates new techniques related to the usage of orthopedic biomaterials. The readers would gain knowledge that would broaden their perspective about the recent studies on these biomaterials. This book will prove to be immensely beneficial to students and researchers in this field.

It has been my immense pleasure to be a part of this project and to contribute my years of learning in such a meaningful form. I would like to take this opportunity to thank all the people who have been associated with the completion of this book at any step.

Editor

1

Application of Zr and Ti-Based Bulk Metallic Glasses for Orthopaedic and Dental Device Materials

Kazuhiro Imai *, Xiao Zhou and Xiaoxuan Liu

Department of Life Sciences, Graduate School of Arts and Sciences, The University of Tokyo, Tokyo 153-8902, Japan; syuusyou1988@yahoo.co.jp (X.Z.); luluxxliu@gmail.com (X.L.)
* Correspondence: imai@idaten.c.u-tokyo.ac.jp

Abstract: Conventional orthopaedic and dental device materials are made of metallic materials such as stainless steel (SUS316L), titanium alloy (Ti-6Al-4V), and cobalt-chrome (Co-Cr). Those materials have the disadvantage of mechanical properties and anti-corrosion behavior. Bulk metallic glasses (BMGs), which are also called amorphous alloys, are metallic materials with metastable glassy states and have a higher strength, higher elasticity, higher failure resistance, and lower Young's modulus compared with crystalline alloys. There are several types of BMGs. Among them, Zr-based BMGs and Ti-based BMGs have excellent mechanical properties. In addition, they have good corrosion resistance and are promising for orthopaedic and dental device materials. In this review article, *in vitro* and *in vivo* studies regarding Zr and Ti-based BMGs applications as biomaterials, especially in orthopaedic and dental device materials, are reviewed.

Keywords: amorphous alloy; bulk metallic glasses; orthopaedic device; dental device; implant; anti-corrosion; biocompatibility

1. Introduction

Biomaterials are materials that are used for therapy and interact with biological systems. They are often used and adapted for medical and dental applications, and are in contact with body fluids, tissues, and cells. In case of organ or tissue damage, degeneration, or dysfunction, biomaterials are used as functional replacements. There are many device materials in which biomaterials are used, i.e., joint replacements, bone fixation devices, tooth fixation implants, blood vessel prostheses, and heart valves. Those device materials need to be non-toxic, anti-corrosion, strong, and tough because they are continuously receiving a reaction from biological systems and bearing daily loadings. In those conditions, metals as well as polymers or ceramics are used as biomaterials. Metals including stainless steel (SUS316L), titanium alloy (Ti-6Al-4V), and cobalt-chrome (Co-Cr) have the advantages of strength, toughness, and elasticity and are used in joint replacements, bone fixation devices, tooth implants, and heart pacemakers. Ceramics, including alumina, zirconia, and hydroxyapatite, have the advantages of strength and anti-abrasion and are used in joint replacements and tooth implants. Polymers, including polymethylmethacrylate (PMMA), silicone, and polyurethanes, have the advantages of workability and are lightweight. These polymers are used in catheters, vascular grafts, and intraocular lenses.

Some types of biomaterials have been made and applied as implanted device materials in medical and dental practice. Especially in orthopaedic fields, load bearing is essential and metallic materials mainly consist of SUS316L, Ti-6Al-4V, and Co-Cr, which are widely used because metals have high mechanical strength. However, there are several limitations when metallic implants are used for orthopaedic and dental device materials. When biomaterials are implanted into patients for bone fracture repairs, they are loaded repeatedly in daily activities. In addition, implanted biomaterials are in direct contact with body fluids and tissues. In those conditions, the implants are sometimes failed or broken by fretting corrosion fatigue [1,2]. To prevent failure or breakage, the devices or implants, such as bone plates or nails, have been made bulky enough. During surgery, long incision is needed to implant a bone plate. After the implantation, closing the skin wound is sometimes difficult. Likewise, to prevent nail failure, an intramedullary nail needs to have a large diameter. Such nails with a large diameter occupy a large area of the medullary canal and block the blood supply, which may incur fracture healing delay. In this way, strength deficiency of the conventional metallic devices is one of the disadvantages and limitations. Another limitation is that Young's moduli of conventional metallic devices are too high. Those metallic devices have the Young's modulus of 100–110 GPa, which is much higher than cortical bone of 15–20 GPa. Stress shielding occurs from the Young's modulus discrepancy between the osteo-synthetic device made of these materials and human bone, and sometimes leads to absorption of the bone around the material [3–7]. Regarding dental root implants, pure Ti and Ti-6Al-4V are universally used, but shielding effect is incurred by significant Young's modulus discrepancy between the Ti alloy and human bone. The stress shielding effect because of the implant's high Young's modulus has been shown as one of the major reasons of implant failure. In addition, SUS316L and Co-Cr release the toxic elements, such as Ni, Cr, and Co. Titanium alloys including Ti-6Al-4V have the disadvantage of low hardness and sometimes suffer from poor wear resistance.

Bulk metallic glasses (BMGs), which are also called amorphous alloys, are another type of metallic materials with metastable glassy states. Most metals are crystalline, which have an atomic structure with a highly ordered arrangement. On the other hand, BMGs have a glass-like structure and a state of non-crystalline. BMGs are prepared by extremely rapid cooling and solidification of melting liquid alloys. The speed of cooling and solidification is high enough. Therefore, the nucleation of crystals can be suppressed without a long-range atomic order. Due to their amorphous atomic structures, BMGs show unique mechanical, physical, and chemical properties and are superior to conventional metallic alloys, i.e., crystalline alloys. On the other hand, the crystalline alloy has grain boundaries, dislocations, and segregations, which are disadvantageous. When the crystalline alloy is subjected to loading, it can easily fail because of its grain boundaries and dislocations. The crystalline alloy has slip planes. Shear stress can move the atomic structure alongside the slip plane and lead to plastic deformation. The plastic deformation can also be enhanced by the dislocations.

In contrast, BMGs have a random and disordered atomic structure without segregations. In BMGs, there are no slip planes generated, and mass movement of the constituent atoms causes elastic deformation until it is under high stresses (Figure 1). As such, BMGs have higher strength, higher elasticity, higher failure resistance, and lower Young's modulus compared to crystalline alloys. With the combination of unique mechanical, physical, and chemical properties, BMGs have a wide range of potential applications including using biomaterials. In this review article, studies regarding Zr-based and Ti-based BMGs applications as biomaterials, especially in orthopaedic and dental device materials, are reviewed.

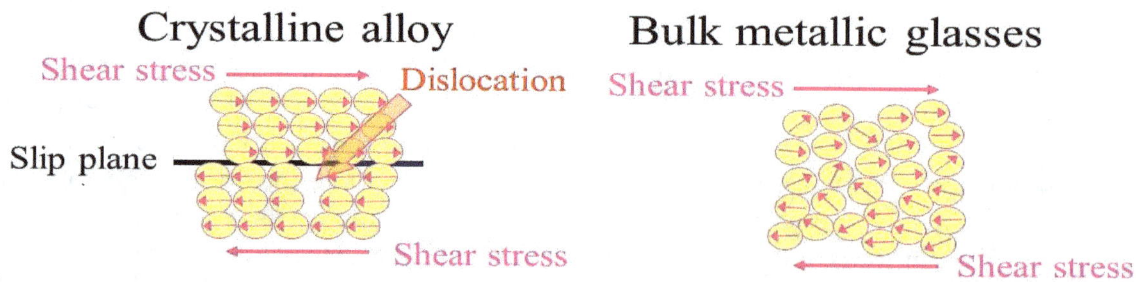

Figure 1. Atomic structures of crystalline alloy and bulk metallic glasses (BMGs). With shear stress, dislocation in a crystalline alloy causes plastic transformation. In BMGs, movement of the mass of atoms induces elastic transformation.

2. Classification of BMGs

BMGs with an amorphous atomic structure is formed as an alloy rather than a pure metal. Three basic rules to form BMGs have been reported [8]. The BMGs alloy constituent materials are made of at least three components. The components' atomic radiuses have to be significantly different to achieve low free volume and high packing density. Among the main constituent materials, the atomic radius of each other should have more than a 12% difference. Based on these basic rules of choosing the appropriate compositions, Mg, Ca, Sr, lanthanide metal (Ln), Ti, Zr, Hf, Fe, Co, Ni, Pd, Pt, Cu, and Au-based BMGs have been produced. Samples with more than 20 mm diameters have been produced based on Mg, Ln, Zr, Fe, Ni, Pd, Pt, and Cu-based BMGs [9–16].

The BMGs are classified into seven groups based on the main component, atomic size difference, and constituent elements [17], and G-I to G-VII (Table 1). Each group has several alloys. The representative of G-I is Zr-Al-Ni-Cu, G-II is Co-Fe-Ta-B, G-III is Fe-Al-Ga-P-C-B, G-IV is Zr-Ti-Be-Ni-Cu, G-V is Pd-Cu-Ni-P, G-VI is Ti-Zr-Cu-Ni, and G-VII is Ca-Mg-Cu, respectively. The radius of the main atom is the smallest in G-VI. In G-II and G-IV, the atomic radius of the main element is intermediate, and it is the largest in G-I, G-V, and G-VII. Properties of BMGs are dependent on the main constituent. The BMGs showed excellent corrosion resistance, high tensile strength, high elastic energy, high impact fracture energy, and excellent ductility for Zr-based BMGs [18] and good soft magnetic properties with high saturation magnetization and low coercivity for Fe-based and Co-based BMGs [19].

Table 1. Classification of bulk metallic glasses (BMGs).

Group	Representatives
I	Zr-Al-Ni, Zr-Al-Cu, Ln-Al-Ni, Ln-Al-Cu Zr-Al-Ni-Cu, Ln-Al-Ni-Cu, Zr-Ti-Al-Ni-Cu Zr-Ga-Ni, Ln-Ga-Ni, Ln-Ga-Cu
II	Fe-Zr-B, Fe-Hf-B Fe-Zr-Hf-B, Fe-Co-Ln-B Co-Zr-Nb-B, Co-Fe-Ta-B
III	Fe-(Al, Ga)-Metalloid
IV	Mg-Ln-Ni, Mg-Ln-Cu Zr-Ti-Be-Ni-Cu, Ti-Cu-Ni-Sn-Be, Ti-Cu-Ni-Sn-Be-Zr
V	Pd-Ni-P, Pd-Cu-Ni-P, Pt-Ni-P
VI	Cu-Zr-Ti, Ni-Nb-Ta, Ni-Nb-Sn Ti-Zr-Cu-Ni, Ti-Ni-Cu-Sn, Ti-Cu-Ni-Mo-Fe
VII	Ca-Mg-Cu, Ca-Mg-Zn

3. Mechanical Properties of Zr and Ti-Based BMGs

Zr-based BMGs have excellent corrosion resistance and wear resistance, high tensile strength, high elastic energy, and relatively low Young's modulus [20–23]. The ultimate tensile strengths of Zr-based BMGs are 1500–1700 MPa, which is approximately twice that of Ti-6Al-4V alloy and three times that of SUS316L [18,24–27]. The Young's moduli of Zr-based BMGs are 70–80 GPa, and are closer to Young's modulus of bone than conventional materials [28–31]. Zr-based BMGs show the fatigue strengths ranging from 560 to 980 MPa and the yield strengths ranging from 1500 to 1900 MPa [32]. The fatigue behavior was affected by the fabrication process, Poisson's ratio, and surface condition [33,34]. Mechanical properties, corrosion resistance, and cytotoxicity of Ni-free Zr-based BMGs were examined [35–37]. The ultimate compression strengths of $Zr_{60}Nb_5Cu_{22.5}Pd_5Al_{7.5}$ BMGs and $Zr_{60}Nb_5Cu_{20}Fe_5Al_{10}$ BMGs were 1724 and 1795 MPa, respectively. The Young's moduli of the BMGs were 70–85 GPa, and closer to Young's modulus of bone than conventional materials [35]. Yield strengths of $Zr_{50}Cu_{35}Al_7Nb_5Pd_3$ BMGs and $Zr_{55}Cu_{30}Al_7Nb_5Pd_3$ BMGs were 1806 and 1664 MPa, respectively. The Young's moduli of them were 88 and 86 GPa, respectively. The Zr-Cu-Al-Nb-Pd BMGs exhibited high Vickers hardness values (HV) above 4700 MPa [36]. $Zr_{60.14}Cu_{22.31}Fe_{4.85}Al_{9.7}Ag_3$ BMGs, sample rods of 2 mm diameter, also showed high fracture tensile strength of 1720 MPa, a relative low Young's modulus of 82 GPa, and high hardness values of 4200 MPa [37].

Mechanical properties of 316L stainless steel, Ti-6Al-4V alloy, Zr-based BMGs, and human bone are summarized in Table 2.

Table 2. Mechanical properties of 316L stainless steel, Ti-6Al-4V alloy, Zr-based bulk metallic glasses (BMGs), and human bone.

Mechanical Properties	Yield Strength (MPa)	Fracture Strength (MPa)	Young's Modulus (GPa)	Hardness (MPa)
316L stainless steel [25–27]	>175	190–690	200–203	3580
Ti-6Al-4V alloy [24,26,27]	853	950	108–116	3138
$Zr_{65}Al_{7.5}Ni_{10}Cu_{17.5}$ BMGs [18]	-	1500–1700	70–80	-
$Zr_{60}Nb_5Cu_{22.5}Pd_5Al_{7.5}$ BMGs [35]	1378	1724	70–85	-
$Zr_{60}Nb_5Cu_{20}Fe_5Al_{10}$ BMGs [35]	1393	1795	70–85	-
$Zr_{50}Cu_{35}Al_7Nb_5Pd_3$ BMGs [36]	1806	-	88	5060
$Zr_{55}Cu_{30}Al_7Nb_5Pd_3$ BMGs [36]	1664	-	86	4790
$Zr_{60.14}Cu_{22.31}Fe_{4.85}Al_{9.7}Ag_3$ BMGs [37]	-	1720	82	4200
Human bone (femur) [28–31]	80	120	15–20	-

Ti-based BMGs also have superior mechanical properties compared to crystalline Ti alloys (Table 3). The yield strengths of Ti-based BMGs are 2000 ± 78 MPa, which is approximately 2.5 times as much as the yield strength of pure titanium and Ti-6Al-4V alloy. The Young's moduli of Ti-based BMGs are 80 ± 12 GPa, and are closer to Young's modulus of bone than conventional biomaterials [38].

Table 3. Mechanical properties comparison of Ti-based BMGs, conventional biomaterials, and human bone.

Mechanical Properties	Yield Strength (MPa)	Young's Modulus (GPa)
316L stainless steel	>175	200–203
Ti-6Al-4V alloy	853	108–116
Pure titanium	800 ± 50	100 ± 7
Ti-based BMGs	2000 ± 78	80 ± 12
Human bone (femur)	80	15–20

4. *In Vitro* Studies for Biomaterial Applications

4.1. Zr-Based BMGs

Due to the properties with excellent corrosion resistance, high strength, high fatigue limit, and relative low modulus, Zr-based BMGs are promising for biomaterial applications. As *in vitro* experiments, $Zr_{65}Al_{7.5}Ni_{10}Cu_{17.5}$ BMGs in a phosphate buffered solution (PBS) were investigated to assess the effect of chloride-ion concentration and dissolved oxygen pressure on the polarization behavior. Zr-based BMGs showed high anti-corrosion performance in physiological environments [39–44]. To show biocompatibility, the electrochemical interactions, which result in the release of metal ions into the surrounding tissue, have been evaluated. Electrochemical characterization was performed at 37 °C in PBS electrolyte simulating conditions similar to *in vivo* [45]. Electrochemical cyclic-anodic-polarization tests were conducted and the corrosion penetration rate (CPR) values were estimated for $Zr_{52.5}Cu_{17.9}Ni_{14.6}Al_{10.0}Ti_{5.0}$ BMG, SUS316L, Co-Cr-Mo alloy, and Ti-6Al-4V [46]. The mean (±95% CIs) CPR values of $Zr_{52.5}Cu_{17.9}Ni_{14.6}Al_{10.0}Ti_{5.0}$ BMGs was 0.8 ± 0.4 μm/year, and significantly lower than the mean CPR values of SUS316L, which was 1.5 ± 0.4 μm/year. The result indicated that $Zr_{52.5}Cu_{17.9}Ni_{14.6}Al_{10.0}Ti_{5.0}$ BMGs demonstrated better corrosion resistance compared to SUS316L. However, CPR values of the Co-Cr-Mo alloy and Ti-6Al-4V were much lower (Co-Cr-Mo alloy, 0.3 ± 0.2 μm/year, Ti-6Al-4V; 0.3 ± 0.2 μm/year) and showed better corrosion resistance [45].

In vitro biocompatibility of $Zr_{41}Ti_{14}Cu_{12}Ni_{10}Be_{23}$ BMGs, $Zr_{44}Ti_{11}Cu_{10}Ni_{10}Be_{25}$ BMGs, and $Zr_{57}Nb_5Cu_{15.4}Ni_{12.6}Al_{10}$ BMGs were investigated by *in vitro* corrosion resistance evaluation and cytotoxicity evaluation with pure Ti and pure Zr as controls [47]. The BMGs were immersed in pH 7.4 simulated body fluid (SBF) and pH 6.3 artificial saliva (AS). As the result, all the immersed BMGs samples had better anti-corrosion properties in AS than in SBF, and corrosion resistance of $Zr_{44}Ti_{11}Cu_{10}Ni_{10}Be_{25}$ BMGs was comparable with pure Ti and pure Zr. The pitting corrosion potentials of $Zr_{44}Ti_{11}Cu_{10}Ni_{10}Be_{25}$ BMGs were much higher than that of pure Zr. The experiment to assess direct cytotoxicity showed that cells could adhere well on the Zr-based BMGs sample surface [47]. Most Zr-based BMGs contain Ni, which is commonly blamed of possible allergy occurrence and a possible carcinogenic factor for the human [48]. Therefore, Ni-free Zr-based BMGs might be more appropriate for biomaterial use.

Zr-based BMGs' corrosion behaviors in phosphate buffered solution were evaluated by electrochemical polarization and the excellent corrosion resistance was revealed [35–37]. The excellent corrosion resistance might come from the passive film formation on the surface. X-ray photoelectron spectroscopy (XPS) was used to assess the chemical compositions on the surface, and the oxide film formed on the surface of the Zr-based BMGs. The oxide film that consisted of ZrO_2, Al_2O_3, and Nb_2O_5 were observed [36,37]. The results indicated that the enriched oxides on the Zr-based BMGs surface might provide excellent anti-corrosion performance and prevention of corrosive reactions in phosphate buffered solution.

The Zr-based BMGs cytotoxicity evaluation by a one-week cell culture showed a good biocompatibility as Ti-6Al-4V [18,35]. Cell adhesions and morphologies after four hours of incubation showed the biocompatibility and biosafety [36]. Ni-free Zr-based BMGs showed good biocompatibility and biocorrosion *in vitro* study [49,50]. Powder consolidated $Zr_{76.6}Al_{3.5}Ni_{7.6}Cu_{12.3}$ BMGs, which showed fatigue strength equivalent to that of pure Ti [26]. An *in vitro* biocompatibility assessment of $Zr_{61}Ti_2Cu_{25}Al_{12}$ BMGs and cylindrical rods 6 mm in diameter for a potential application in dental implants showed that the in-cellular response for $Zr_{61}Ti_2Cu_{25}Al_{12}$ BMGs biocompatibility was comparable to Ti and Ti alloys [51]. The good biocompatibility and good corrosion-resistance in the physiological environment of $Zr_{61}Ti_2Cu_{25}Al_{12}$ BMGs was associated with the zirconium oxide layer formation on the surface.

4.2. *Ti-Based BMGs*

Rod-shaped $Ti_{40}Zr_{10}Cu_{38}Pd_{12}$ BMGs, which are 2.5 mm in diameter, showed a hardness value of 9400 MPa, which was much larger than that of the Ti-6Al-4V alloy of 3138 MPa [52]. *In vitro* test in Hank's solution of the $Ti_{40}Zr_{10}Cu_{38}Pd_{12}$ BMGs rod showed anti-corrosion performance as good as Ti-6Al-4V alloy. The performance of the $Ti_{40}Zr_{10}Cu_{38}Pd_{12}$ BMGs rod in the anodic region suggested the existence of wide passive regions, which were related to protective passive film formation. The mechanism of the high anti-corrosion performance of Ti-based BMGs was connected to the rapid formation of protective oxide films, mainly TiO_2, which were stable, continuous, and highly adherent on metal surfaces in a wide range of the corrosive region.

In vitro biocompatibility assessment of $Ti_{40}Cu_{38}Zr_{10}Pd_{12}$ BMGs, 3 mm in diameter for a potential application in orthopaedic implants, showed differentiation into osteoblasts and Cu ion release [53]. The low levels of inflammatory cytokines secretion showed the absence of an immunogenic response to the $Ti_{40}Cu_{38}Zr_{10}Pd_{12}$ BMGs. The biocompatibility assessment suggested that the $Ti_{40}Cu_{38}Zr_{10}Pd_{12}$ BMGs rod allow pre-osteoblasts to adhere to a mirror-like surface and to differentiate into osteoblasts under the appropriate culture conditions, which prevented the inflammatory response.

In vitro anti-corrosion and cytotoxicity assessment of $Ti_{41.5}Zr_{2.5}Hf_5Cu_{37.5}Ni_{7.5}Si_1Sn_5$ BMGs was investigated, with cylindrical rods 3 mm in diameter and a mirror-like surface for potential application in dental implants [54]. $Ti_{41.5}Zr_{2.5}Hf_5Cu_{37.5}Ni_{7.5}Si_1Sn_5$ BMGs showed great corrosion resistance in electrochemical measurements due to the oxide film that formed on its surface. Regarding pitting corrosion, anti-corrosion properties in artificial saliva (AS) solution were much higher than those in SBF solution. The cytotoxicity results showed that $Ti_{41.5}Zr_{2.5}Hf_5Cu_{37.5}Ni_{7.5}Si_1Sn_5$ BMGs had low cell viability on murine fibroblast cells. The BMGs have better anti-corrosion properties because of the lack of grain boundaries. In addition, $Ti_{41.5}Zr_{2.5}Hf_5Cu_{37.5}Ni_{7.5}Si_1Sn_5$ BMGs has a stable surface in the same level of pure Ti, which was attributed to the oxide film formed on the surface. As a promising dental implant material, $Ti_{41.5}Zr_{2.5}Hf_5Cu_{37.5}Ni_{7.5}Si_1Sn_5$ BMGs was found safe in the human body [54].

5. *In Vivo* Studies for Biomaterial Applications

Compared to abundant *in vitro* studies for BMGs biomedical applications, *in vivo* animal tests of BMGs are currently limited. However, the results of *in vivo* studies have shown that Zr-based BMGs and Ti-based BMGs are promising materials for orthopaedic and dental applications. All the animal tests were approved by the ethics committee of the institute based on the *in vitro* studies to prove the safety, anti-corrosion, and non-cytotoxicity of BMGs.

5.1. Animal Tests of Zr-Based BMGs

There are three types of Zr-based BMGs animal tests. The first type is the intramedullary nails in rat femora [55]. $Zr_{65}Al_{7.5}Ni_{10}Cu_{17.5}$ BMGs rods 2 mm in diameter and 40 mm in length were implanted as osteosynthesis intramedullary nails in rat femora after osteotomy (Figure 2). After 12 weeks implantation, systemic effects were investigated using the blood test. Local effects were investigated using graphite furnace atomic absorption spectroscopy. Removed implants were investigated using scanning electron microscopy (SEM) and energy dispersion X-ray spectroscopy (EDS). Osteotomy healings were investigated and compare $Zr_{65}Al_{7.5}Ni_{10}Cu_{17.5}$ BMGs with Ti-6Al-4V alloy using mechanical testing and peripheral quantitative computed tomography (pQCT) evaluation. From the results of systemic effects and local effects, there were no harmful effects after 12 weeks of implantation. The SEM (Figure 3) and EDS (Figure 4) results of the removed implants indicated that $Zr_{65}Al_{7.5}Ni_{10}Cu_{17.5}$ BMGs were almost biologically inert. The results of mechanical testing and pQCT evaluation indicated that $Zr_{65}Al_{7.5}Ni_{10}Cu_{17.5}$ BMGs had the tendency to get better osteotomy healing than the Ti-6Al-4V alloy even though the difference did not reach significance.

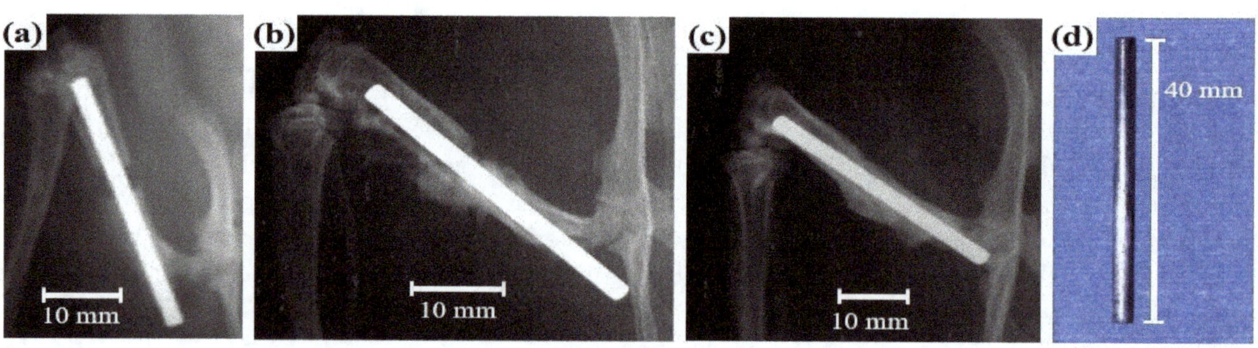

Figure 2. $Zr_{65}Al_{7.5}Ni_{10}Cu_{17.5}$ bulk metallic glasses (BMGs) rod implantation in rat femora after osteotomy as an intramedullary nail. (**a**) X-ray image of femoral bone immediately after osteotomy and BMGs intramedullary nail implantation. (**b**) X-ray image after implantation for six weeks. (**c**) X-ray image after implantation for 12 weeks. (**d**) Removed $Zr_{65}Al_{7.5}Ni_{10}Cu_{17.5}$ BMGs rod after 12 weeks of implantation.

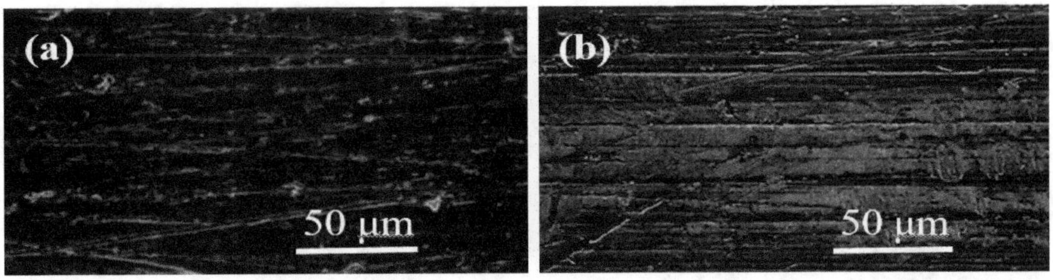

Figure 3. Scanning electron microscopy (SEM) images of $Zr_{65}Al_{7.5}Ni_{10}Cu_{17.5}$ BMGs rod (**a**) before and (**b**) after 12 weeks of implantation. Polishing scars were observed in both images. No reactions nor changes were observed after the *in vivo* experiment.

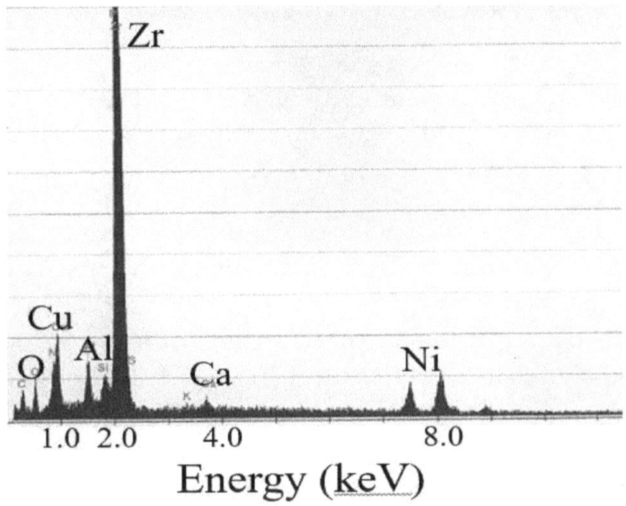

Figure 4. Energy dispersion X-ray spectroscopy (EDS) image of $Zr_{65}Al_{7.5}Ni_{10}Cu_{17.5}$ BMGs rod after 12 weeks of implantation. Oxygen (O) and calcium (Ca) were noted with the exception of Zr, Al, Ni, Cu. No element of corrosion was noted, which showed anti-corrosion behaviour.

The second type is the embedded samples in the rabbit femora [56]. Zr-Cu-Al-Ag BMGs cylindrical rods 2 mm in diameter and 6 mm in length were implanted to evaluate the *in vivo* biocompatibility. After four weeks, eight weeks, and 12 weeks of implantation, removed implants were observed via SEM equipped with EDS. Tissues around the implant were investigated through a histological examination. After eight weeks and 12 weeks of implantation, no gap could be observed between the bone tissue and implant samples, which indicated that Zr-Cu-Al-Ag BMGs exhibits new bone formation and excellent *in vivo* biocompatibility. There were no inflammatory reactions or osteonecrosis changes.

The third type is the sub-periosteal implanted on the bone surface of rat femora [57,58]. $Zr_{65}Al_{7.5}Ni_{10}Cu_{17.5}$ BMGs ribbons 10 mm in length, 2 mm in width, and 0.5 mm in thickness were implanted on the bone surface for six weeks (Figure 5). After the implantation, systemic effects were investigated using a blood test. Femur and soft tissues around the implant were investigated through a histological examination. Removed implants were investigated using SEM equipped with EDS. The results show that blood levels of Cu and Ni did not increase, and no findings of the biological effects were recognized including cell necrosis or dysplasia, infiltration of inflammatory cells, bone resorption, and wear debris of the alloy. Regarding removed implants, there were no findings of breakage nor pitting corrosion.

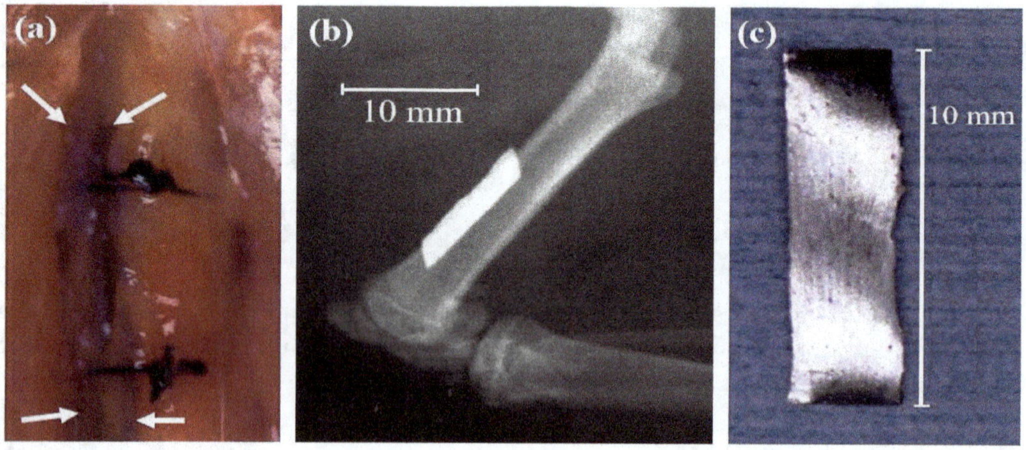

Figure 5. $Zr_{65}Al_{7.5}Ni_{10}Cu_{17.5}$ BMGs ribbon sub-periosteal implantation on the bone surface of rat femoral bone. (**a**) BMGs ribbon (arrows) was implanted and tied to the femoral bone with 4-0 nylon suture string. (**b**) The X-ray image after implantation for six weeks. (**c**) Removed $Zr_{65}Al_{7.5}Ni_{10}Cu_{17.5}$ BMGs ribbon after six weeks of implantation.

Among the three types of Zr-based BMGs *in vivo* animal tests, there were no sign of systemic effects, local inflammatory reactions or osteonecrosis changes, and breakage or pitting corrosion of the implants. The first study and the second study revealed that Zr-based BMGs had good biocompatibility. The first study showed the Zr-based BMGs implant as an osteosynthesis device. Osteotomy healing occurred as fast as the Ti-6Al-4V alloy. The first and the third study concluded that Zr-based BMGs implants were nearly biologically inert and were promising for eventually removed osteosynthesis devices. On the other hand, the second study concluded that the Zr-based BMGs implant shows excellent new bone formation around the implant, which might be suitable for osteosynthesis devices that are implanted eternally. Zr-based BMGs implants are promising, especially in orthopaedic and dental device materials, but further investigation will be needed to know whether Zr-based BMGs implants should be implanted temporally or eternally.

5.2. Animal Tests of Ti-Based BMGs

There are three types of Ti-based BMG animal tests. The first type is the dental material in beagle dog's mandible [54]. $Ti_{41.5}Zr_{2.5}Hf_5Cu_{37.5}Ni_{7.5}Si_1Sn_5$ BMGs samples 3 mm in diameter and 5 mm in length were implanted in one side of the beagle dogs' mandible for one month. There was no inflammation observed around the BMGs sample. The histological examination and EDS analysis showed that the $Ti_{41.5}Zr_{2.5}Hf_5Cu_{37.5}Ni_{7.5}Si_1Sn_5$ BMGs samples are well integrated with the bone tissue and new bone was formed around the samples, which proved the *in vivo* biocompatibility [54].

The second type is the $Ti_{40}Zr_{10}Cu_{34}Pd_{14}Sn_2$ BMGs alloy bar in rat femora implanted for three months [59]. The Ti-based BMGs sample showed good compatibility with bone integration ability, and no component material ion diffusion, which indicated that the Ti-based BMGs is promising for bone implants.

The third type is the implanted material in the cavity of rat tibial tubercle [60]. $Ti_{45}Zr_{40}Si_{15}$, $Ti_{40}Zr_{40}Si_{15}Cu_5$, and $Ti_{45}Zr_{20}Cu_{35}$ BMGs ribbons with 6 mm in length, 3 mm in width, and 1.0-1.5 mm in thickness were implanted for 3, 6, and 12 weeks. There were no findings of septic or inflammatory reactions. The X-ray photographs showed that the thin callus layer and woven bone were formed directly on the BMGs ribbons, which explained good biocompatibility. The SEM images of $Ti_{45}Zr_{20}Cu_{35}$ BMGs ribbons showed the presence of significant small cavities in the cortical tibial bone. The sample implanted with $Ti_{45}Zr_{40}Si_{15}$ BMGs ribbons had a high cortical bone density. Therefore, Cu-free $Ti_{45}Zr_{40}Si_{15}$ BMGs has good potential for biomaterials in orthopaedic and dental device materials.

5.3. *Animal Tests of Mg-Based, Sr-Substituted, and Nanopatterned Pt-Based BMGs*

Besides Zr and Ti-based BMGs that are non-biodegradable, there are Mg, Zn, Ca, and Sr-based BMGs, which are biodegradable. Biodegradable materials are useful to apply as orthopaedic materials such as absorbable screws and artificial bones. However, biodegradable materials inevitably cause reactions between the implants and the tissues. Therefore, biocompatibility of biodegradable BMGs should be evaluated by *in vivo* animal tests.

$Mg_{60}Zn_{35}Ca_5$ BMGs were implanted in rabbit femur as a tendon-bone interference fixation model for 24 weeks [61] compared to the Ti-6Al-4V alloy and polylactic acid (PLA). After 24 weeks of implantation, no inflammatory cells such as leukocytes or macrophages were observed in all of $Mg_{60}Zn_{35}Ca_5$ BMGs, Ti-6Al-4V alloy, and PLA, which indicates the good biocompatibility of $Mg_{60}Zn_{35}Ca_5$ BMGs. Micro-CT images and histology observation showed new bone formation surrounding the $Mg_{60}Zn_{35}Ca_5$ BMGs and the Ti-6Al-4V alloy. In addition, more sustainable osteo-promoting effects were found in $Mg_{60}Zn_{35}Ca_5$ BMGs when compared to the Ti-6Al-4V alloy after 24 weeks of implantation.

Strontium-substituted SiO_2-Al_2O_3-P_2O_5-CaO-CaF_2 BMGs were implanted in bone defects of rabbit femur for 26 weeks [62]. There was no finding of an adverse effect including inflammation or necrosis. There was some evidence of good bone regeneration and a remodeling process in bone defects. Newly formed bone is integrated between Strontium-substituted BMGs and the host bone. These findings indicated the good biocompatibility of Strontium-substituted BMGs and the possibility of application as artificial bone or a bioactive implant-like hydroxyapatite (HA) implant.

Nanopatterned Pt-based BMGs biomaterials were implanted subcutaneously in mice for two weeks and four weeks, with the nano-patterned side facing the dermis [63]. After two weeks of implantation, the ratio of Arg-1 to iNOS expression of macrophages adjacent to 55 nanometer (nm) nano-patterned BMGs (BMG-55) implants increased significantly compared to flat BMGs. Macrophage fusion with fibrous capsule thickness declined after four weeks of implantation. In addition, the vessel's number and size in tissues surrounding BMG-55 implants increased in two weeks of implantation and decreased in four weeks of implantation. The results indicated nano-patterning of BMG implants as a promising method to modulate macrophage polarization for the immune response. Surface roughness and biochemical composition of BMGs might affect biocompatibility, cell responses, and immune response.

6. Anti-Corrosion Behavior and Biocompatibility of a BMGs Implant for Biomaterial Applications

To apply the BMGs' implant for orthopaedic and dental biomaterials, anti-corrosion behavior and biocompatibility are greatly important and should be evaluated. When the implant of particular material is contact with tissues, the cell biological activity for the implant and material degradation in the body environment may occur. These could lead the constituent metal ions or implant particles to release into the body and cause reactions including allergic and toxic ones. Through *in vitro* tests and *in vivo* animal tests, Zr-based BMGs and Ti-based BMGs have been shown to have excellent anti-corrosion behavior and biocompatibility. Based on these *in vitro* tests and *in vivo* animal tests, Zr-based BMGs and Ti-based BMGs may be promising biomaterials.

7. Biomaterials for Dental Device Materials

When dealing with biomaterials for dental implants, adhesiveness of the implant surfaces to oral bacteria should be reviewed. In the oral environment, dental implants are easily accessible to microbial contamination. Key points regarding bacterial adherence is biofilm formation on biomaterial implants [64]. Biofilm formation functions to protect from antibiotics, which causes threats of infecting the biomaterial implants. Biofilm growth is controlled by physical, chemical, and biological factors. Extra polysaccharide substances control the binding and cell adhesion to the implant surface. The extra polysaccharide substances act as a barrier and protects the microbes during adverse conditions. The biological behavior depends on the chemical composition as well as morphology of the implant surface. To improve surface properties of biomedical implants, various trials using physical and chemical techniques have been attempted. These trials aim to facilitate bio-integration and prevent bacterial adhesion. Controlling bacterial adhesion, biofilm formation, and biofilm-associated infection are essential to prevent infection surrounding dental implants.

Biofilm formation is directly influenced by electrostatic interactions between bacteria and chemical composition of the implant surface. ZrO_2 and Ti are hydrophobic materials, which attract forces and electrostatic charge interactions between bacteria and the implant surface and prevent bacterial adhesion. The influence of physical and chemical characteristics of ZrO_2 and Ti surfaces on bacterial adhesion were investigated when compared to bovine enamel simulating human oral tooth [65]. In the study, Streptococcus mutans (S. mutans) and Porphyromonas gingivalis (P. gingivalis) were used as common pathogens of the oral cavity. The results of surface hydrophobicity on bacterial adhesion indicated that ZrO_2 and Ti surfaces could prevent bacterial adhesion more than bovine enamel for both S. mutans and P. gingivalis. Accordingly, Zr-based and Ti-based BMGs are good candidates for dental device materials or implant abutment surfaces. Further *in vitro* and *in vivo* tests using Zr-based and Ti-based BMGs are needed to discuss the prevention of infection surrounding dental implants.

8. Conclusions and Prospects for the Future

A recent article showed potentials of Ti, Zr, Fe, Mg, Zn, Ca, and Sr-based BMGs in biomedical applications [66]. This article specializes in Zr-based and Ti-based BMGs, which are non-biodegradable, higher strength, higher elasticity, higher failure resistance, and lower Young's modulus compared with crystalline alloys. This article also refers to dental applications including adhesiveness of material surfaces to oral bacteria. BMGs have great potentials in biomedical applications especially as orthopaedic and dental device materials. Zr-based BMGs and Ti-based BMGs have both excellent mechanical properties and corrosion resistance. Those BMGs can be used as orthopaedic and dental device materials, such as implanted pins, screws, plates, nails, and dental implants. They can also be used as minimally invasive surgical devices. Orthopaedic and dental device materials are needed to survive in a harsh human body environment for a long time. Anti-corrosion behavior and biocompatibility of Zr-based BMGs and a Ti-based BMGs implant have been proven through *in vitro* tests and *in vivo* animal tests.

One of the problems of the current BMGs, the limited diameter sizes restrain the design and types of biomedical devices using BMGs. One promising measure to solve the limited components size of BMGs is a thin film form of Zr-based and Ti-based BMGs. Metallic glass coating using thin film form onto the substrate of biomedical devices might widen the design and types of implants. A thin film form of Zr-based and Ti-based BMGs can exhibit a combination of large mechanical properties with good biocompatibility [67] and cytocompatibility [68]. In addition, a thin film form of Zr-based BMGs showed size effects on mechanical properties, which can be used as coatings for biomedical applications [69,70]. In addition, future technology might overcome the size limitation. When BMGs with larger sizes are obtained, further *in vivo* animal tests of BMGs pins, screws, plates, nails, and dental implants can be proceeded, which may lead to clinical application as orthopaedic and dental device materials.

The other problem of BMGs is the localization of deformation within shear bands reporting a brittle-like failure behavior. This limitation is extremely important especially for *in vivo* applications, which directly connects with clinical application as orthopaedic and dental device materials. This mechanical property of BMGs could restrain the clinical application. To coat a metallic glass with a thin film form of BMGs onto the substrate of biomedical devices might solve this problem. For future work in this field, metallic glass coating techniques with a thin film form of BMGs including *in vitro* and *in vivo* studies are recommended.

Author Contributions: K.I. designed the study. K.I. and X.Z. contributed to data acquisition. K.I. drafted the manuscript. X.Z. checked and revised the manuscript. X.L. contributed to the English proofreading. All authors have read and agreed to the published version of the manuscript.

Acknowledgments: The authors are grateful to Takao Hanawa, Sachiko Hiromoto and Isao Ohnishi for valuable discussions.

References

1. Antunes, R.A.; de Oliveira, M.C. Corrosion processes of physical vapor deposition-coated metallic implants. *Crit. Rev. Biomed. Eng.* **2009**, *37*, 425–460. [CrossRef] [PubMed]
2. Whitaker, R.A. Environmental effects on the life of bone-plate-type surgical implants. *Rev. Environ. Health* **1982**, *4*, 63–82.
3. Molster, A.O. Biomechanical effects of intramedullary reaming and nailing on intact femora in rats. *Clin. Orthop.* **1986**, *202*, 278–285.
4. Bradley, G.W.; McKenna, G.B.; Dunn, H.K.; Daniels, A.U.; Statton, W.O. Effects of flexural rigidity of plates on bone healing. *J. Bone Joint Surg. Am.* **1979**, *61*, 866–872. [CrossRef] [PubMed]
5. Woo, S.L.; Akeson, W.H.; Coutts, R.D.; Rutherford, L.; Doty, D.; Jemmott, G.F.; Amiel, D. A comparison of cortical bone atrophy secondary to fixation with plates with large differences in bending stiffness. *J. Bone Joint Surg. Am.* **1976**, *58*, 190–195. [CrossRef] [PubMed]
6. Tonino, A.J.; Davidson, C.L.; Klopper, P.J.; Linclau, L.A. Protection from stress in bone and its effects. Experiments with stainless steel and plastic plates in dogs. *J. Bone Joint Surg. Br.* **1976**, *58*, 107–113. [CrossRef]
7. Uhthoff, H.K.; Dubuc, F.L. Bone structure changes in the dog under rigid internal fixation. *Clin. Orthop.* **1971**, *81*, 165–170. [CrossRef]
8. Inoue, A. Stabilization of supercooled liquid and opening-up of bulk glassy alloys. *Proc. Jpn. Acad. Ser. B* **1997**, *73*, 19–24. [CrossRef]
9. Inoue, A.; Zhang, T. Fabrication of Bulk Glassy $Zr_{55}Al_{10}Ni_5Cu_{30}$ Alloy of 30 mm in Diameter by a Suction Casting Method. *Mater. Trans.* **1996**, *37*, 185–187. [CrossRef]
10. Inoue, A.; Nishiyama, N.; Kimura, H. Preparation and thermal stability of bulk amorphous $Pd_{40}Cu_{30}Ni_{10}P_{20}$ alloy cylinder of 72 mm in diameter. *Mater. Trans.* **1997**, *38*, 179–183. [CrossRef]
11. Zhang, W.; Inoue, A. Formation and mechanical strength of new Cu-based bulk glassy alloys with large supercooled liquid region. *Mater. Trans.* **2004**, *45*, 1210–1213. [CrossRef]
12. Schroers, J.; Johnson, W.L. Highly processable bulk metallic glass-forming alloys in the Pt–Co–Ni–Cu–P system. *Appl. Phys. Lett.* **2004**, *84*, 3666–3668. [CrossRef]
13. Zheng, Q.; Xu, J.; Ma, E. High glass-forming ability correlated with fragility of Mg–Cu(Ag)–Gd alloys. *J. Appl. Phys.* **2007**, *102*, 113519-1–113519-5. [CrossRef]
14. Li, R.; Pang, S.; Ma, C.; Zhang, T. Influence of similar atom substitution on glass formation in (La–Ce)–Al–Co bulk metallic glasses. *Acta Mater.* **2007**, *55*, 3719–3726. [CrossRef]
15. Yokoyama, Y.; Mund, E.; Inoue, A.; Schultz, L. Production of $Zr_{55}Cu_{30}Ni_5Al_{10}$ glassy alloy rod of 30 mm in diameter by a cap-cast technique. *Mater. Trans.* **2007**, *48*, 3190–3192. [CrossRef]
16. Zeng, Y.; Nishiyama, N.; Yamamoto, T.; Inoue, A. Ni-Rich bulk metallic glasses with high glass-forming ability and good metallic properties. *Mater. Trans.* **2009**, *50*, 2441–2445. [CrossRef]
17. Takeuchi, A.; Inoue, A. Classification of bulk metallic glasses by atomic size difference, heat of mixing and period of constituent elements and its application to characterization of the main alloying element. *Mater. Trans.* **2005**, *46*, 2817–2829. [CrossRef]
18. Inoue, A.; Zhang, T.; Masumoto, T. Preparation of bulky amorphous Zr-Al-Ni-Cu alloys by copper mold casting and their thermal and mechanical properties. *Mater. Trans. JIM* **1995**, *36*, 391–398. [CrossRef]
19. Wang, W.H. Roles of minor additions in formation and properties of bulk metallic glasses. *Prog. Mater. Sci.* **2007**, *52*, 540–596. [CrossRef]
20. Gilbert, C.J.; Ritchie, R.O.; Johnson, W.L. Fracture toughness and fatigue-crack propagation in a Zr-Ti-Ni-Cu-Be bulk metallic glass. *Appl. Phys. Lett.* **1997**, *71*, 476–478. [CrossRef]

21. Pang, S.J.; Zhang, T.; Kimura, H.; Asami, K.; Inoue, A. Corrosion behavior of Zr-(Nb-)Al-Ni-Cu glassy alloys. *Mater. Trans. JIM* **2000**, *41*, 1490–1494. [CrossRef]
22. Wang, J.G.; Choi, B.M.; Nieh, T.G.; Liu, C.T. Nano-scratch behavior of a bulk Zr-10Al-5Ti-17.9Cu-14.6Ni amorphous alloy. *J. Mater. Res.* **2000**, *15*, 913–922. [CrossRef]
23. Liu, L.; Qiu, C.L.; Zou, H.; Chan, K.C. The effect of the microalloying of Hf on the corrosion behavior of ZrCuNiAl bulk metallic glass. *J. Alloys Compd.* **2005**, *399*, 144–148. [CrossRef]
24. Boyer, R.; Welsch, G.; Collings, E.W. Titanium Alloys. In *Materials Properties Handbook*; ASM International: Materials Park, OH, USA, 1994.
25. Hanawa, T.; Yoneyama, T. Metals. In *Biomaterials*; Corona Publishing CO., LTD.: Tokyo, Japan, 2007.
26. Long, M.; Rack, H.J. Titanium alloys in total joint replacement—A materials science perspective. *Biomaterials* **1998**, *19*, 1621–1639. [CrossRef]
27. Niinomi, M. Mechanical properties of biomedical titanium alloys. *Mater. Sci. Eng. A* **1998**, *243*, 231–236. [CrossRef]
28. Katsamanis, F.; Raftopoulos, D.D. Determination of mechanical properties of human femoral cortical bone by the Hopkinson bar stress technique. *J. Biomech.* **1990**, *23*, 1173–1184. [CrossRef]
29. Choi, K.; Kuhn, J.L.; Ciarelli, M.J.; Goldstein, S.A. The elastic moduli of human subchondral, trabecular, and cortical bone tissue and the size-dependency of cortical bone modulus. *J. Biomech.* **1990**, *23*, 1103–1113. [CrossRef]
30. Kopperdahl, D.L.; Keaveny, T.M. Yield strain behavior of trabecular bone. *J. Biomech.* **1998**, *31*, 601–608. [CrossRef]
31. Turner, C.H.; Wang, T.; Burr, D.B. Shear strength and fatigue properties of human cortical bone determined from pure shear tests. *Calcif. Tissue Int.* **2001**, *69*, 373–378. [CrossRef]
32. Wang, G.Y.; Liaw, P.K.; Yokoyama, Y.; Inoue, A.; Liu, C.T. Fatigue behavior of Zr-based bulk-metallic glasses. *Mater. Sci. Eng. A* **2008**, *494*, 314–323. [CrossRef]
33. Maruyama, N.; Nakazawa, K.; Hanawa, T. Fatigue properties of Zr-based amorphous alloy in phosphate buffered saline solution. *Mater. Trans.* **2002**, *43*, 3118–3121. [CrossRef]
34. Wang, G.; Liaw, P.K.; Yokoyama, Y.; Freels, M.; Inoue, A. Investigations of the factors that affected fatigue behavior of Zr-based bulk-metallic glasses. *Adv. Eng. Mater.* **2008**, *10*, 1030–1033. [CrossRef]
35. Liu, L.; Qiu, C.L.; Chen, Q.; Chan, K.C.; Zhang, S.M. Deformation behavior, corrosion resistance, and cytotoxicity of Ni-free Zr-based bulk metallic glasses. *J. Biomed. Mater. Res. Part A* **2008**, *86*, 160–169. [CrossRef] [PubMed]
36. Huang, L.; Yokoyama, Y.; Wu, W.; Liaw, P.K.; Pang, S.; Inoue, A.; Zhang, T.; He, W. Ni-free Zr-Cu-Al-Nb-Pd bulk metallic glasses with different Zr/Cu ratios for biomedical applications. *J. Biomed. Mater. Res. Part B Appl. Biomater.* **2012**, *100*, 1472–1482. [CrossRef] [PubMed]
37. Liu, Y.; Wang, Y.M.; Pang, H.F.; Zhao, Q.; Liu, L. A Ni-free ZrCuFeAlAg bulk metallic glass with potential for biomedical applications. *Acta Biomater.* **2013**, *9*, 7043–7053. [CrossRef]
38. Inoue, A.; Wang, X.M.; Zhang, W. Developments and applications of bulk metallic glasses. *Rev. Adv. Mater. Sci.* **2008**, *18*, 1–9.
39. Hiromoto, S.; Tsai, A.-P.; Sumita, M.; Hanawa, T. Effect of chloride ion on the polarization behavior of the $Zr_{65}Al_{7.5}Ni_{10}Cu_{17.5}$ amorphous alloy in phosphate buffered solution. *Corr. Sci.* **2000**, *42*, 1651–1660. [CrossRef]
40. Hiromoto, S.; Tsai, A.-P.; Sumita, M.; Hanawa, T. Effect of surface finishing and dissolved oxygen on the polarization behavior of $Zr_{65}Al_{7.5}Ni_{10}Cu_{17.5}$ amorphous alloy in phosphate buffered solution. *Corr. Sci.* **2000**, *42*, 2167–2185. [CrossRef]
41. Hiromoto, S.; Tsai, A.-P.; Sumita, M.; Hanawa, T. Effect of pH on the polarization behavior of $Zr_{65}Al_{7.5}Ni_{10}Cu_{17.5}$ amorphous alloy in a phosphate-buffered solution. *Corr. Sci.* **2000**, *42*, 2193–2200. [CrossRef]
42. Hiromoto, S.; Asami, K.; Tsai, A.-P.; Sumita, M.; Hanawa, T. Surface composition and anodic polarization behavior of zirconium-based amorphous alloy with various alloying elements in a phosphate buffered saline solution. *J. Electrochem. Soc.* **2002**, *149*, B117–B122. [CrossRef]
43. Hiromoto, S.; Hanawa, T. Re-passivation current of amorphous $Zr_{65}Al_{7.5}Ni_{10}Cu_{17.5}$ alloy in a Hanks' balanced solution. *Electrochim. Acta* **2002**, *47*, 1343–1349. [CrossRef]

44. Hiromoto, S.; Tsai, A.-P.; Sumita, M.; Hanawa, T. Surface characterization of Zr-Al-(Ni, Cu) amorphous alloys immersed in a cell-culture medium. *Mater. Trans. JIM* **2002**, *43*, 261–266. [CrossRef]
45. Morrison, M.L.; Buchanan, R.A.; Leon, R.V.; Liu, C.T.; Green, B.A.; Liaw, P.K.; Horton, J.A. The electrochemical evaluation of a Zr-based bulk metallic glass in a phosphate-buffered saline electrolyte. *J. Biomed. Mater. Res. Part A* **2005**, *74*, 430–438. [CrossRef] [PubMed]
46. Stansbury, E.E.; Buchanan, R.A. Faraday's Law. In *Fundamentals of Electrochemical Corrosion*; ASM International: Materials Park, OH, USA, 2000; pp. 147–149.
47. Wang, Y.B.; Zheng, Y.F.; Wei, S.C.; Li, M. In vitro study on Zr-based bulk metallic glasses as potential biomaterials. *J. Biomed. Mater. Res. Part B* **2011**, *96*, 34–46. [CrossRef] [PubMed]
48. Wataha, J.C.; Lockwood, P.E.; Schedle, A. Effect of silver, copper, mercury, and nickel ions on cellular proliferation during extended, low-dose exposures. *J. Biomed. Mater. Res.* **2000**, *52*, 360–364. [CrossRef]
49. Liu, L.; Qiu, C.L.; Huang, C.Y.; Yu, Y.; Huang, H.; Zhang, S.M. Biocompatibility of Ni-free Zr-based bulk metallic glasses. *Intermetallics* **2009**, *17*, 235–240. [CrossRef]
50. Monfared, A.; Vali, H.; Faghihi, S. Biocorrosion and biocompatibility of Zr–Cu–Fe–Al bulk metallic glasses. *Surf. Interface Anal.* **2013**, *45*, 1714–1720. [CrossRef]
51. Li, J.; Shi, L.L.; Zhu, Z.D.; He, Q.; Ai, H.J.; Xu, J. $Zr_{61}Ti_2Cu_{25}Al_{12}$ metallic glass for potential use in dental implants; Biocompatibility assessment by in vitro cellular responses. *Mater. Sci. Eng. C* **2013**, *33*, 2113–2121. [CrossRef]
52. Fornell, J.; Van Steenberge, N.; Varea, A.; Rossinyol, E.; Pellicer, E.; Suriñach, S.; Baró, M.D.; Sort, J. Enhanced mechanical properties and in vitro corrosion behavior of amorphous and devitrified $Ti_{40}Zr_{10}Cu_{38}Pd_{12}$ metallic glass. *J. Mech. Behav. Biomed. Mater.* **2011**, *4*, 1709–1717. [CrossRef]
53. Blanquer, A.; Pellicer, E.; Hynowska, A.; Barrios, L.; Ibáñez, E.; Baró, M.D.; Sort, J.; Nogués, C. In vitro biocompatibility assessment of $Ti_{40}Cu_{38}Zr_{10}Pd_{12}$ bulk metallic glass. *J. Mater. Sci. Mater. Med.* **2014**, *25*, 163–172. [CrossRef]
54. Wang, Y.B.; Li, H.F.; Cheng, Y.; Zheng, Y.F.; Ruan, L.Q. In vitro and in vivo studies on Ti-based bulk metallic glass as potential dental implant material. *Mater. Sci. Eng. C* **2013**, *33*, 3489–3497. [CrossRef] [PubMed]
55. Imai, K.; Hiromoto, S. In vivo evaluation of Zr-based bulk metallic glass alloy intramedullary nails in rat femora. *J. Mater. Sci. Mater. Med.* **2014**, *25*, 759–768. [CrossRef] [PubMed]
56. Sun, Y.; Huang, Y.; Fan, H.; Wang, Y.; Ning, Z.; Liu, F.; Feng, D.; Jin, X.; Shen, J.; Sun, J.; et al. In vitro and in vivo biocompatibility of an Ag-bearing Zr-based bulk metallic glass for potential medical use. *J. Non-Cryst. Solids* **2015**, *419*, 82–91. [CrossRef]
57. Imai, K.; Hiromoto, S. In vivo evaluation of bulk metallic glasses for osteosynthesis devices. *Materials* **2016**, *9*, 676. [CrossRef] [PubMed]
58. Imai, K. In vivo investigation of Zr-based bulk metallic glasses sub-periosteally implanted on the bone surface. *J. Mater. Sci. Chem. Eng.* **2016**, *4*, 46–51. [CrossRef]
59. Kokubun, R.; Wang, W.; Zhu, S.; Xie, G.; Ichinose, S.; Itoh, S.; Takakuda, K. In vivo evaluation of a Ti-based bulk metallic glass alloy bar. *Bio-Med. Mater. Eng.* **2015**, *26*, 9–17. [CrossRef]
60. Lin, C.H.; Chen, C.H.; Huang, Y.S.; Huang, C.H.; Huang, J.C.; Jang, J.S.C.; Lin, Y.S. In-vivo investigations and cytotoxicity tests on Ti/Zr-based metallic glasses with various Cu contents. *Mater. Sci. Eng. C* **2017**, *77*, 308–317. [CrossRef]
61. Wong, C.C.; Wong, P.C.; Tsai, P.H.; Jang, J.S.; Cheng, C.K.; Chen, H.H.; Chen, C.H. Biocompatibility and osteogenic capacity of Mg-Zn-Ca bulk metallic glass for rabbit tendon-bone interference fixation. *Int. J. Mol. Sci.* **2019**, *20*, 2191. [CrossRef]
62. Basu, B.; Sabareeswaran, A.; Shenoy, S.J. Biocompatibility property of 100% strontium-substituted SiO_2-Al_2O_3-P_2O_5-CaO-CaF_2 glass ceramics over 26 weeks implantation in rabbit model: Histology and micro-Computed Tomography analysis. *J. Biomed. Mater. Res. Part B Appl. Biomater.* **2015**, *103*, 1168–1179. [CrossRef]
63. Shayan, M.; Padmanabhan, J.; Morris, A.H.; Cheung, B.; Smith, R.; Schroers, J.; Kyriakides, T.R. Nanopatterned bulk metallic glass-based biomaterials modulate macrophage polarization. *Acta Biomater.* **2018**, *75*, 427–438. [CrossRef]
64. Veerachamy, S.; Yarlagadda, T.; Manivasagam, G.; Yarlagadda, P.K. Bacterial adherence and biofilm formation on medical implants: A review. *Proc. Inst. Mech. Eng. Part H* **2014**, *228*, 1083–1099. [CrossRef] [PubMed]

65. Avila, E.D.; Molon, R.S.; Lima, B.P.; Lux, R.; Shi, W.; Junior, M.J.; Spolidorio, D.M.; Vergani, C.E.; Assis Mollo Junior, F. Impact of physical chemical characteristics of abutment implant surfaces on bacteria adhesion. *J. Oral Implantol.* **2016**, *42*, 153–158. [CrossRef] [PubMed]
66. Li, H.F.; Zheng, Y.F. Recent advances in bulk metallic glasses for biomedical applications. *Acta Biomater.* **2016**, *36*, 1–20. [CrossRef] [PubMed]
67. Subramanian, B.; Maruthamuthu, S.; Rajan, S.T. Biocompatibility evaluation of sputtered zirconium-based thin film metallic glass-coated steels. *Int. J. Nanomed.* **2015**, *10*, 17–29. [CrossRef] [PubMed]
68. Thanka, R.S.; Bendavid, A; Subramanian, B. Cytocompatibility assessment of Ti-Nb-Zr-Si thin film metallic glasses with enhanced osteoblast differentiation for biomedical applications. *Colloids Surf. B Biointerfaces* **2019**, *173*, 109–120. [CrossRef] [PubMed]
69. Ghidelli, M.; Gravier, S.; Blandin, J.J.; Djemia, P.; Mompiou, F.; Abadias, G.; Raskin, J.P.; Pardoen, T. Extrinsic mechanical size effects in thin ZrNi metallic glass films. *Acta Mater.* **2015**, *90*, 232–241. [CrossRef]
70. Ghidelli, M.; Idrissi, H.; Gravier, S.; Blandin, J.J.; Raskin, J.P.; Schryvers, D.; Pardoen, T. Homogeneous flow and size dependent mechanical behavior in highly ductile Zr65Ni35 metallic glass films. *Acta Mater.* **2017**, *131*, 246–259. [CrossRef]

2

Antimicrobial and Osseointegration Properties of Nanostructured Titanium Orthopaedic Implants

Marcus Jäger [1,*], Herbert P. Jennissen [1,2], Florian Dittrich [1], Alfons Fischer [3] and Hedda Luise Köhling [4]

1 Department of Orthopaedics and Trauma Surgery, University of Duisburg-Essen, Hufelandstrasse 55, D-45147 Essen, Germany; hp.jennissen@uni-due.de (H.P.J.); florian.dittrich@uk-essen.de (F.D.)
2 Institute of Physiological Chemistry, University Hospital, University of Duisburg Essen, Hufelandstrasse 55, D-45147 Essen, Germany
3 Institute of Metal Engineering, University of Duisburg-Essen, Campus Duisburg, Lotharstraße 1, D-47057 Duisburg, Germany; alfons.fischer@uni-due.de
4 Institute of Medical Microbiology, University of Duisburg-Essen, Virchowstr. 179, D-45147 Essen, Germany; Hedda-Luise.Koehling@uk-essen.de
* Correspondence: marcus.jaeger@uk-essen.de

Abstract: The surface design of titanium implants influences not only the local biological reactions but also affects at least the clinical result in orthopaedic application. During the last decades, strong efforts have been made to improve osteointegration and prevent bacterial adhesion to these surfaces. Following the rule of "smaller, faster, cheaper", nanotechnology has encountered clinical application. It is evident that the hierarchical implant surface micro- and nanotopography orchestrate the biological cascades of early peri-implant endosseous healing or implant loosening. This review of the literature gives a brief overview of nanostructured titanium-base biomaterials designed to improve osteointegration and prevent from bacterial infection.

Keywords: nanostructure; implants; bone; antimicrobial; titanium; protein layer

---

1. Introduction

Titanium (Ti) is a bioinert metal which is frequently applied in orthopaedic surgery for decades. In contrast to other metals such as cobalt-chrome-molybdenum (CoCrMo) or surgical steel (CrNiMo), it has almost no allergenic or immunogenic potential in vivo, showed excellent corrosion resistance and promotes osseointegration when applied to and fixed with osseous tissue. In addition, the low Young's modulus of titanium and its alloys has biomechanical advantages since it results in smaller stress shielding compared to other biometals (Table 1). In contrast to pure commercial titanium (cp-Ti), the alloy Ti-6Al-4V is commonly used in orthopaedic implants. One prominent candidate is total joints. Here, it was shown, that the macro- and microsurface structure influences the behaviour of protein adsorption as well as local cell adherence, proliferation and differentiation. Aiming for a high initial stability at the bone–implant interface, different manufacturers have modified and optimized surface structures. Typical examples are:

- the increase of the surface area by sandblasting;
- the surface coating with hydroxyapatite (HA) deposit; and
- the increase of macroporosity such as "metal spongiosa".

To date, the variety of surface modifications for titanium is extensive including mechanical (gritt blasting and attrition), chemical (acid etching and electrochemical depositions) and physical techniques (plasma-spraying) or a combination of these [1] (Table 2).

In contrast to its excellent osteoconductive properties, the low hardness of titanium exhibits a low wear resistance and limits its application for articulating parts of artificial joints. Another major disadvantage of most Ti surface designs is that they do only promote initial cell adherence followed by osseointegration but also promote bacterial adherence. The winner in the "race for the surface" (cell versus bacteria) decides if biomineralization leads to a solid anchoring of a total joint or bacterial growth and biofilm deposit leads to the clinical incidence of a periprosthetic infection (PI). The treatment of PI is demanding for both the orthopaedic surgeon and the patient. Even in uncomplicated cases, it is associated with two or more operations and requires mid-term immobilization of the patient. Moreover, PI results in relevant bone loss and soft tissue defects leading to reduced muscular function and may result in poor implant survivorship and disability of the patient. Especially multiresistant bacteria are problematic since their escape from eradication by antibiotics. Therefore, strong efforts have been made to develop innovative implant surface structures, which promote osseointegration as well as prevent PI. Since nanopatterning with dimensions smaller than 100 nm has entered orthopaedic research, one alternative is to design surface structures at the nanoscale, which are promising to reach these aims. This review of the literature summarizes recent data of nanostructured titanium implants with emphasis on orthopaedics.

Table 1. Different metal alloys and their density and Young's modulus in comparison to bone [2–6].

Material	Density (Mg/m^3)	Young's Modulus, E (GPa)
Cp-Ti grade II	4.2	100–110
Ti-6Al-4V	4.5	100–130
Ti-6Al-7Nb	4.52	110–130
Surgical CrNiMo-Steel 316L	7.8	195–210
CoCrMo alloys	8.5	210–230
Cortical bone	1.19–1.85	18.6–20.7

Table 2. Commonly applied methods to modify titanium surface structures into the nanoscale in the orthopaedic field [7–24].

	Technique	Modified Layer	Objective
Mechanical	• Grinding • Polishing • Machining • Blasting	Rough or smooth surface formed by the subtraction process	Produce specific surface topographies; Clean and roughen surface; Improve adhesion in bonding
	• Attrition	To fabricate nanophase surface layers on Ti of commercial purity which improve the tensile properties and surface hardness of Ti	Produce materials with nanometre size grains (1–100 nm); To produce rough morphology and higher hydrophilicity
Chemical	• Acidic treatment • Alkaline treatment • Hydrogen peroxide treatment	<10 nm of surface oxide layer ~1 µm of sodium titanate gel ~5 nm of dense inner oxide and porous outer layer	Remove oxide scales and contamination. Improve biocompatibility, bioactivity or bone conductivity. Improve biocompatibility, bioactivity or bone conductivity
	• Sol-gel	~10 µm of thin film, such as calcium phosphate, TiO_2 and silica	Improve biocompatibility, bioactivity or bone conductivity
	• CVD	~1 µm of TiN, TiC, TiCN, diamond and diamond-like carbon thin film	Improve wear resistance, corrosion resistance and blood compatibility
	• Anodic oxidation	~10 nm–40 µm of TiO_2 layer, adsorption and incorporation of electrolyte anions	Produce specific surface topographies; improve corrosion resistance; improve biocompatibility, bioactivity or bone conductivity
	• Biochemical methods	Coating deposition; modification through silanized Ti, photochemistry, self-assembled monolayers, protein-resistance, etc.	Induce specific cell and tissue response by means of surface immobilized peptides, proteins, or growth factors

Table 2. *Cont.*

	Technique	Modified Layer	Objective
Physical	• Thermal spray ✓ *flame spray* ✓ *plasma spray* ✓ *high velocity oxy-fuel spray* ✓ *others*	~30 to ~200 μm of coatings, such as titanium, HA, calcium silicate, Al_2O_3, ZrO_2, TiO_2	Improve wear resistance, corrosion resistance and biological properties (osteoblast adhesion)
	• Physical vapour deposition ✓ *Evaporation* ✓ *Ion plating* ✓ *Sputtering*	~1 μm of TiN, TiC, TiCN, diamond and diamond-like carbon thin film Hydroxyapatite coating by sputtering	Improve wear resistance, corrosion resistance and blood compatibility.
	• Ion implantation and deposition	~10 nm of surface modified layer and/or um of thin film	Modify surface composition; improve wear, corrosion resistance, and biocompatibility
	• Glow discharge plasma treatment	~1 nm to ~100 nm of surface modified layer	Cleaning, sterilizing or oxidizing the surface; surface nitridation; removal of the native oxide layer

2. Bone Cells and Their Interactions

To predict the response of an osseous microenvironment to nanostructured titanium biomaterial in vivo, it is essential to get a brief insight into the complexity of the osseous cellular interactions in general and in the cell–surface interface in detail. Bones have multiple and various functions. The vital bone structure, by definition a rigid organ, is part of the hematopoietic system, stores minerals, supports and protects vulnerable organs, provides structure for the human skeleton and enables mobility. Depending on the constantly changing biomechanical requirements, bone adapts its structure. This is physiologically conditioned by a continuous balance of bone formation and degradation. This bone remodelling process is influenced by systemic (e.g., calcitonin and oestrogens) as well as local (e.g., growth factors and cytokines) stimuli [25]. Moreover, osteocytes act as mechanosensors and orchestrators of this homeostasis. Osteoblasts are able to produce osteoid (a collagen I rich matrix) and additional capable of osteoid calcification (hydroxyapatite). An adequate stimulus derives the active osteoblast, characterized by a large amount of endoplasmatic reticulum as well as a large Golgi apparatus, from its mesenchymal progenitor cell which is mainly localized in the bone marrow [26].

In contrast, osteoclasts maintain the homeostasis between bone formation and resorption as antagonists of the osteoblasts. They are characterized by multiple nuclei and are derived from the hematopoietic cell line. The homeostasis of bone formation and degradation is complex and predominantly regulated by the receptor activator of nuclear factor κβ (RANK) and its associated ligand. Receptor activator of nuclear factor κβ ligand (RANKL) does not only activate downstream pathways of osteoclastogenesis, but also modulates the homoeostasis of physiological as well as pathological osseous processes by linking to other signal paths [27]. During differentiation, the osteoblast progenitor cells express stimuli of osteoclastogenesis factors like macrophage colony stimulating factor (M-CSF) and RANKL. In contrast, osteoprotegerin can antagonize RANKL by preventing binding to the receptor RANK.

In addition to the primarily bone forming cells, the osseous milieu contains its genuine and high specialized immune system. Nevertheless, the transition between immune and bone forming cells is fluent. The formation of osteolysis is commonly associated with the activity of osteoclasts as primarily bone-resorbing cells. In contrast, some studies showed that macrophages or multinuclear giant cells, which are ontogenetically closely linked to osteoclasts, are also capable of low-grade bone resorption [28]. The macrophages' dual function as both immune and bone degrading cells is just an exemplary demonstration of the complexity and tight interaction of the osseous milieu.

3. Titanium Surface Properties and Osteointegration

It is evident that the osseous response depends not only on the biochemical composition of a biomaterial but also on the biomechanical characteristics of the implants surface. Topographical factors such as size, surface texture, macro- and microstructure, and shape of the implant play a crucial role in the cellular reaction [29]. The biomaterial effects in terms of bioinertness, bioactivity, and biocompatibility are important in implantology as well as biomechanical characteristics. Biocompatibility means the ability of a material to induce an adequate reaction in the host (human, animal, organ, and cell) in a specific situation [30].

Titanium (Ti) as a feedstock and Ti-based alloys have been widely used as implant biomaterials in orthopaedic surgery in the last sixty years because of their genuine biomechanical and biocompatible characteristics. In comparison with CrNiMo stainless steel, Ti has a 50% greater strength to weight ratio and, in contrast to CoCrMo, it has almost no allergenic or immunogenic potential in vivo. Moreover, the rapidly forming durable dielectric titanium dioxide layer on the implant surface induces cell integration, enabling a much stronger contact between Ti-based implants and bone tissue after implantation compared to steel [31]. The cause of this continuous protective and thermodynamically stable oxide layer is a very high affinity of titanium for oxygen (so called "passive film"). Thus, disruptions or damages are repaired immediately when bioliquid surrounds the metal [32]. The detailed composition of this passive film in vivo is mostly based on TiO_2 while any small content of Ti_2O_3 and TiO depends on the local micro-environment [33,34].

The thickness and quality of the passive condition in titanium can be controlled by thermal treatment. High temperatures (up to 800 °C) and longer thermal oxidation times cause oxide de-bonding, whereas oxide layers obtained at lower temperatures and shorter times are also not sufficiently thick.

In aqueous solutions such as body fluids, the passive film under mechanical stress is not a static condition but might be characterized by continuous depassivation and repassivation. Here, alloying elements and impurities such as molybdenum (Mo), niobium (Nb), vanadium (V) or chromium (Cr) are probably not involved to significant content. Nevertheless, dissolution of alloying elements during time is possible, as well as incorporation of different elements from surrounding solutions into the passive film. These effects might play a role in orthopaedic implants since "repassivation of titanium" at the osseous implantation site led to the adsorption of calcium and phosphate ions into the film, whereas at the outermost surface calcium phosphate and calcium titanium phosphate were formed [35–37]. In contrast to cp-Ti, the alloy Ti-6Al-4V is commonly used in orthopaedic implants for its better mechanical properties [38].

It is generally accepted that the biocompatibility of titanium can be improved by the coating with bioactive titanium dioxide and by the presence of structures at micro- and nanoscales [39]. Especially plasma spraying, chemical vapour deposition, atomic layer deposition anodic oxidation, sol-gel and other methods have been established for nano-designs [40]. However, osteointegration is in first turn conditioned by osteoconduction (adaptive bone tissue growth/ingrowth). Therefore, not only nano-scale structures but also surface topography at the macro- and microscale are relevant for the success of an orthopaedic implant.

3.1. Local Biomolecular Reactions to Titanium Surfaces

The detailed cellular mechanisms on the bone–implant interface during osteogenesis are still largely unknown. The first response after application of titanium to an osseous environment is wetting followed by rapid protein adsorption to its surface [41].

The capacity of an implant surface to adsorb small proteins depends on its physicochemical characteristics such as hydrophobicity or surface energy and the local milieu (pH, temperature, concentrations of ions, composition and functional groups of proteins, strength of solution) [42].

The first proteins that rapidly adsorb at the solid–liquid interface in vivo usually derive from blood. These interact with the surface structure and undergo conformational changes, such as fibrinogen adopting a fibrin-like structure, depending on the surface type and the exposure time. Here, it is evident that the composition of the adsorbed protein layer varies and proteins with stronger adsorption are favoured.

During the next minutes and hours this initial phase is replaced by a formation of a resident protein layer, which influences the interaction of platelets, activation of intrinsic coagulation, adhesion as well as aggregation of platelets and activation of the complement system [43]. Especially the Arg-Gly-Asp (RGD) sequences of the proteins fibronectin and vitronectin play a crucial role as chemotactic or adhesive stimuli in biomineralization and matrix maturation [44,45]. In addition, the implant surface has a strong impact on the platelet activation level. Here, some blood coagulation factors are triggering formation of thrombin followed by converting fibrinogen into insoluble fibrin. Fibrin is retained by titanium surface structures as a transient matrix. The fibrin retention forces are strongly influenced by the local topography of the implant surface. Therefore, fibrin is not only involved in initial cellular adherence but also concomitant with cell traction.

Once the biomaterial is coated with a transitory protein layer, different cell types attach rapidly to the protein-conditioned surface [46]. This initial attachment follows an adhesion phase, dominated by interactions of the extracellular matrix (ECM) proteins and adjacent cells. Integrins play a crucial role as "molecular bridges" between adherence proteins and adsorbed ECM proteins of the biomaterials surface and are able to transduce information about biomechanical load from ECM proteins to the peripheral cytoskeleton. This interaction leads to the activation of gene promotors via nuclear matrix architectural transcription factors (NMATF) and finally to the release of chemotactical signals [47]. Osteogenic cell migration, proliferation and differentiation follow in the next phase. One can highlight that bone cells align along defined morphologies but the underlying interactions with the nanotopography are complex and not fully understood in detail. Mainly responsible for the final osseointegration of titanium biomaterial and bone formation are osteoblasts. However, under pathological conditions, protein adsorption can be reversible, especially if the local pH value decreases, as in inflammation [48–50].

Figure 1 gives more detailed information on the different interactions between Ti surfaces and its in vivo microenvironment which can divided into the following five phases:

Phase I: Adsorption of low and higher molecular molecules. The positive charge of titanium is responsible for an initial binding of negative charged small molecules followed by negatively loaded functionalized groups of high molecular weight molecules. In this dynamic stage, local proteins (e.g., fibronectin, albumin, fibrinogen, IgG, complement C3 from blood and bone marrow, and vitronectin) are mainly involved, whereas lipids play a subordinate role. The type of binding is non-covalent (hydrophobic interactions, electrostatic forces, hydrogen bonding, and Van der Waals forces). With time, molecules with greater affinity for the surface but slower diffusion rates replace the smaller molecules (*"Vroman effect"*) [42]. This protein adsorption is associated with conformational change of the tertiary protein structures and changes the initial surface characteristics of the titanium implant [51]. This affects parameters such as wettability, surface energy, and hydrophilic qualities. The result in vivo is a more or less (polar) functionalized interface, which is ready now for cellular attachment ("conditioning film"). Fibronectin and collagen promotes osteoblast adhesion and osteointegration whereas albumin inhibits cellular attachment and spreading [52]. Typical example of the influence of titanium surfaces on protein adsorption are increased albumin adsorption rates in laser-engineered porous titanium [53] or higher fibronectin adsorption and lower albumin adsorption rates in magnesium-incorporated anodized titanium surfaces compared to blasted surfaces [54]. However, the detailed sequence and kinetics of competitive protein adsorption in vivo remains unclear. From 218 identified human serum proteins, 30 were detected to be associated with bone metabolism. Of these, Apo E, antithrombin and protein C are found predominantly on sand-blasted or acid-etched Ti, whereas proteins of the complement system (C3) prefer adsorption onto smooth Ti surfaces [55].

Phase II: In this stage, it is crucial for local cells or bacteria bind to the protein film ("the race for the surface"). Most nanostructured titanium surfaces promote both cellular and bacterial attachment. At this level, a preliminary decision of the further fate of the implant is determined (PI vs. osteointegration). Recently wound healing macrophages (M2) have been implicated as crucial for initiation of osseointegration of implants.

Phase III: The cells attached initially are fixed by extracellular matrix anchoring proteins to the surface of the titanium implant (non-specific cellular adhesion).

Besides mesenchymal cells, neutrophils and macrophages colonize the implant, leading to the foreign body covering process and releasing cytokines and growth factors including BMP-2 to attract fibroblasts and osteoblasts. This phase is also accompanied with a quantitative and qualitative change of the protein layer between the cell and titanium surface. The interface biology of implants is complex. Especially the ubiquitous dimetric glycoprotein fibronectin (FN), with its two subunits, is involved in this process since it binds to cellular transmembrane integrins (e.g., integrin $\alpha_5\beta_1$ binds the arg-gly-asp [RGD]-containing repeat of FN and acts as a primary receptor). FN also has growth factor binding regions and is able to fix growth factors for the corresponding receptors of the cellular membrane, e.g., synergistic effects on FN and bone morphogenic proteins (BMPs). Although rough titanium surfaces exhibit a better cellular attachment, some data indicate that smooth surfaces promote cellular spreading more than rough topography [56–58].

The initial layer of predominantly negatively charged proteins onto the titanium surface neutralizes its charge during phase I and II. Afterwards also positive loaded extra- or intracellular proteins and ions (e.g., Ca^{2+}) bind to the negatively charged functional groups of the protein layer. One prominent example are the positive loaded histones from cellular fragments or from cytosol that bind to the interface of nanostructured titanium [59,60]. The epigenetic function of these proteins remains unclear.

Phase IV: Controlled by titanium surface structures and its interface molecules and mediated by focal cellular contacts, local growth factors and intercellular cytokine proliferation and differentiation are induced. Focal adhesions (contacts) are dynamic structures and link the cytoskeletal network to the ECM, allowing cells to respond to the external environment (feedback loop: inside-outside-inside signalling). Therefore, mechanical forces at the implant-cellular interface can be translated by the cytoskeleton and second messenger activities into gene expression and posttranscriptional modification of expressed proteins [61]. At this stage, it is evident that much of the natural environment surrounding osteoblasts and osteoclasts consist of structures with nano-scale topography. Following bionic principles, nanoscale surface architectures of grain sizes less than 100 nm attempt to recapitulate the physiological environment of growing bone. This results in enhanced osteoblasts spreading and filopodial extension. The detailed cellular response is sophisticated and varies according to the level of differentiation of the cell. While osteoblasts show enhanced differentiation on nanorough titanium, the effect of mesenchymal stem cells is controversy discussed. In a meta-analysis, Goldman et al. summarize the results of different investigators [62]. Especially the cellular Ca^{2+} influx, which is regulated by connexion 43 (Cx43), initiates similar cellular signals via gap junctions and is involved in osteoblast differentiation of MSCs [63].

Phase V: Local changes of the pH and accumulation of Ca and PO4 lead to biomineralization and osteointegration of the titanium implant. Here, osteoblasts and osteoclasts are mainly involved. At last biomechanical forces induce bone remodelling.

The detailed effects of micro- and nanoscale implant surface structures are not known and controversy discussed in the literature [64]. Most in vitro and in vivo studies suggest the minimal pore size required for bone tissue regeneration should be around 100 μm and pore sized below can lead to fibrous tissue formation or overgrowth with ossein. Especially pore sizes above 150 μm and functionally graded scaffolds favour bone formation and cell proliferation [65–68]. The influence of additive manufacturing to pore geometry, orientation and arrangement should also be considered in Ti implants. These procedures may affect mechanical strength as well as surface topography [69–72].

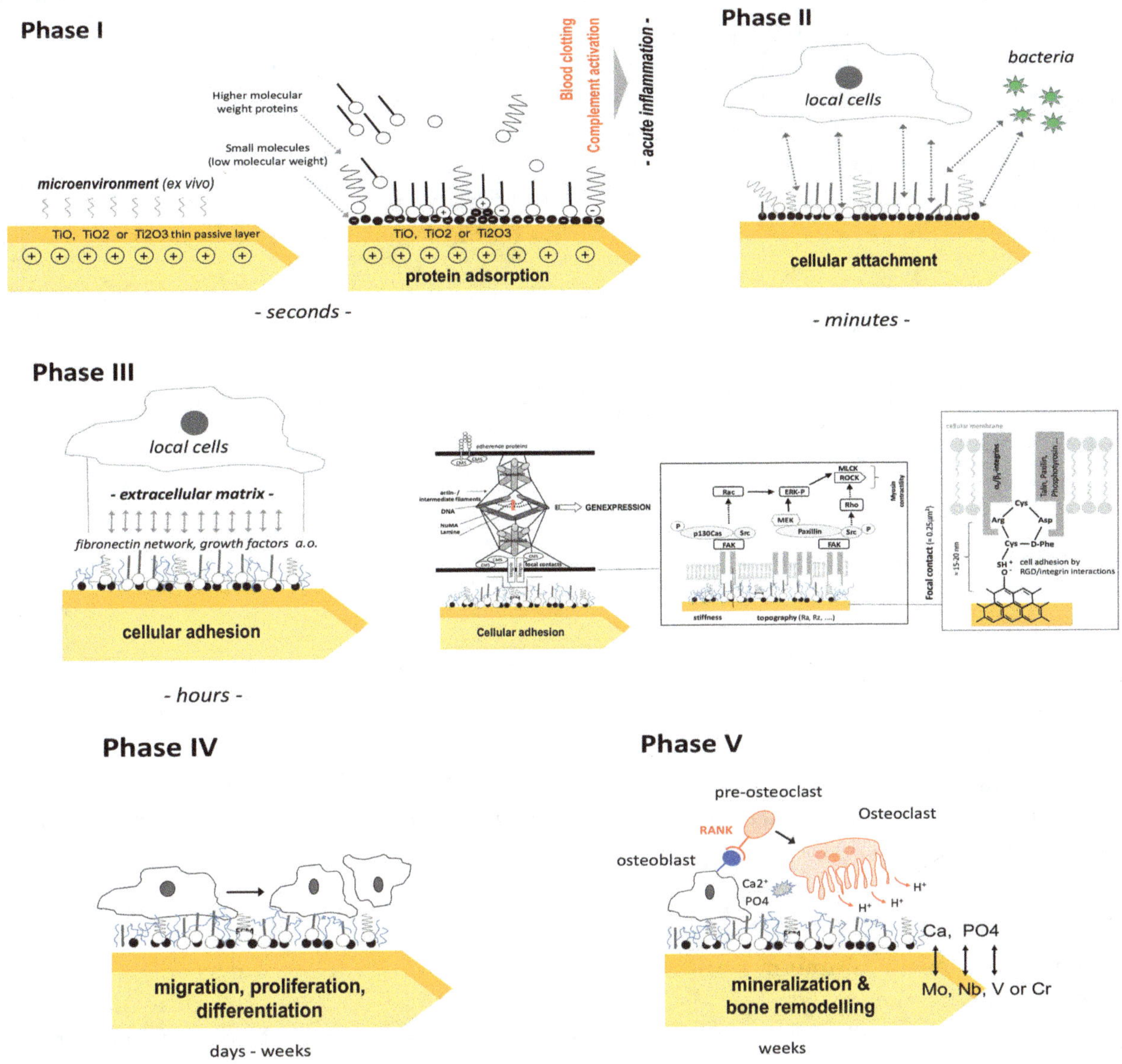

Figure 1. Local reactions onto titanium surfaces after in vivo application.

Regardless of the type of biomaterial, an initial inflammation response occurs in vivo but subsides within few days postoperatively. In contrast to this, the foreign body reaction, the extent of fibrosis and the potency for cellular or bacterial adherence is dependent on the biomaterial properties (Figure 2).

The reaction of osteogenic bone cells to micro- and nanoscaled structured surfaces must first be elucidated in order to design the adequate coating for orthopaedic implants. In the following, the effects of microtopography, nanotopography, surface roughness, porosity and surface energy on osteogenic cell function and their consecutive influence on osseointegration are further described.

The bone cells surrounded by physiological osseous milieu and its connected topographical architecture consist of nanoscaled structures. Osteocytes, hydroxyapatite crystals and collagen fibrils, as predominant elements of the bone matrix, are in the range of 50–300 nm in length and 0.5–5 nm in width. Therefore, the design of nanoscaled implant surfaces is derived from its organic standard and simulates equal growing conditions for osteogenic cells [73].

However, even titanium implants are integrated close to the mineralized tissue. Some data suggest that titanium is separated by a very thin soft-tissue layer as a result of a weak foreign body reaction that prevents a direct contact its surface to the bone [7]. In well osteointegrated implants, these layers are missing (direct bone contact) [46] or have microscopic dimension leading to contact forces which are stronger than that of adjacent bone (Figure 3).

Nevertheless, the extent of this fibrosis is crucial for the clinical result: since encapsulation of titanium implants is not desirable for orthopaedic implants as it cannot withstand the physical stresses of daily activities, micromovements may result in chronic implant loosening or fracture. Therefore, there is enough room for further improvements of titanium surface properties to decrease inflammatory response, avoid foreign body reaction and promote cellular attachment and biomineralization. Nanostructures are one promising technology to reach these aims.

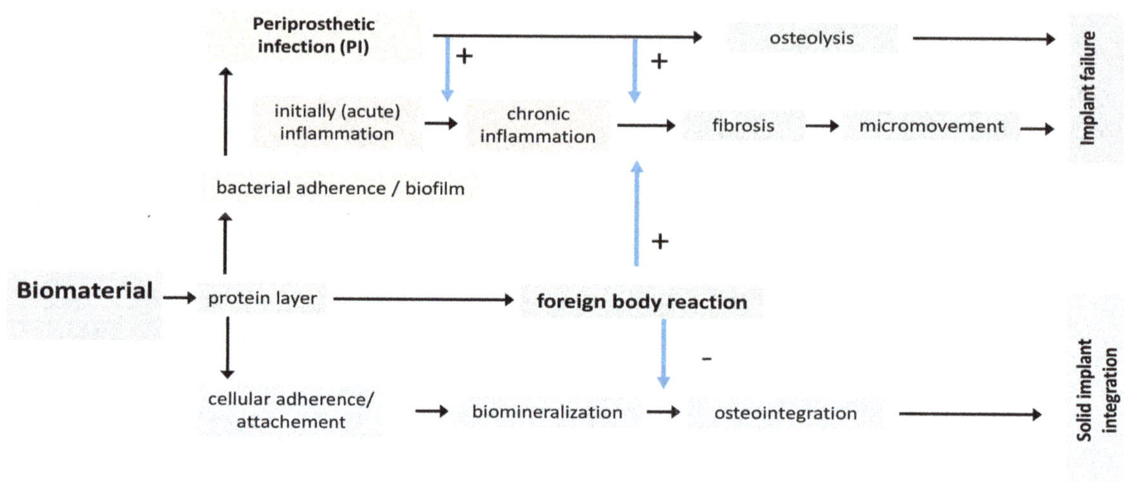

Figure 2. Local and systemic response after biomaterial application. The type of biomaterial and its surface structure dominantly influence osteointegration whereas an initial acute inflammatory reaction occurs independently and is based on the local surgical trauma.

3.2. Titanium Nanostructures and Osteointegration

Cellular reactions (attachment, proliferation, differentiation, and protein synthesis) in vivo relay not only on the micrometre scale but also on the nanometre scale. Here, modifications of surface structures at the nanoscale level can improve the bioactivity and performance of titanium without changing its bioinert properties. Some of these effects are related to initial protein binding: shifting topography from the micro to the nanoscale increased surface energy leading to higher protein adsorption rates. In addition, nano-roughness alone influences the adhesion of osteoblasts and their spreading and proliferation ("rapid bone regeneration") [74].

In vivo, microstructured surfaces provided a better implant surface–bone contact and an increased mechanical stability. The higher is the roughness, the higher are the local surface eletrostatic charge density and adhesion energy. Thus, it is possible to generate nanostructured titanium surfaces with superhydrophilic properties which can accelerate bone healing in early stages [75–79].

Meanwhile a large amount of diverse methods has been established to modify the surface structure of titanium implants. A typical example is the inorganic apatite coating, which can be controlled by plasmaspray techniques, electrodeposition or biomimetic precipitation of calcium phosphate (CaP immersion). During the last years, much more emphasis was put on the development of functionalized biomolecules onto titanium surfaces (e.g., collagen, fibronectin, protein fragments).

One example is the immobilization of ECM proteins such as fibronectin, collagen, osteopontin or laminin by plasma polymerized and crosslinked allylamine (pp-AA) [80] or the covalent binding of RGD-peptides [81]. In addition, polylactide (PLLA) coating and bound bone morphogenic protein (BMP) 2 seems to be one option for titanium surface structures with increased osteoinductive potential [82]. However, the critical point is the technical immobilization of these molecules to titanium and also the ability of the molecules to survive sterilization as well as surgical procedures.

Aiming for both optimization of osteointegration and prevention of bacterial adherence, a tremendous amount of research has been carried out into nanorough titanium implants. Especially defined nanostructures (nanotubes, nanorods, mesosponges, nanochannels, microcones, etc.) are promising candidates to improve implant properties [83]. To design these nanoscale structures electrochemical anodization, template method patterns, sol-gel processes or hydrothermal treatments are available. However, electrochemical anodization is one of the most established methods since it allows the formation of controlled surface structures such as nanotubes, pillar-like nanostructures, nanospikes and nanodots. The self-organization of Ti nanotubes in organic electrolytes depends strongly on its water content. Finally, this critical factor determinates whether self-ordered TiO_2 nanopores or nanotubes were formed (*"pore wall splitting mechanism"*). Modifications in anodization conditions (voltage, anodization time, and concentration of chemicals) control the morphology such as diameter (15 nm–300 nm) or length of generated TiO_2 tanotubes [84].

The growth rate and mechanical strength can be improved by high-voltage (HV) hard anodization (growth rate in HV: 1.2 $\mu mh^{-1} \cdot V^{-1}$ vs. ~20 $nmh^{-1} \cdot V^{-1}$ in LV regime) [85,86].

If the applied voltage exceeds the dielectric breakdown limit of the titanium oxide, the oxide will no longer be resistive to prevent further current flow and oxide growth. This leads to more gas evolution and sparking known as "Anodic Spark Deposition" (ASD), and "Micro-Arc Oxidation" (MAO) [87].

Among all electrolytes, the anodic oxide thickness is highest in H_2SO_4, but fluoride solutions seem to be more useful by producing biologically-inspired nano-tubular structures. Another major advantage of anodization is that nanotubes from almost all Ti alloys can be generated (e.g., Ti-6Al-7Nb, Ti-6Al-4V, Ti-6Al-4Zr). Interestingly nanotubes formed on Ti-6Al-4V by anodic oxidation have mainly been referred to as TiO_2 nanotubes, while pure titanium oxide nanotubes are formed only on pure Ti [88–90]. Some impurities (e.g., V, Fe, F, C, N) derived from chemical etching solutions before anodizing. The detailed surface structure of nanotitanium processed by etching techniques is dependent on the etchant (e.g., acidic or basic Piranha solutions) and on the exposure time [40]. In contrast to anodization, where predominantly TiO_2 nanotubes are created, the nanotubes formed on Ti-6Al-4V by thermal oxidation were referred to as Ti-Al-V-O nanotubes.

Besides morphological parameters, the degree of crystallinity changes the hydrophilic character of the nanotube. This has an impact on cell proliferation and osteointegration since nanostructured/hydrophilic surfaces show advantages [91–95]. Moreover, the formation of crystallic islands in the TiO_2 nanotube structure accelerates growth in eukaryotic cells and reduces the ability of staphylococcal aggregate/biofilm formation. Nanotubes have a relevant size-effect on bone and other cells: Whereas diameters of 15–20 nm are optimal for increased cell adhesion, proliferation as well as for alkaline phosphatase (ALP) activity and bone matrix deposition [96–100], nanotobe diameters of approximately 100 nm led to programmed cell death (apoptosis). The hypothesis that hierarchical surfaces with smaller micro- and nanostructures mimicking nanoscale topography of the bone and thus promoting cell proliferation and osteoblast differentiation was confirmed by different investigators during the last decade [101–104].

Typical structures are bone apatite which forms 10–20 nm long and 2–3 nm wide plates, whereas type I collagen fibres are ~200 nm long and 2–3 nm thick [105,106].

This size-effect is valid for different substrate materials (e.g., TiO_2 or ZrO_2), for different crystallization states (amorphous and annealed) and is also unchanged in different fluoride contents in the tubes. It was confirmed on several cell types such as mesenchymal stem cells, haematopoietic stem cells, endothelial cells, osteoblasts and osteoclasts [84]. Nevertheless, alternative methods for anodization have been established to design and modify nanostructures (e.g., by ultrasonic fabrication of β-type Ti-Nb-Ta-Zr or by electrospinning of $BaTiO_3$) [107,108].

The cause of the size effect is probably based on integrin clustering in the cell membrane leading to focal adhesion complexes. These have a diameter of about 10 nm which perfectly fit to nanotubular diameters of about 15 nm. In vivo, the cytotoxic effect of 100 nm is mitigated because larger nanotube dimensions show higher interaction energies, thus leading to higher protein adsorption which obviously influences cell behaviour [109]. Even in sharp nanorough titanium surfaces, the attraction between the negatively charged titanium and a negatively charged osteoblast is mediated by charged proteins with a distinctive quadrupolar internal charge distribution [75,76].

In addition, the cation-mediated attraction between extracellular matrix proteins (e.g., fibronectin) and the titanium surface is expected to be more efficient for a high surface charge density. This facilitated integrin-mediated osteoblast adhesion along the sharp convex edges or spikes of nanorough titanium surfaces where the magnitude of the negative surface charge density is the highest. In summary, Ti nanotubes with sharp edges and a diameter of approximately 15 nm should be the preferred surface for orthopaedic nanostructured implant. However, there are only few studies on whether in vitro effects of nanorough titanium can be transplanted to the in vivo situation.

Some other investigators described improved bone bonding strength and osteointegration in nanotubular surfaces compared with grit blasted surfaces [79,110]. These results were confirmed for TiO_2 nanotubes (diameter: 37 ± 11 nm, thickness: 160 nm thick) by pull-out experiments in rabbits [111,112]. Moreover, the osteointegrative nature of Ti nanotubes can be improved by further modifications such as Si-doped TiO_2 (TiO_2-NT) [113] or Ti-24Nb-4Zr-7.9Sn [114].

In summary, most in vivo data suggest that especially the initial bone formation is enhanced in nanorough titanium surfaces [111]. This statement has a relevant clinical impact because patients with poor bone quality (e.g., elderly people) might benefit from earlier full weight bearing after cementless fixed total joint.

One further option for changing surface properties of titanium is the implantation of bioactive ions such as Ca, Zn, H and Sr. Hegedus et al. found improved cell viability for Ti with implanted Ca or dual Ca + Si ion compared to pristine Ti substrate [115]. This corresponds to the findings of Wang et al. who showed advantages in osteointegration for Ca and Ta entangled porous titanium (EPT) by plasma immersion ion implantation and deposition [116]. It is believed that Ta–OH groups can facilitate the adsorption of calcium and phosphate ions, thus enhancing osteoblasts adhesion. Gold (Au) is also qualified to optimize Ti surfaces aiming for osteointegration as shown for gold ion implantation, thin Au layer deposition and thermal annealing [117–119].

More complex for getting official approval as a medical device is the covalent immobilization of biomolecules e.g., BMP-2 onto nanostructured Ti surfaces. Experimental data have shown that this can be a useful tool to control differentiation of mesenchymal stem cells (MSCs). Typical examples are:

- immobilization of epidermal growth factor (EGF) on 100 nm diameter TiO_2 nanotubes (prevention of apoptosis, promotion of attachment and proliferation) [120];
- immobilization of bone BMP-2 onto TiO nanotubes:
    - higher osteocalcin and osteopontin levels at 30 nm diameter [121]; and
    - enhanced osteogenic differentiation 15 nm diameter, chondrogenic differentiation on 100 nm [98]; and
- vascular endothelial growth factor (VEGF) [122].

This functionalization could be performed directly, but usually is realized via self-assembled monolayers (SAMs), antibodies or peptides on the surface of nanostructures [123]. The concept of bio-functionalization of metal surface structures is not new but still an increasing area of research [124].

Especially the pharmacokinetics of Ti-bound BMPs is hard to control in vivo. This is relevant, since extensive concentration of local released BMP can induce osteolysis [125–128]. Aiming for steady release over a longer period, Ti surfaces coated with graphene oxide through layer-by-layer assembly of positively and negatively charged grapheme oxide sheets guarantees high load dosages of BMP-2. This and biodegradable-loaded BMP-2 carriers have shown promising results in vitro and in animal experiments [129–133].

However, it has been taken into account that the secondary structure of rhBMP-2 can change significantly dependent on the modified surface (e.g., decreased percentage of α-helix structure in acid alkali-treated Ti). These conformational changes will also influence the BMP-2 activity [134]. Another strategy is to improve the osteoinductive properties of Ti implants to activate the TGF-β/BMP and non-canonicalWNT/Ca^{2+} (WNT5A, FZD6) pathways directly by modified surface structures as shown by Chakravorty et al. [135]. Especially in vitro results require highly standardized animal models to receive reliable data [136].

The latest development of nanostructured titanium aims at osteopromotion and prevention of bacterial adhesion. One example is to design hierarchical architectures by a "layer-by-layer" (LbL) concept. Here, chitosan coated BSA nanoparticles (CBSA NPs) and oxidized alginate (OSA) showed features of nanostructures on titanium. The functional groups provide active sites for BMP-2-immobilization and promote bone formation. Furthermore, it was shown that the antibiotic vancomycin binds on the OSA. Therefore, these assembling nanoparticles might prevent infection during the bone healing process [137].

However, the application of local antibiotics to nanostructured titanium for clinical application seems to be critical regarding pharmacological side effects including bacterial resistance, limitations in implant sterilization and official approval.

More promising is the combination of a titanium surface structure with other agents such as HA or iodine as described by Tsuchiya et al. [138,139]. The authors report good clinical results (osteointegration and infection treatment) in 222 patients using an iodine filled nanopore titanium surface with an oxide film of 5 and 10 μm (>50,000 pores/mm^2).

The following section summarizes further anti-microbiological effects of nanotitanium structured surfaces and clinical strategies to treat infections.

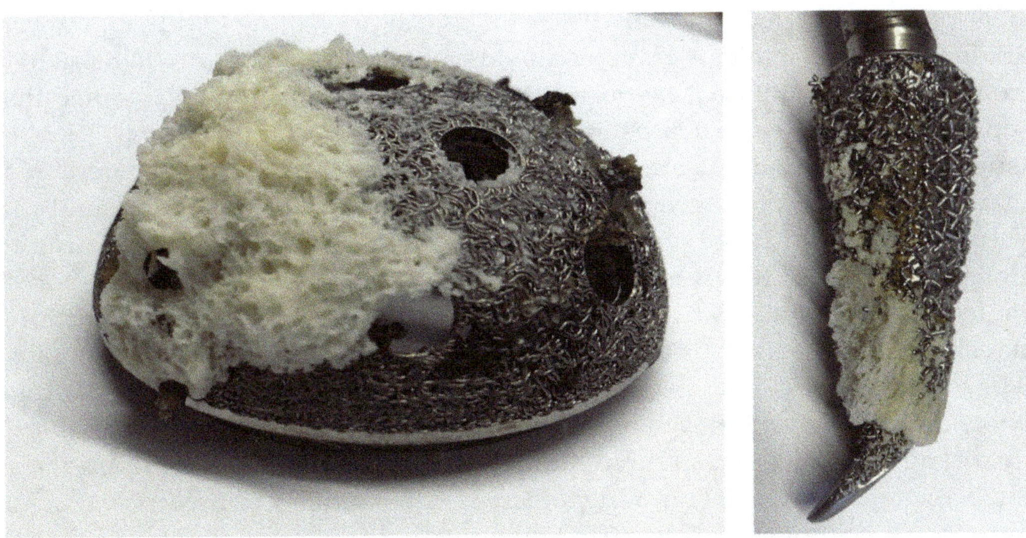

Figure 3. Macro- and microstrucured titanium implants show excellent biomechanical integration into bone in long-term. This implant-to-bone strength is higher than within the adjacent cancellous bone leading to intra-bone fracture during explantation. Here, de novo bone formation (contact osteogenesis) is based on micro-mechanical interdigitation of the surface with the material surface. It is believed that nanostructure titanium surfaces accelerate the initial phase of osteointegration leading to early full weight bearing even in poor bone quality. In contrast, the "bone-bonding phenomenon" is based on a chemical interaction of collagen, from the adjacent bone interdigitating with the chemically active surface of the implant [46,140].

4. Periprosthetic Infections and Biofilm

The demographic change in the Western world and prolonged life expectance have increased the rate of total joint revision operations dramatically [141]. Implant failures due to PI or surgical site infections (SSI) are the third most common cause in total hip arthroplasty (15%) and the most common cause in total knee arthroplasty (25%) [142,143].

The consequences of PI are an imprinting and traumatic experience for the patient. Radical debridement of soft tissue and bone during revision surgery leads to progressive bone loss and therefore loss of biomechanical stability. The revision operation increases the complication rate compared to primary implantation significantly [144]. Furthermore, the cases of infections with multiresistant bacteria are increasing and the pharmacological options are stretched to its limit. In addition to the physical and psychological impairment of the patient, there is an economic burden on the health system caused by PI revision surgery that cannot be neglected.

The pathogenesis of PI or septic loosening is due to intraoperative contamination of the implant or the periprosthetic interface, which may become apparent in an early-onset acute local putrid infection, a Systemic Inflammatory Response Syndrome (SIRS) or in a "low-grade infection". In addition to the direct contamination, a secondary infection of the prosthetic joint by bacteraemia e.g., after soft tissue infection, pneumonia or tooth extraction is also possible [145].

The initial contamination of the biomaterials surface is followed by the development of a biofilm on the colonized surfaces. Biofilms are "aggregates of microorganisms in which cells are frequently embedded in a self-produced matrix of extracellular polymeric substances that are adherent to each other and/or a surface". Typically, biofilms comprise many species and are complex systems with high cell densities [146]. This biofilm is critically influencing the implants function itself and initiates an periprosthetic inflammation [147].

Innovative solutions for biofilm absorbing or antibacterial Ti surfaces were achieved by permanent binding of antibiotics [148], antimicrobial peptides [149], antibacterial nanoparticles [150] and nanosilver or sputtered silver compounds [151]. Indeed, more effective in preventing PIs are topographical changes of the biomaterials surfaces on a micro- or nanoscaled level to prevent the growing risk of antimicrobial resistance without using any additional chemicals or antibiotics. It is generally accepted that nanoscaled Ti with 20–80 nm surface features decreases the bacterial adhesion significantly [152].

Mechanisms for these inherent antimicrobial properties are part of current research. It is hypothesised that defined nanotopographies are able to disrupt bacterial cell membranes and lead to a decreased bacterial viability. An effective microbial lysis is achieved by creating topographies which generate an adequate local stress across the microbial cell membrane. Dickson et al. defined the ideal space in between nanopillars in the range of 130–380 nm [153]. In addition, Gorth et al. pointed out that sharp edges on grains of Si_3N_4 surfaces are also capable of bacterial lysis. Thus, the topographical bactericidal effect is primarily dominated by its surface nanotopography and not only by its surface biochemistry [154]. Sjöström et al. underlined this hypothesis by using thermal oxidation to manufacture a range of nanospikes with a diameter of approximately 20 nm on the surfaces of Ti alloy beads. The nanospikes in the 20 nm range decrease the viability of *Escherichia coli* on the surface by 40% in comparison with polished Ti in vitro [155].

Mathew et al. showed that greater nanoscale surface roughness led to significantly decreased bacterial colonisation. In detail, implants coated with electrophoretic-deposited hydroxyapatite inhibited the growth of *Staphylococcus aureus* more effectively compared to less nanoscaled Ti surfaces [156].

Recently, a new potential antibacterial phenomenon based on solely nanotopographical properties has been found in locus-like insects. The wings of Clanger cicada (*Psaltoda claripennis*) are covered by hexagonal arrays of nanopillars which are able to eliminate Gram-negative bacteria by its physical surface structure consistently [157]. The antimicrobial effect is again due to rupture of the bacterial cell membrane and independent from its biochemistry. The nanopillars' height and spacing is about 200 nm and 100 nm in diameter at its base and covered by a self-cleaning wax layer, which leads to a super hydrophobic surface [158]. The "cicada wing effect" can be translated into titanium biomaterials by imitating the nanocolumnar structures using glancing angle sputter deposition (GLAD). In conclusion, a selective antimicrobial effect, using the GLAD technique, against Gram-negative bacteria, e.g., *Escherichia coli*, could be shown, whereas Gram-positive bacteria, e.g., *Staphylococcus aureus*, were not affected [159]. Table 3 summarized different Ti surface structures and its effects on prokaryotes.

Table 3. Nanostructured antibacterial titanium surfaces (Ag: silver, Zn: zinc, Fe: iron, TiN: titanium nitride, MRSA: Methicillin-resistant *Staphyloccus aureus*) [160].

	Method	Effect	
Coating	• Ag-nanoparticle modified Ti by silanization	Decreased viabilitiy and adhesion of *Escherichia coli* and *Staphylococcus aureus* in vitro	[161]
	• Poly(quaternary ammonium)-modified gold and TiO_2 nanoparticles	Decreased viability of *Escherichia coli* (5 logs in 10 min) in vitro	[162]
Surface structure	• Nanophased ZnO and TiO_2	Decreased adhesion of *Staphylococcus epidermidis* in vitro	[163]
	• Nanoscaled TiN/Ag multi-layered films on Fe (modulation period 7.5 nm)	Bactericidal in *Escherichia coli* in vitro	[164]
	• Electrospun TiO_2 nanorods by sol-gel electrospinning technique	Disruption of cell membrane in *Escherichia coli*, *Salmonella* Typhimurium, *Klebsiella pneumoniae*, *Staphylococcus aureus* in vitro	[165]
	• Zn-doped Ti nanofibers	Disruption of cell membrane in *Escherichia coli*, *Staphylococcus aureus* in vitro	[166]
	• Nanopillars/Nanotubes on Ti "cicada wing effect"	Disruption of cell membrane in *Escherichia coli* in vitro	[159]
	• Nanostructured Zn-incorporated TiO_2	Decreased growth of *Escherichia coli* and *Staphylococcus aureus* in vitro	[167]
	• Ag/TiO_2 nanocomposite powder by one-pot sol-gel technique (Np < 2 nm)	Complete growth inhibition of *Escherichia coli* in vitro	[168]
	• Nanostructured sodium silver titanate (nanotube) thin films	Antibacterial against MRSA in vitro	[169]

Another example how surface topography can affect bacterial growth are "rose stem-like constructs": The combination of anisotropic branched-shaped zinc oxide (ZnO) nanoparticles with fibrous scaffolds such as polycaprolactone (PCL) fabricated by electrospinning lead to protrusions mimicking the architecture of a rose stem. The branched nanoparticles (spikes length: 1–5 μm; diameter: 50–200 nm) induced heterogeneous crystallization of the polymeric matrix. This three-dimensional composite enhances the mechanical strain and strength and offers excellent antibacterial activity, while supporting the growth of eukaryote cells [170]. Bounded to Ti surfaces these structures might improve osteocondutivity and inhibit proliferation of prokaryotes. In addition, at the micoporous level prototypes of such hierarchical microspikes have shown excellent osteopromoting properties in vitro and in vivo [171]. However, if the bactericidal activity of the micro- and nanoscale structure itself is not potent enough, other mechanisms are required to accelerate the antimicrobial properties of Ti surfaces. Embedding of additional ions such as Ag, Cu, Arg or Ga is one promising option. The major challenge is to create surfaces that are harmless to eukaryotic cells but show antimicrobial activity.

The bactericidal effect of silver is based on interactions of Ag^+ with bacterial membrane constituents. This causes structural changes, interrupts transmembrane electron transfer, oxidizes bacterial components and may at least induce bacterial death. In addition, Ag^+ shows also cytotoxic effects such as mitochondrial dysfunction, disturbed membrane integrity, induction of reactive oxygen species, and interrupted adenosine triphosphate synthesis resulting in DNA lesions. The cytotoxic effects of Ag^+ depend on the instability of Ag-based bactericides, such as the high mobility of Ag nanoparticles (NPs) or Ag-containing calcium titanate. This can be avoided by silver plasma immersion ion implantation (Ag-PIII) with atomic-scale heating (ASH). The three-dimensional, hierarchical structure of sand-blasted, large grit, and acid-etched (SLA) Ti surfaces showed optimal preconditions for silver plasma immersion ion implantation. These techniques showed not only a sufficient defence against multiple cycles of bacterial attacks, independently from silver release, but they are also nontoxic to eukaryotic cells such as bone marrow mesenchymal stem cells [172–175].

Another strategy to combine antimicrobial and osteoprotective properties is the incorporation of gallium (Ga) ions in Ti surfaces. In contrast to Ag, Ga showed higher cytocompatibility since it can substitute Fe in many biological systems (same charge 3+, similarities in ionic radius and electronic configuration) and inhibits bone resorption. In bacteria Ga^{3+} acts also as a "Trojan horse" competiting with Fe^{3+} for binding to siderophores, thus interrupting crucial Fe-dependent metabolic pathways. One method embedding Ga into Ti surfaces is based on chemical and heating treatments resulting in a Ga-containing calcium titanate (Ga–CT) or gallium titanate (GT) surface. It was demonstrated that Ga–CT and GT interfaces exhibited very high antibacterial activity against multidrug resistant *Acinetobacter baumannii* (MRAB12) and inhibits bone resorption [176–179]. However, there are no clinical trials with the "Two-in-One Biointerface" available so far. Other authors are embedding Ti nanoparticles to improve the antimicrobial effects of polymers, which have a potential for orthopaedic application. Typical examples are carbon-fibre-reinforced polyetheretherketone (CFRPEEK) [180] or poly lactic acid (PLA) [181].

Inspired by bacteriophages that use nanostructured proteins to invade bacteria, other investigators study the antibiotic role of nanostructures. Mimicking the two basic structural motifs of bacteriophages, spherical and rod-like polymer molecular brushes (PMBs) have been designed. However, the impact of these techniques for Ti implants is unclear in future [182,183]. However, for the practical performances the two-dimensional surface structures such as nano-grits, nano-tube, or nano-ripple are critical (Figure 4 and Table 4).

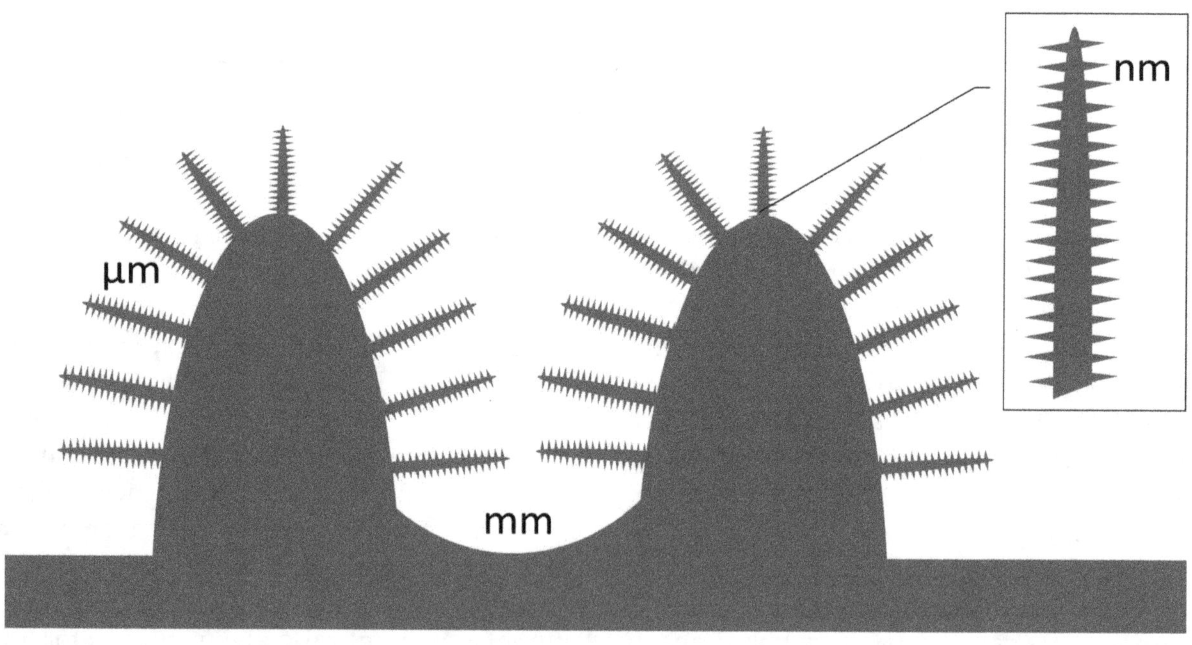

Figure 4. The hierarchical structure of a typical implant surface includes different levels of roughness. The morphology of each dimension is dependent from the material composition, the manufacturing process and post processed changes. Defined rose stock, brush-like or multi-spike topographies showed osteoconductive and bactericidal properties. It is hypothesized that these bioinspired nanospikes designs will deform or rupture the bacterial cell wall and lead to death (physical killing mechanism) [184].

Table 4. Natural nanostructures and bio-inspired Ti structures modified from [155,184–187]. In contrast to hydrophilic surfaces hydrophobic surfaces prohibit bacterial growth as the bacteria cannot stick to the surface. Defined nanostructured surfaces can stretch and rupture the relatively thin bacterial cell wall. This rapid morphological change of the adhered bacteria induce its death within a few minutes (approximately 3–5 min, "contact killing mechanism"). However, the peptidoglycan layer of the cell wall of Gram-positive (G+) bacteria is 4–5 times thicker than that of Gram-negative (G−). Here, defined surface textures of the nanostructure are required to enfold its bacteriostatic effects which are based on reduced adhesion forces. A special challenge and exception are mycobacteria. In contrast to many other bacteria their cell wall is thicker, hydrophobic, and rich in mycolic acids. It is believed that, for this reason, there has not been any study on the bactericidal efficiency of nanostructured surfaces. HY: hydrophobic, HP: hydrophilic, CA: contact angle.

Surface	Surface Feature	Method	Wettability (CA)	Bactericidal and Fungicidal Efficacy
Cicada wing	Nanoneedles, height 200 nm, diameter 60 nm size at the top, 100 nm at the base of the pillar, and spacing 170 nm	natural	HY [159°]	Lethal to *P. aeruginosa* (G−)
Gecko skin	Hair (spinules) like structures with sub-micron spacing and a tip radius of curvature <20 nm	natural	HY [151°–155°]	Lethal to *Porphyromonas gingivalis* (G−)
Dragon fly wing	Nanograss, diameter 50–70 nm, height 240 nm	natural	HY [153°]	Lethal to *P. aeruginosa* (G−), *S. aureus* (G+), *B. subtilis* (G+)
Periodical cicada	Hemispherical nano features with height 83.5 nm, diameter 167 nm, pitch 252 nm	natural	HP [80.1°]	Caused cell wall rupturing of *Saccharomyces cerevisiae*
Annual DD cicada	Spherical nanocones with height 183 nm, base diameter 104 nm, cap diameter 104 nm, pitch 175 nm	natural	HY [132°]	Caused cell wall rupturing of *Saccharomyces cerevisiae*
Sanddragon dragonfly	High-aspect ratio spherical capped nanocylinders with height 241 nm, diameter 53 nm, pitch 123 nm	natural	HY [119°]	Caused cell wall rupturing of *Saccharomyces cerevisiae*
Megapomponia intermedia	Nanopillars with height 241 nm, diameter 156 nm, pitch 165 nm	natural	HY [135.5°]	Bactericidal against *Pseudomonas fluorescens* (G−)
Cryptotympana aguila	Nanopillars with height 182 nm, diameter 159 nm, pitch 187 nm	natural	HY [113.2°]	Bactericidal against G− *P. fluorescens*
Ayuthia spectabile	Nanopillars with height 182 nm, diameter 207 nm, pitch 251 nm	natural	HY [95.65°]	Bactericidal against *P. fluorescens* (but more than *Megapomponia intermedia* and *Cryptotympana aguila)*
Titania nanowire arrays	Nanowires, brush type: Diameter 100 nm	Hydrothermal	-	Effective in killing motile bacteria (*P. aeruginosa*, *Escherichia coli* (G−), *B. subtilis*), less lethal against non-motile bacteria (*S. aureus*, *Enterococcus faecalis* (G+), *K. pneumoniae (G−))*
Titania nanowire arrays	Nanowires, niche type: Diameter 10–15 µm	Hydrothermal	-	Effective in killing motile bacteria (*P. aeruginosa*, *Escherichia coli* and *B. subtilis*), less lethal against non-motile bacteria (*S. aureus*, *Enterococcus faecalis*, and *Klebsiella pneumoniae*)
Ti nanopatterned arrays	Nanopatterned arrays, average diameter 40.3 nm	Hydrothermal etching	*HP [73°]*	Effective in killing *P. aeruginosa*, less lethal against *S. aureus*
Ti alloy nanospike surface	Nanospikes, average diameter 10 nm, spacing 2 µm, height 2 µm	Anodization	-	Lethal to *S. aureus*
Ti alloy anospike surface	Nanospikes, average diameter 20 nm	Thermal oxidation	-	Lethal to *E. coli*

However, for practical performance in orthopaedic surgery, the narrow valleys or slots of nanomaterials might be filled up with adsorbed proteins and other molecules within few minutes. Therefore, it also seems to be questionable if the antimicrobial effects of the nanostructures (e.g., nano-grits, nano-tube, or nano-ripple) will have a relevant and persisting effect on prokaryotes. Besides, appropriate mechanical strength of nanostructures is a requirement for clinical application. For some materials infinite element analysis is available to predict the mechanical behaviour [188]. Especially in press fit implants, these structures have to withstand relevant shear forces during application and also load bearing.

5. Outlook and Recent Trends in Nanostructured Ti

From our point of view, the future in nano-based orthopaedic Ti implants will stronger focus on NPs composites such as PLA electrospun fiber-TiO_2 nanoparticle [189] and also on custom-made scaffolds fabricated by additive manufacturing (AM) methods. Besides composites, also coating techniques such as sialinisation-mediated binding have a strong potential to improve cellular binding and biomineralization as well as infection prophylaxis. In this context we doubt that antibiotics are promising coating candidates for Ti implants [190]. Besides regulatory burdens, clinical effects might be complicated by molecule instabilities (sterilization, storage, and shelf life), biomechanical forces (in vivo application), and local bacterial resistances. Nevertheless, from the evolution point of view there is also evidence that biological systems respond to novel materials and develop ion escape strategies. Some investigators emphasize that their surface modification decrease the release of cytotoxic metal ions, but there are no data available yet on the possible role of metal ions in the development of bacterial resistance in sub-minimal inhibitory concentrations (MIC).

Many bacteria express metal-sensing transcriptional regulators allowing them to adapt to their environment rather quickly. Within minutes to hours, bacteria are able to escape toxic metals such as Ag^+, Cd^{2+}, Hg^{2+}, Ni^{2+}, etc. (physiological acclimation). These species and strain dependent strategies include:

- energy dependent efflux of toxic metals e.g., enzymatic transformations (oxidation, reduction, methylation, and demethylation);
- the expression of metal-binding proteins (metallothionein, SmtA, chaperone CopZ, SilE);
- inhibition of ions to enter the cell (downregulated expression of membrane transport proteins); and
- persisting phenotypes with slower growth or ceasing cell division [191].

In contrast to these initial physiological responses to toxins, which is described for *E. coli* and Ag^+ [192], there is always genetic variation among the microbes leading to natural selection. The result is an evolutionary adaption which occurs rapidly.

In contrast to today's implants, future Ti surfaces will have more controlled surface design with less variation on the macro-, micro- and nanoscale. For many years, the pharmaceutical industry designed drugs on a molecular level. Future medical devices such as Ti implants might follow these developments to the benefit of orthopaedic patients. Rapid Prototyping (RP) Technologies (e.g., 3D fibre deposition), electron beam melting (EBM), selective laser melting (SLM) or 3D printing can fabricate porous Ti scaffolds with fully interconnected porous network and highly controllable porosity and pore size [193–199].

Understanding the molecular principles and interactions at the tissue-surface interface at different dimensional levels (porosity gradient) might help closing the gap between promising new designed Ti structures of the research stage ("valley of dreams") and the so-called "valley of death" of further translational and preclinical stages of implants. One example is to control cell performance to a certain extent by varying pore sizes [69,200]. Smart, multicomponent surface systems capable of delivering both local osteoinductive and bactericidal stimuli will make the breakthrough and revolutionize orthopaedic implants.

Abbreviations

AM	additive manufacturing
ASH	atomic-scale heating
Ag	argentum (silver)
Al	aluminium
ALP	alkaline phosphatase
B.	Bacillus
Ba	barium
BMP	bone morphogenic protein
BSA	bovine serum albumin anoparticles
C	carbon
Ca	calcium
CA	contact angle
CFRPEEK	carbon-fiber-reinforced polyetheretherketone
Cd	cadmium
copZ	copper transport protein, metallochaperone, Crk-associated substrate
cp	commercial pure
Cr	chromium
E.	*Escherichia*
EFG	epidermal growth factor
EPT	entangled porous titanium
F	flour
FAK	fokal adhesion kinase
FN	fibronectin
ECM	extracellular matrix
G−	gram negative
G+	gram positive
Ga	gallium
Ga–CT	Ga-containing calcium titanate
GT	gallium titanate
ERK	extracellular signal-regulated kinase
Fe	ferrum (iron)
GLAD	glancing angle sputter deposition
H	hydrogen
Hg	hydrargyrum (mercury)
HA	hydroxyapatite
Hf	hafnium
HP	hydrophilic
HV	high voltage
HY	hydrophobic
K.	*Klebsiella*
LV	low voltage
Mo	molybdenum
MEK	MAPK/Erk kinase
MIC	minimal inhibitory concentration
MLC	myosin light chain
N	nitrogen
Nb	niobium
NMATF	nuclear matrix architectural transcription factors
NPs	nanoparticles
O	oxygen

OSA	oxidized alginate
P	phosphorus/phosphate
P.	*Pseudomonas*
PCL	polycaprolactone
PI	periprosthetic infection
PLLA	polylactide
PMB	polymer molecular brushes
RANKL	receptor activator of nuclear factor kappa-B ligand
Rho	Ras (Rat sarcom) homologue
RGD	Arginylglycylaspartic acid (tripeptide composed of L-arginine, glycine, and L-aspartic)
ROCK	Rho-associated protein kinase
S.	*Staphylococcus*
SAMs	self-assembled monolayers
SLA	sand-blasted, large grit, and acid-etched
Si	silicium
SilE	periplasmic Ag(I)-binding protein expressed by a sensor/responder two-component transcriptional regulatory system
SIRS	systemic inflammatory response syndrome
Sr	strontium
Ta	tantalum
Ti	titanium
V	vanadium, vascular endothelial growth factor (VEGF)
Zn	zinc
Zr	zirkonium

References

1. Wang, X.; Xu, S.; Zhou, S.; Xu, W.; Leary, M.; Choong, P.; Qian, M.; Brandt, M.; Xie, Y.M. Topological design and additive manufacturing of porous metals for bone scaffolds and orthopaedic implants: A review. *Biomaterials* **2016**, *83*, 127–141. [CrossRef] [PubMed]
2. Park, J.; Lakes, R.S. *Biomaterials. An Introduction*; Springer: New York, NY, USA, 2007.
3. Black, J.; Hastings, G. *Handbook of Biomaterial Properties*; Springer: New York, NY, USA, 1998.
4. Tassani, S.; Ohman, C.; Baruffaldi, F.; Baleani, M.; Viceconti, M. Volume to density relation in adult human bone tissue. *J. Biomech.* **2011**, *44*, 103–108. [CrossRef] [PubMed]
5. Cuppone, M.; Seedhom, B.B.; Berry, E.; Ostell, A.E. The longitudinal young's modulus of cortical bone in the midshaft of human femur and its correlation with CT scanning data. *Calcif. Tissue Int.* **2004**, *74*, 302–309. [PubMed]
6. Rho, J.Y.; Ashman, R.B.; Turner, C.H. Young's modulus of trabecular and cortical bone material: Ultrasonic and microtensile measurements. *J. Biomech.* **1993**, *26*, 111–119. [CrossRef]
7. Brunette, D.M.; Tengvall, P.; Textor, M.; Thomsen, P. *Titanium in Medicine: Material Science, Surface Science, Engineering, Biological Responses and Medical Applications*; Springer: Berlin/Heidelberg, Germany, 2001.
8. Bagno, A.; Di Bello, C. Surface treatments and roughness properties of Ti-based biomaterials. *J. Mater. Sci. Mater. Med.* **2004**, *15*, 935–949. [CrossRef] [PubMed]
9. Kim, K.H.; Ramaswamy, N. Electrochemical surface modification of titanium in dentistry. *Dent. Mater. J.* **2009**, *28*, 20–36. [CrossRef] [PubMed]
10. Yoshida, K.; Kamada, K.; Sato, K.; Hatada, R.; Baba, K.; Atsuta, M. Thin sol-gel-derived silica coatings on dental pure titanium casting. *J. Biomed. Mater. Res.* **1999**, *48*, 778–785. [CrossRef]
11. Sul, Y.T.; Johansson, C.B.; Jeong, Y.; Albrektsson, T. The electrochemical oxide growth behaviour on titanium in acid and alkaline electrolytes. *Med. Eng. Phys.* **2001**, *23*, 329–346. [CrossRef]
12. Nanci, A.; Wuest, J.D.; Peru, L.; Brunet, P.; Sharma, V.; Zalzal, S.; McKee, M.D. Chemical modification of titanium surfaces for covalent attachment of biological molecules. *J. Biomed. Mater. Res.* **1998**, *40*, 324–335. [CrossRef]

13. Schliephake, H.; Scharnweber, D.; Dard, M.; Sewing, A.; Aref, A.; Roessler, S. Functionalization of dental implant surfaces using adhesion molecules. *J. Biomed. Mater. Res. B Appl. Biomater.* **2005**, *73*, 88–96. [CrossRef] [PubMed]
14. Morra, M. Biochemical modification of titanium surfaces: Peptides and ECM proteins. *Eur. Cells Mater.* **2006**, *12*, 1–15. [CrossRef]
15. Rautray, T.R.; Narayanan, R.; Kwon, T.Y.; Kim, K.H. Surface modification of titanium and titanium alloys by ion implantation. *J. Biomed. Mater. Res. B Appl. Biomater.* **2010**, *93*, 581–591. [CrossRef] [PubMed]
16. Shibata, Y.; Miyazaki, T. Anode glow discharge plasma treatment enhances calcium phosphate adsorption onto titanium plates. *J. Dent. Res.* **2002**, *81*, 841–844. [CrossRef] [PubMed]
17. Chen, Y.M.; Yu, G.P.; Huang, J.H. Role of process parameters in the texture evolution of tin films deposited by hollow cathode discharge ion plating. *Surf. Coat. Technol.* **2001**, *141*, 156–163. [CrossRef]
18. Liu, X.; Chu, P.; Ding, C. Surface modification of titanium, titanium alloys, and related materials for biomedical applications. *Mater. Sci. Eng.* **2004**, *47*, 49–121. [CrossRef]
19. Jung, M.J.; Nam, K.H.; Shaginyan, L.R.; Han, J.G. Deposition of Ti thin film using the magnetron sputtering method. *Thin Solid Films* **2003**, *435*, 145–149. [CrossRef]
20. Li, P.; Ohtsuki, C.; Kokubo, T.; Nakanishi, K.; Soga, N. Apatite formation induced by silica gel in a simulated body fluid. *J. Am. Ceram. Soc.* **1992**, *75*, 2094–2097. [CrossRef]
21. Li, P.; Kangasniemi, I.; de Groot, K.; Kokubo, T. Bonelike hydroxyapatite induction by a Gel-derived titania on a titanium substrate. *J. Am. Ceram. Soc.* **1994**, *77*, 1307–1312. [CrossRef]
22. LeClair, P.; Berera, G.P.; Moodera, J.S. Titanium nitride thin films obtained by a modified physical vapor deposition process. *Thin Solid Films* **2000**, *376*, 9–15. [CrossRef]
23. Kim, K.H.; Narayanan, R.; Rautray, R.T. *Surface Modification of Titanium for Biomaterial Applications*; Nova Publishers Science Inc.: Hauppauge, NY, USA, 2010.
24. Gardon, M.; Guilemany, J.M. Milestones in functional titanium dioxide thermal spray coatings: A review. *J. Therm. Srpay Technol.* **2014**, *23*, 577–595. [CrossRef]
25. Florencio-Silva, R.; Sasso, G.R.; Sasso-Cerri, E.; Simoes, M.J.; Cerri, P.S. Biology of bone tissue: Structure, function, and factors that influence bone cells. *Biomed. Res. Int.* **2015**, *2015*, 421746. [CrossRef] [PubMed]
26. Schmidt, C.; Kaspar, D.; Sarkar, M.R.; Claes, L.E.; Ignatius, A.A. A scanning electron microscopy study of human osteoblast morphology on five orthopedic metals. *J. Biomed. Mater. Res.* **2002**, *63*, 252–261. [CrossRef] [PubMed]
27. Leibbrandt, A.; Penninger, J.M. Rank(L) as a key target for controlling bone loss. *Adv. Exp. Med. Biol.* **2009**, *647*, 130–145. [PubMed]
28. Athanasou, N.A.; Quinn, J.; Bulstrode, C.J. Resorption of bone by inflammatory cells derived from the joint capsule of hip arthroplasties. *J. Bone Jt. Surg. Br.* **1992**, *74*, 57–62.
29. Beauvais, S.; Drevelle, O.; Jann, J.; Lauzon, M.A.; Foruzanmehr, M.; Grenier, G.; Roux, S.; Faucheux, N. Interactions between bone cells and biomaterials: An update. *Front. Biosci. (Sch. Ed.)* **2016**, *8*, 227–263.
30. Williams, D.F. On the mechanisms of biocompatibility. *Biomaterials* **2008**, *29*, 2941–2953. [CrossRef] [PubMed]
31. Prasad, K.; Bazaka, O.; Chua, M.; Rochford, M.; Fedrick, L.; Spoor, J.; Symes, R.; Tieppo, M.; Collins, C.; Cao, A.; et al. Metallic biomaterials: Current challenges and opportunities. *Materials* **2017**, *10*, 884. [CrossRef] [PubMed]
32. Donachie, M.J. *Titanium: A Technical Guide*, 2nd ed.; ASM International: Cleveland, OH, USA, 2000.
33. Hanawa, T.; Asami, K.; Asaoka, K. Repassivation of titanium and surface oxide film regenerated in simulated bioliquid. *J. Biomed. Mater. Res.* **1998**, *40*, 530–538. [CrossRef]
34. Brown, S.A. *Medical Applications of Titanium and Its Alloys: The Material and Biological Issues*; ASTM Special Technical Publication: Ann Arbor, MI, USA, 1996.
35. Kulkarni, M.M.A.; Schmuki, P.; Iglič, A. Biomaterial surface modification of titanium and titanium alloys for medical applications. In *Nanomedicine*; Seifalian, A.D., Kalaskar, D.M., Eds.; One Central Press: Cheshire, UK, 2014; pp. 112–130.
36. Hiromoto, S.; Inoue, M.; Taguchi, T.; Yamane, M.; Ohtsu, N. In vitro and in vivo biocompatibility and corrosion behaviour of a bioabsorbable magnesium alloy coated with octacalcium phosphate and hydroxyapatite. *Acta Biomater.* **2015**, *11*, 520–530. [CrossRef] [PubMed]
37. Hiromoto, S.; Hanawa, T.; Asami, K. Composition of surface oxide film of titanium with culturing murine fibroblasts L929. *Biomaterials* **2004**, *25*, 979–986. [CrossRef]

38. Saini, M.; Singh, Y.; Arora, P.; Arora, V.; Jain, K. Implant biomaterials: A comprehensive review. *World J. Clin. Cases* **2015**, *3*, 52–57. [CrossRef] [PubMed]
39. Li, B.E.; Li, Y.; Min, Y.; Hao, J.Z.; Liang, C.Y.; Li, H.P.; Wang, G.C.; Liu, S.M.; Wang, H.S. Synergistic effects of hierarchical hybrid micro/nanostructures on the biological properties of titanium orthopaedic implants. *RSC Adv.* **2015**, *5*, 49552–49558. [CrossRef]
40. Nazarov, D.V.; Zemtsova, E.G.; Valiev, R.Z.; Smirnov, V.M. Formation of micro- and nanostructures on the nanotitanium surface by chemical etching and deposition of titania films by atomic layer deposition (ALD). *Materials* **2015**, *8*, 8366–8377. [CrossRef] [PubMed]
41. Andrade, J.D.; Hlady, V. Plasma protein adsorption: The big twelve. *Ann. N. Y. Acad. Sci.* **1987**, *516*, 158–172. [CrossRef] [PubMed]
42. Vroman, L. The importance of surfaces in contact phase reactions. *Semin. Thromb. Hemost.* **1987**, *13*, 79–85. [CrossRef] [PubMed]
43. Bakir, M. Haemocompatibility of titanium and its alloys. *J. Biomater. Appl.* **2012**, *27*, 3–15. [CrossRef] [PubMed]
44. Meyer, U.; Meyer, T.; Jones, D.B. Attachment kinetics, proliferation rates and vinculin assembly of bovine osteoblasts cultured on different pre-coated artificial substrates. *J. Mater. Sci. Mater. Med.* **1998**, *9*, 301–307. [CrossRef] [PubMed]
45. Rezania, A.; Healy, K.E. The effect of peptide surface density on mineralization of a matrix deposited by osteogenic cells. *J. Biomed. Mater. Res.* **2000**, *52*, 595–600. [CrossRef]
46. Davies, J.E. Understanding peri-implant endosseous healing. *J. Dent. Educ.* **2003**, *67*, 932–949. [PubMed]
47. Jager, M.; Zilkens, C.; Zanger, K.; Krauspe, R. Significance of nano- and microtopography for cell-surface interactions in orthopaedic implants. *J. Biomed. Biotechnol.* **2007**, *2007*, 69036. [CrossRef] [PubMed]
48. Delcroix, M.F.; Laurent, S.; Huet, G.L.; Dupont-Gillain, C.C. Protein adsorption can be reversibly switched on and off on mixed PEO/PAA brushes. *Acta Biomater.* **2015**, *11*, 68–79. [CrossRef] [PubMed]
49. Delcroix, M.F.; Demoustier-Champagne, S.; Dupont-Gillain, C.C. Quartz crystal microbalance study of ionic strength and pH-dependent polymer conformation and protein adsorption/desorption on PAA, PEO, and mixed PEO/PAA brushes. *Langmuir* **2014**, *30*, 268–277. [CrossRef] [PubMed]
50. Delcroix, M.F.; Huet, G.L.; Conard, T.; Demoustier-Champagne, S.; Du Prez, F.E.; Landoulsi, J.; Dupont-Gillain, C.C. Design of mixed PEO/PAA brushes with switchable properties toward protein adsorption. *Biomacromolecules* **2013**, *14*, 215–225. [CrossRef] [PubMed]
51. Soria, J.; Soria, C.; Mirshahi, M.; Boucheix, C.; Aurengo, A.; Perrot, J.-Y.; Bernadou, A.; Samama, M.; Rosenfeld, C. Conformational change in fibrinogen induced by adsorption to a surface. *J. Colloid Interface Sci.* **1985**, *107*, 204–208. [CrossRef]
52. Kusakawa, Y.; Yoshida, E.; Hayakawa, T. Protein adsorption to titanium and zirconia using a quartz crystal microbalance method. *Biomed. Res. Int.* **2017**, *2017*, 1521593. [CrossRef] [PubMed]
53. Cei, S.; Karapetsa, D.; Aleo, E.; Graziani, F. Protein adsorption on a laser-modified titanium implant surface. *Implant Dent.* **2015**, *24*, 134–141. [CrossRef] [PubMed]
54. Jimbo, R.; Ivarsson, M.; Koskela, A.; Sul, Y.T.; Johansson, C.B. Protein adsorption to surface chemistry and crystal structure modification of titanium surfaces. *J. Oral Maxillofac. Res.* **2010**, *1*, e3. [CrossRef] [PubMed]
55. Romero-Gavilan, F.; Gomes, N.C.; Rodenas, J.; Sanchez, A.; Azkargorta, M.; Iloro, I.; Elortza, F.; Garcia Arnaez, I.; Gurruchaga, M.; Goni, I.; et al. Proteome analysis of human serum proteins adsorbed onto different titanium surfaces used in dental implants. *Biofouling* **2017**, *33*, 98–111. [CrossRef] [PubMed]
56. Nishimoto, S.K.; Nishimoto, M.; Park, S.W.; Lee, K.M.; Kim, H.S.; Koh, J.T.; Ong, J.L.; Liu, Y.; Yang, Y. The effect of titanium surface roughening on protein absorption, cell attachment, and cell spreading. *Int. J. Oral Maxillofac. Implants* **2008**, *23*, 675–680. [PubMed]
57. Paredes, J.A.; Polini, A.; Chrzanowski, W. Protein-based biointerfaces to control stem cell differentiation. In *Biointerfaces: Where Material Meets Biology*; Hutmacher, D.C.W., Ed.; Royal Society of Chemistry: London, UK, 2005.
58. Biao, M.N.; Chen, Y.M.; Xiong, S.B.; Wu, B.Y.; Yang, B.C. Synergistic effects of fibronectin and bone morphogenetic protein on the bioactivity of titanium metal. *J. Biomed. Mater. Res. A* **2017**, *105*, 2485–2498. [CrossRef] [PubMed]

59. Kulkarni, M.; Mazare, A.; Park, J.; Gongadze, E.; Killian, M.S.; Kralj, S.; von der Mark, K.; Iglic, A.; Schmuki, P. Protein interactions with layers of TiO_2 nanotube and nanopore arrays: Morphology and surface charge influence. *Acta Biomater.* **2016**, *45*, 357–366. [CrossRef] [PubMed]
60. Huber-Lang, M.; Ignatius, A.; Brenner, R.E. Role of complement on broken surfaces after trauma. *Adv. Exp. Med. Biol.* **2015**, *865*, 43–55. [PubMed]
61. Hoon, J.L.; Tan, M.H.; Koh, C.G. The regulation of cellular responses to mechanical cues by Rho GTPases. *Cells* **2016**, *5*, 17. [CrossRef] [PubMed]
62. Goldman, M.; Juodzbalys, G.; Vilkinis, V. Titanium surfaces with nanostructures influence on osteoblasts proliferation: A systematic review. *J. Oral Maxillofac. Res.* **2014**, *5*, e1. [CrossRef] [PubMed]
63. Park, J.; Mazare, A.; Schneider, H.; von der Mark, K.; Fischer, M.J.; Schmuki, P. Electric field-induced osteogenic differentiation on TiO_2 nanotubular layer. *Tissue Eng. Part C Methods* **2016**, *22*, 809–821. [CrossRef]
64. Uskokovic, V. When 1 + 1 > 2: Nanostructured composites for hard tissue engineering applications. *Mater. Sci. Eng. C Mater. Biol. Appl.* **2015**, *57*, 434–451. [CrossRef] [PubMed]
65. Karageorgiou, V.; Kaplan, D. Porosity of 3D biomaterial scaffolds and osteogenesis. *Biomaterials* **2005**, *26*, 5474–5491. [CrossRef] [PubMed]
66. Hollander, D.A.; von Walter, M.; Wirtz, T.; Sellei, R.; Schmidt-Rohlfing, B.; Paar, O.; Erli, H.J. Structural, mechanical and in vitro characterization of individually structured Ti-6AL-4V produced by direct laser forming. *Biomaterials* **2006**, *27*, 955–963. [CrossRef] [PubMed]
67. Warnke, P.H.; Douglas, T.; Wollny, P.; Sherry, E.; Steiner, M.; Galonska, S.; Becker, S.T.; Springer, I.N.; Wiltfang, J.; Sivananthan, S. Rapid prototyping: Porous titanium alloy scaffolds produced by selective laser melting for bone tissue engineering. *Tissue Eng. Part C Methods* **2009**, *15*, 115–124. [CrossRef] [PubMed]
68. Van Bael, S.; Chai, Y.C.; Truscello, S.; Moesen, M.; Kerckhofs, G.; Van Oosterwyck, H.; Kruth, J.P.; Schrooten, J. The effect of pore geometry on the in vitro biological behavior of human periosteum-derived cells seeded on selective laser-melted Ti6AL4V bone scaffolds. *Acta Biomater.* **2012**, *8*, 2824–2834. [CrossRef] [PubMed]
69. Wysocki, B.; Idaszek, J.; Szlazak, K.; Strzelczyk, K.; Brynk, T.; Kurzydlowski, K.J.; Swieszkowski, W. Post processing and biological evaluation of the titanium scaffolds for bone tissue engineering. *Materials* **2016**, *9*, 197. [CrossRef] [PubMed]
70. Choren, J.A.; Heinrich, S.M.; Silver-Thorn, M.B. Young's modulus and volume porosity relationships for additive manufacturing applications. *J. Mater. Sci.* **2013**, *48*, 5103–5112. [CrossRef]
71. Ahmadi, S.M.; Campoli, G.; Amin Yavari, S.; Sajadi, B.; Wauthle, R.; Schrooten, J.; Weinans, H.; Zadpoor, A.A. Mechanical behavior of regular open-cell porous biomaterials made of diamond lattice unit cells. *J. Mech. Behav. Biomed. Mater.* **2014**, *34*, 106–115. [CrossRef] [PubMed]
72. Heinl, P.; Muller, L.; Korner, C.; Singer, R.F.; Muller, F.A. Cellular Ti-6AL-4V structures with interconnected macro porosity for bone implants fabricated by selective electron beam melting. *Acta Biomater.* **2008**, *4*, 1536–1544. [CrossRef] [PubMed]
73. Zhang, B.G.; Myers, D.E.; Wallace, G.G.; Brandt, M.; Choong, P.F. Bioactive coatings for orthopaedic implants-recent trends in development of implant coatings. *Int. J. Mol. Sci.* **2014**, *15*, 11878–11921. [CrossRef] [PubMed]
74. Dale, G.R.; Hamilton, J.W.; Dunlop, P.S.; Lemoine, P.; Byrne, J.A. Electrochemical growth of titanium oxide nanotubes: The effect of surface roughness and applied potential. *J. Nanosci. Nanotechnol.* **2009**, *9*, 4215–4219. [CrossRef] [PubMed]
75. Gongadze, E.; Kabaso, D.; Bauer, S.; Slivnik, T.; Schmuki, P.; van Rienen, U.; Iglic, A. Adhesion of osteoblasts to a nanorough titanium implant surface. *Int. J. Nanomed.* **2011**, *6*, 1801–1816.
76. Gongadze, E.; Kabaso, D.; Bauer, S.; Park, J.; Schmuki, P.; Iglic, A. Adhesion of osteoblasts to a vertically aligned TiO_2 nanotube surface. *Mini Rev. Med. Chem.* **2013**, *13*, 194–200. [PubMed]
77. Ueno, T.; Yamada, M.; Suzuki, T.; Minamikawa, H.; Sato, N.; Hori, N.; Takeuchi, K.; Hattori, M.; Ogawa, T. Enhancement of bone-titanium integration profile with UV-photofunctionalized titanium in a gap healing model. *Biomaterials* **2010**, *31*, 1546–1557. [CrossRef] [PubMed]
78. Schwarz, F.; Herten, M.; Sager, M.; Wieland, M.; Dard, M.; Becker, J. Bone regeneration in dehiscence-type defects at chemically modified (slactive) and conventional SLA titanium implants: A pilot study in dogs. *J. Clin. Periodontol.* **2007**, *34*, 78–86. [CrossRef] [PubMed]

79. Zhao, G.; Schwartz, Z.; Wieland, M.; Rupp, F.; Geis-Gerstorfer, J.; Cochran, D.L.; Boyan, B.D. High surface energy enhances cell response to titanium substrate microstructure. *J. Biomed. Mater. Res. A* **2005**, *74*, 49–58. [CrossRef] [PubMed]
80. Heller, M.; Kammerer, P.W.; Al-Nawas, B.; Luszpinski, M.A.; Forch, R.; Brieger, J. The effect of extracellular matrix proteins on the cellular response of HUVECS and HOBS after covalent immobilization onto titanium. *J. Biomed. Mater. Res. A* **2015**, *103*, 2035–2044. [CrossRef] [PubMed]
81. Jager, M.; Boge, C.; Janissen, R.; Rohrbeck, D.; Hulsen, T.; Lensing-Hohn, S.; Krauspe, R.; Herten, M. Osteoblastic potency of bone marrow cells cultivated on functionalized biometals with cyclic RGD-peptide. *J. Biomed. Mater. Res. A* **2013**, *101*, 2905–2914. [CrossRef] [PubMed]
82. Haversath, M.; Hulsen, T.; Boge, C.; Tassemeier, T.; Landgraeber, S.; Herten, M.; Warwas, S.; Krauspe, R.; Jager, M. Osteogenic differentiation and proliferation of bone marrow-derived mesenchymal stromal cells on PDLLA + BMP-2-coated titanium alloy surfaces. *J. Biomed. Mater. Res. A* **2016**, *104*, 145–154. [CrossRef] [PubMed]
83. Mas-Moruna, C.E.M.; Montufar, E.; Mestres, G.; Aparicio, D.; Javier, G.F.; Ginebra, M. *Biomaterials Surface Science*; Wiley-VCH Verlag: Weinheim, Germany, 2013.
84. Roy, P.; Berger, S.; Schmuki, P. TiO_2 nanotubes: Synthesis and applications. *Angew. Chem. Int. Ed. Engl.* **2011**, *50*, 2904–2939. [CrossRef] [PubMed]
85. Yin, L.; Ji, S.; Liu, G.; Xu, G.; Ye, C. Understanding the growth behavior of titania nanotubes. *Electrochem. Commun.* **2011**, *13*, 454–457. [CrossRef]
86. Schultze, J.W.; Lohrengel, M.M. Stability, reactivity and breakdown of passive films. Problems of recent and future research. *Electrochim. Acta* **2000**, *45*, 2499–2513. [CrossRef]
87. Webster, T.J.; Yao, C. *Anodizaton: A Promising Nano-Modification Technique of Titanium-Based Implants for Orthopedic Application*; Springer: Heidelberg, Germany, 2007; pp. 21–47.
88. Li, Y.; Ding, D.; Ning, C.; Bai, S.; Huang, L.; Li, M.; Mao, D. Thermal stability and in vitro bioactivity of Ti-Al-V-O nanostructures fabricated on Ti6AL4V alloy. *Nanotechnology* **2009**, *20*, 065708. [CrossRef] [PubMed]
89. Wang, L.; Zhao, T.T.; Zhang, Z.; Li, G. Fabrication of highly ordered TiO_2 nanotube arrays via anodization of Ti-6AL-4V alloy sheet. *J. Nanosci. Nanotechnol.* **2010**, *10*, 8312–8321. [CrossRef] [PubMed]
90. Moon, S.H.; Lee, S.J.; Park, I.S.; Lee, M.H.; Soh, Y.J.; Bae, T.S.; Kim, H.S. Bioactivity of Ti-6AL-4V alloy implants treated with ibandronate after the formation of the nanotube TiO_2 layer. *J. Biomed. Mater. Res. B Appl. Biomater.* **2012**, *100*, 2053–2059. [CrossRef] [PubMed]
91. Kang, K.; Lim, H.; Yun, K.D.; Park, S.; Jeong, C.; Lee, K. Effect of viscosities on the surface morphology and crystallographic properties of hydroxyapatite coated titanium dioxide nanotubes. *J. Nanosci. Nanotechnol.* **2015**, *15*, 5310–5313. [CrossRef] [PubMed]
92. Lewandowska, Z.; Piszczek, P.; Radtke, A.; Jedrzejewski, T.; Kozak, W.; Sadowska, B. The evaluation of the impact of titania nanotube covers morphology and crystal phase on their biological properties. *J. Mater. Sci. Mater. Med.* **2015**, *26*, 163. [CrossRef] [PubMed]
93. Lotz, E.M.; Olivares-Navarrete, R.; Berner, S.; Boyan, B.D.; Schwartz, Z. Osteogenic response of human mscs and osteoblasts to hydrophilic and hydrophobic nanostructured titanium implant surfaces. *J. Biomed. Mater. Res. A* **2016**, *104*, 3137–3148. [CrossRef] [PubMed]
94. Lattner, D.; Jennissen, H.P. Preparation and properties of ultra-hydrophilic surfaces on titanium and steel. *Mater. Sci. Eng. Technol.* **2009**, *40*, 109–116. [CrossRef]
95. Jennissen, H.P.; Lüers, S. Lotus-effect and inverse lotus-effect in connection with extremely rough titanium surfaces. *Mater. Sci. Eng. Technol.* **2010**, *41*. [CrossRef]
96. Park, J.; Bauer, S.; von der Mark, K.; Schmuki, P. Nanosize and vitality: TiO_2 nanotube diameter directs cell fate. *Nano Lett.* **2007**, *7*, 1686–1691. [CrossRef] [PubMed]
97. Park, J.; Bauer, S.; Schmuki, P.; Schlegel, K.; Neukam, F.; von der Mark, K. Nanotube diameter directs stem cell fate. *J. Stem Cells Regen. Med.* **2007**, *2*, 168. [PubMed]
98. Park, J.; Bauer, S.; Pittrof, A.; Killian, M.S.; Schmuki, P.; von der Mark, K. Synergistic control of mesenchymal stem cell differentiation by nanoscale surface geometry and immobilized growth factors on TiO_2 nanotubes. *Small* **2012**, *8*, 98–107. [CrossRef] [PubMed]
99. Von Wilmowsky, C.; Bauer, S.; Roedl, S.; Neukam, F.W.; Schmuki, P.; Schlegel, K.A. The diameter of anodic TiO_2 nanotubes affects bone formation and correlates with the bone morphogenetic protein-2 expression in vivo. *Clin. Oral Implants Res.* **2012**, *23*, 359–366. [CrossRef] [PubMed]

100. Fagan, J.A.; Bauer, B.J.; Hobbie, E.K.; Becker, M.L.; Hight Walker, A.R.; Simpson, J.R.; Chun, J.; Obrzut, J.; Bajpai, V.; Phelan, F.R.; et al. Carbon nanotubes: Measuring dispersion and length. *Adv. Mater.* **2011**, *23*, 338–348. [CrossRef] [PubMed]
101. Iwata, N.; Nozaki, K.; Horiuchi, N.; Yamashita, K.; Tsutsumi, Y.; Miura, H.; Nagai, A. Effects of controlled micro-/nanosurfaces on osteoblast proliferation. *J. Biomed. Mater. Res. A* **2017**, *105*, 2589–2596. [CrossRef] [PubMed]
102. Palin, E.; Liu, H.; Webster, T.J. Mimicking the nanofeatures of bone increases bone-forming cell adhesion and proliferation. *Nanotechnology* **2005**, *16*, 1828–1835. [CrossRef]
103. Gao, L.; Feng, B.; Wang, J.; Lu, X.; Liu, D.; Qu, S.; Weng, J. Micro/nanostructural porous surface on titanium and bioactivity. *J. Biomed. Mater. Res. B Appl. Biomater.* **2009**, *89*, 335–341. [CrossRef] [PubMed]
104. Zinger, O.; Anselme, K.; Denzer, A.; Habersetzer, P.; Wieland, M.; Jeanfils, J.; Hardouin, P.; Landolt, D. Time-dependent morphology and adhesion of osteoblastic cells on titanium model surfaces featuring scale-resolved topography. *Biomaterials* **2004**, *25*, 2695–2711. [CrossRef] [PubMed]
105. Kane, R.; Ma, P.X. Mimicking the nanostructure of bone matrix to regenerate bone. *Mater. Today* **2013**, *16*, 418–423. [CrossRef] [PubMed]
106. Weiner, S.; Wagner, H.D. The material bone: Structure-mechanical function relations. *Annu. Rev. Mater. Sci.* **1998**, *28*, 271–298. [CrossRef]
107. Kheradmandfard, M.; Kashani-Bozorg, S.F.; Kim, C.L.; Hanzaki, A.Z.; Pyoun, Y.S.; Kim, J.H.; Amanov, A.; Kim, D.E. Nanostructured beta-type titanium alloy fabricated by ultrasonic nanocrystal surface modification. *Ultrason. Sonochem.* **2017**, *39*, 698–706. [CrossRef] [PubMed]
108. Li, Y.; Dai, X.; Bai, Y.; Liu, Y.; Wang, Y.; Liu, O.; Yan, F.; Tang, Z.; Zhang, X.; Deng, X. Electroactive $BaTiO_3$ nanoparticle-functionalized fibrous scaffolds enhance osteogenic differentiation of mesenchymal stem cells. *Int. J. Nanomed.* **2017**, *12*, 4007–4018. [CrossRef] [PubMed]
109. Yang, W.; Xi, X.; Shen, X.; Liu, P.; Hu, Y.; Cai, K. Titania nanotubes dimensions-dependent protein adsorption and its effect on the growth of osteoblasts. *J. Biomed. Mater. Res. A* **2014**, *102*, 3598–3608. [CrossRef] [PubMed]
110. Bauer, S.; Park, J.; Faltenbacher, J.; Berger, S.; von der Mark, K.; Schmuki, P. Size selective behavior of mesenchymal stem cells on ZrO_2 and TiO_2 nanotube arrays. *Integr. Biol.* **2009**, *1*, 525–532. [CrossRef] [PubMed]
111. Salou, L.; Hoornaert, A.; Louarn, G.; Layrolle, P. Enhanced osseointegration of titanium implants with nanostructured surfaces: An experimental study in rabbits. *Acta Biomater.* **2015**, *11*, 494–502. [CrossRef] [PubMed]
112. Bjursten, L.M.; Rasmusson, L.; Oh, S.; Smith, G.C.; Brammer, K.S.; Jin, S. Titanium dioxide nanotubes enhance bone bonding in vivo. *J. Biomed. Mater. Res. A* **2010**, *92*, 1218–1224. [PubMed]
113. Zhao, X.; Wang, T.; Qian, S.; Liu, X.; Sun, J.; Li, B. Silicon-doped titanium dioxide nanotubes promoted bone formation on titanium implants. *Int. J. Mol. Sci.* **2016**, *17*, 292. [CrossRef] [PubMed]
114. Li, X.; Chen, T.; Hu, J.; Li, S.; Zou, Q.; Li, Y.; Jiang, N.; Li, H.; Li, J. Modified surface morphology of a novel Ti-24Nb-4Zr-7.9Sn titanium alloy via anodic oxidation for enhanced interfacial biocompatibility and osseointegration. *Colloids Surf. B Biointerfaces* **2016**, *144*, 265–275. [CrossRef] [PubMed]
115. Hegedus, C.; Ho, C.C.; Csik, A.; Biri, S.; Ding, S.J. Enhanced physicochemical and biological properties of ion-implanted titanium using electron cyclotron resonance ion sources. *Materials* **2016**, *9*, 25. [CrossRef] [PubMed]
116. Wang, Q.; Qiao, Y.; Cheng, M.; Jiang, G.; He, G.; Chen, Y.; Zhang, X.; Liu, X. Tantalum implanted entangled porous titanium promotes surface osseointegration and bone ingrowth. *Sci. Rep.* **2016**, *6*, 26248. [CrossRef] [PubMed]
117. Heo, D.N.; Ko, W.K.; Lee, H.R.; Lee, S.J.; Lee, D.; Um, S.H.; Lee, J.H.; Woo, Y.H.; Zhang, L.G.; Lee, D.W.; et al. Titanium dental implants surface-immobilized with gold nanoparticles as osteoinductive agents for rapid osseointegration. *J. Colloid Interface Sci.* **2016**, *469*, 129–137. [CrossRef] [PubMed]
118. Csarnovics, I.; Hajdu, P.; Biri, S.; Hegedus, C.; Kökényesi, S.; Rácz, R.; Csik, A. Preliminary studies of creation of gold nanoparticles on titanium surface towards biomedical applications. *Vaccum* **2017**, *126*, 55–58. [CrossRef]
119. Zainali, K.; Danscher, G.; Jakobsen, T.; Baas, J.; Moller, P.; Bechtold, J.E.; Soballe, K. Assessment of modified gold surfaced titanium implants on skeletal fixation. *J. Biomed. Mater. Res. A* **2013**, *101*, 195–202. [CrossRef] [PubMed]

120. Bauer, S.; Park, J.; Pittrof, A.; Song, Y.; von der Mark, K.; Schmuki, P. Covalent functionalization of TiO_2 nanotube arrays with EGF and BMP-2 for modified behavior towards mesenchymal stem cell. *Integr. Biol.* **2011**, *3*, 927–936. [CrossRef] [PubMed]
121. Lai, M.; Cai, K.; Zhao, L.; Chen, X.; Hou, Y.; Yang, Z. Surface functionalization of TiO_2 nanotubes with bone morphogenetic protein 2 and its synergistic effect on the differentiation of mesenchymal stem cells. *Biomacromolecules* **2011**, *12*, 1097–1105. [CrossRef] [PubMed]
122. Hu, X.; Neoh, K.G.; Zhang, J.; Kang, E.T.; Wang, W. Immobilization strategy for optimizing vegf's concurrent bioactivity towards endothelial cells and osteoblasts on implant surfaces. *Biomaterials* **2012**, *33*, 8082–8093. [CrossRef] [PubMed]
123. Kulkarni, M.; Mazare, A.; Gongadze, E.; Perutkova, S.; Kralj-Iglic, V.; Milosev, I.; Schmuki, P.; Iglic, A.; Mozetic, M. Titanium nanostructures for biomedical applications. *Nanotechnology* **2015**, *26*, 062002. [CrossRef] [PubMed]
124. Xiao, M.; Chen, Y.M.; Biao, M.N.; Zhang, X.D.; Yang, B.C. Bio-functionalization of biomedical metals. *Mater. Sci. Eng. C Mater. Biol. Appl.* **2017**, *70*, 1057–1070. [CrossRef] [PubMed]
125. Chrastil, J.; Patel, A.A. Complications associated with posterior and transforaminal lumbar interbody fusion. *J. Am. Acad. Orthop. Surg.* **2012**, *20*, 283–291. [CrossRef] [PubMed]
126. Jennissen, H.P. A macrophage model of osseointegration. *Curr. Dir. Biomed. Eng.* **2016**, *2*, 53–56. [CrossRef]
127. Chatzinikolaidou, M.; Lichtinger, T.K.; Muller, R.T.; Jennissen, H.P. Peri-implant reactivity and osteoinductive potential of immobilized rhbmp-2 on titanium carriers. *Acta Biomater.* **2010**, *6*, 4405–4421. [CrossRef] [PubMed]
128. Becker, J.; Kirsch, A.; Schwarz, F.; Chatzinikolaidou, M.; Rothamel, D.; Lekovic, V.; Laub, M.; Jennissen, H.P. Bone apposition to titanium implants biocoated with recombinant human bone morphogenetic protein-2 (rhbmp-2). A pilot study in dogs. *Clin. Oral Investig.* **2006**, *10*, 217–224. [CrossRef] [PubMed]
129. Lee, H.J.; Koo, A.N.; Lee, S.W.; Lee, M.H.; Lee, S.C. Catechol-functionalized adhesive polymer nanoparticles for controlled local release of bone morphogenetic protein-2 from titanium surface. *J. Control. Release* **2013**, *170*, 198–208. [CrossRef] [PubMed]
130. Ripamonti, U.; Reddi, A.H. Growth and morphogenetic factors in bone induction: Role of osteogenin and related bone morphogenetic proteins in craniofacial and periodontal bone repair. *Crit. Rev. Oral Biol. Med.* **1992**, *3*, 1–14. [CrossRef] [PubMed]
131. Jansen, J.A.; Vehof, J.W.; Ruhe, P.Q.; Kroeze-Deutman, H.; Kuboki, Y.; Takita, H.; Hedberg, E.L.; Mikos, A.G. Growth factor-loaded scaffolds for bone engineering. *J. Control. Release* **2005**, *101*, 127–136. [CrossRef] [PubMed]
132. Kokubo, S.; Mochizuki, M.; Fukushima, S.; Ito, T.; Nozaki, K.; Iwai, T.; Takahashi, K.; Yokota, S.; Miyata, K.; Sasaki, N. Long-term stability of bone tissues induced by an osteoinductive biomaterial, recombinant human bone morphogenetic protein-2 and a biodegradable carrier. *Biomaterials* **2004**, *25*, 1795–1803. [CrossRef] [PubMed]
133. La, W.G.; Park, S.; Yoon, H.H.; Jeong, G.J.; Lee, T.J.; Bhang, S.H.; Han, J.Y.; Char, K.; Kim, B.S. Delivery of a therapeutic protein for bone regeneration from a substrate coated with graphene oxide. *Small* **2013**, *9*, 4051–4060. [CrossRef] [PubMed]
134. Xiao, M.; Biao, M.; Chen, Y.; Xie, M.; Yang, B. Regulating the osteogenic function of rhBMP 2 by different titanium surface properties. *J. Biomed. Mater. Res. A* **2016**, *104*, 1882–1893. [CrossRef] [PubMed]
135. Chakravorty, N.; Ivanovski, S.; Prasadam, I.; Crawford, R.; Oloyede, A.; Xiao, Y. The microrna expression signature on modified titanium implant surfaces influences genetic mechanisms leading to osteogenic differentiation. *Acta Biomater.* **2012**, *8*, 3516–3523. [CrossRef] [PubMed]
136. Babuska, V.; Moztarzadeh, O.; Kubikova, T.; Moztarzadeh, A.; Hrusak, D.; Tonar, Z. Evaluating the osseointegration of nanostructured titanium implants in animal models: Current experimental methods and perspectives. *Biointerphases* **2016**, *11*, 030801. [CrossRef] [PubMed]
137. Han, L.; Wang, M.; Sun, H.; Li, P.; Wang, K.; Ren, F.; Lu, X. Porous titanium scaffolds with self-assembled micro/nano hierarchical structure for dual functions of bone regeneration and anti-infection. *J. Biomed. Mater. Res. A* **2017**. [CrossRef] [PubMed]
138. Tsuchiya, H.; Shirai, T.; Nishida, H.; Murakami, H.; Kabata, T.; Yamamoto, N.; Watanabe, K.; Nakase, J. Innovative antimicrobial coating of titanium implants with iodine. *J. Orthop. Sci.* **2012**, *17*, 595–604. [CrossRef] [PubMed]

139. Shirai, T.; Shimizu, T.; Ohtani, K.; Zen, Y.; Takaya, M.; Tsuchiya, H. Antibacterial iodine-supported titanium implants. *Acta Biomater.* **2011**, *7*, 1928–1933. [CrossRef] [PubMed]
140. Dziedzic, D.M.; Savva, I.H.; Wilkinson, D.S.; Davies, J.E. Osteoconduction on, and bonding to, calcium phosphate ceramic implants. *Mater. Res. Soc. Symp. Proc.* **1996**, *414*, 147–156. [CrossRef]
141. Wengler, A.; Nimptsch, U.; Mansky, T. Hip and knee replacement in germany and the USA: Analysis of individual inpatient data from german and us hospitals for the years 2005 to 2011. *Dtsch. Ärzteblatt Int.* **2014**, *111*, 407–416.
142. Kurtz, S.M.; Ong, K.L.; Lau, E.; Bozic, K.J.; Berry, D.; Parvizi, J. Prosthetic joint infection risk after TKA in the medicare population. *Clin. Orthop. Relat. Res.* **2010**, *468*, 52–56. [CrossRef] [PubMed]
143. Ong, K.L.; Kurtz, S.M.; Lau, E.; Bozic, K.J.; Berry, D.J.; Parvizi, J. Prosthetic joint infection risk after total hip arthroplasty in the medicare population. *J. Arthroplast.* **2009**, *24*, 105–109. [CrossRef] [PubMed]
144. Bohl, D.D.; Samuel, A.M.; Basques, B.A.; Della Valle, C.J.; Levine, B.R.; Grauer, J.N. How much do adverse event rates differ between primary and revision total joint arthroplasty? *J. Arthroplast.* **2016**, *31*, 596–602. [CrossRef] [PubMed]
145. Krenn, V.; Morawietz, L.; Kienapfel, H.; Ascherl, R.; Matziolis, G.; Hassenpflug, J.; Thomsen, M.; Thomas, P.; Huber, M.; Schuh, C.; et al. Revised consensus classification. Histopathological classification of diseases associated with joint endoprostheses. *Z. Rheumatol.* **2013**, *72*, 383–392. [CrossRef] [PubMed]
146. Flemming, H.C.; Wingender, J.; Szewzyk, U.; Steinberg, P.; Rice, S.A.; Kjelleberg, S. Biofilms: An emergent form of bacterial life. *Nat. Rev. Microbiol.* **2016**, *14*, 563–575. [CrossRef] [PubMed]
147. Campoccia, D.; Montanaro, L.; Arciola, C.R. The significance of infection related to orthopedic devices and issues of antibiotic resistance. *Biomaterials* **2006**, *27*, 2331–2339. [CrossRef] [PubMed]
148. Romano, C.L.; Scarponi, S.; Gallazzi, E.; Romano, D.; Drago, L. Antibacterial coating of implants in orthopaedics and trauma: A classification proposal in an evolving panorama. *J. Orthop. Surg. Res.* **2015**, *10*, 157. [CrossRef] [PubMed]
149. Kazemzadeh-Narbat, M.; Kindrachuk, J.; Duan, K.; Jenssen, H.; Hancock, R.E.; Wang, R. Antimicrobial peptides on calcium phosphate-coated titanium for the prevention of implant-associated infections. *Biomaterials* **2010**, *31*, 9519–9526. [CrossRef] [PubMed]
150. Taylor, E.; Webster, T.J. Reducing infections through nanotechnology and nanoparticles. *Int. J. Nanomed.* **2011**, *6*, 1463–1473.
151. Gallo, J.; Panacek, A.; Prucek, R.; Kriegova, E.; Hradilova, S.; Hobza, M.; Holinka, M. Silver nanocoating technology in the prevention of prosthetic joint infection. *Materials* **2016**, *9*, 337. [CrossRef] [PubMed]
152. Ercan, B.; Kummer, K.M.; Tarquinio, K.M.; Webster, T.J. Decreased staphylococcus aureus biofilm growth on anodized nanotubular titanium and the effect of electrical stimulation. *Acta Biomater.* **2011**, *7*, 3003–3012. [CrossRef] [PubMed]
153. Dickson, M.N.; Liang, E.I.; Rodriguez, L.A.; Vollereaux, N.; Yee, A.F. Nanopatterned polymer surfaces with bactericidal properties. *Biointerphases* **2015**, *10*, 021010. [CrossRef] [PubMed]
154. Gorth, D.J.; Puckett, S.; Ercan, B.; Webster, T.J.; Rahaman, M.; Bal, B.S. Decreased bacteria activity on Si(3)N(4) surfaces compared with peek or titanium. *Int. J. Nanomed.* **2012**, *7*, 4829–4840.
155. Sjöström, T.; Nobbs, A.H.; Su, B. Bactericidal nanospike surfaces via thermal oxidation of ti alloy substrates. *Mater. Lett.* **2016**, *167*, 22–26. [CrossRef]
156. Mathew, D.; Bhardwaj, G.; Wang, Q.; Sun, L.; Ercan, B.; Geetha, M.; Webster, T.J. Decreased staphylococcus aureus and increased osteoblast density on nanostructured electrophoretic-deposited hydroxyapatite on titanium without the use of pharmaceuticals. *Int. J. Nanomed.* **2014**, *9*, 1775–1781.
157. Hasan, J.; Webb, H.K.; Truong, V.K.; Pogodin, S.; Baulin, V.A.; Watson, G.S.; Watson, J.A.; Crawford, R.J.; Ivanova, E.P. Selective bactericidal activity of nanopatterned superhydrophobic cicada psaltoda claripennis wing surfaces. *Appl. Microbiol. Biotechnol.* **2013**, *97*, 9257–9262. [CrossRef] [PubMed]
158. Wisdom, K.M.; Watson, J.A.; Qu, X.; Liu, F.; Watson, G.S.; Chen, C.H. Self-cleaning of superhydrophobic surfaces by self-propelled jumping condensate. *Proc. Natl. Acad. Sci. USA* **2013**, *110*, 7992–7997. [CrossRef] [PubMed]
159. Sengstock, C.; Lopian, M.; Motemani, Y.; Borgmann, A.; Khare, C.; Buenconsejo, P.J.; Schildhauer, T.A.; Ludwig, A.; Koller, M. Structure-related antibacterial activity of a titanium nanostructured surface fabricated by glancing angle sputter deposition. *Nanotechnology* **2014**, *25*, 195101. [CrossRef] [PubMed]

160. Campoccia, D.; Montanaro, L.; Arciola, C.R. A review of the biomaterials technologies for infection-resistant surfaces. *Biomaterials* **2013**, *34*, 8533–8554. [CrossRef] [PubMed]
161. Liao, J.; Zhu, Z.; Mo, A.; Li, L.; Zhang, J. Deposition of silver nanoparticles on titanium surface for antibacterial effect. *Int. J. Nanomed.* **2010**, *5*, 261–267.
162. Wan, W.; Yeow, J.T. Antibacterial properties of poly(quaternary ammonium) modified gold and titanium dioxide nanoparticles. *J. Nanosci. Nanotechnol.* **2012**, *12*, 4601–4606. [CrossRef] [PubMed]
163. Colon, G.; Ward, B.C.; Webster, T.J. Increased osteoblast and decreased staphylococcus epidermidis functions on nanophase zno and TiO_2. *J. Biomed. Mater. Res. Part A* **2006**, *78*, 595–604. [CrossRef] [PubMed]
164. Zhao, J.; Cai, X.M.; Tang, H.Q.; Liu, T.; Gu, H.Q.; Cui, R.Z. Bactericidal and biocompatible properties of TiN/Ag multilayered films by ion beam assisted deposition. *J. Mater. Sci. Mater. Med.* **2009**, *20* (Suppl. 1), S101–S105. [CrossRef] [PubMed]
165. Hassan, M.S.; Amna, T.; Mishra, A.; Yun, S.I.; Kim, H.C.; Kim, H.Y.; Khil, M.S. Fabrication, characterization and antibacterial effect of novel electrospun TiO_2 nanorods on a panel of pathogenic bacteria. *J. Biomed. Nanotechnol.* **2012**, *8*, 394–404. [CrossRef] [PubMed]
166. Amna, T.; Hassan, M.S.; Barakat, N.A.; Pandeya, D.R.; Hong, S.T.; Khil, M.S.; Kim, H.Y. Antibacterial activity and interaction mechanism of electrospun zinc-doped titania nanofibers. *Appl. Microbiol. Biotechnol.* **2012**, *93*, 743–751. [CrossRef] [PubMed]
167. Hu, H.; Zhang, W.; Qiao, Y.; Jiang, X.; Liu, X.; Ding, C. Antibacterial activity and increased bone marrow stem cell functions of Zn-incorporated TiO_2 coatings on titanium. *Acta Biomater.* **2012**, *8*, 904–915. [CrossRef] [PubMed]
168. Zhang, H.; Chen, G. Potent antibacterial activities of ag/TiO_2 nanocomposite powders synthesized by a One-Pot Sol-Gel method. *Environ. Sci. Technol.* **2009**, *43*, 2905–2910. [CrossRef] [PubMed]
169. Inoue, Y.; Uota, M.; Torikai, T.; Watari, T.; Noda, I.; Hotokebuchi, T.; Yada, M. Antibacterial properties of nanostructured silver titanate thin films formed on a titanium plate. *J. Biomed. Mater. Res. Part A* **2010**, *92*, 1171–1180. [CrossRef] [PubMed]
170. Nasajpour, A.; Mandla, S.; Shree, S.; Mostafavi, E.; Sharifi, R.; Khalilpour, A.; Saghazadeh, S.; Hassan, S.; Mitchell, M.J.; Leijten, J.; et al. Nanostructured fibrous membranes with rose spike-like architecture. *Nano Lett.* **2017**, *17*, 6235–6240. [CrossRef] [PubMed]
171. Uklejewski, R.; Rogala, P.; Winiecki, M.; Toklowicz, R.; Ruszkowski, P.; Wolun-Cholewa, M. Biomimetic multispiked connecting Ti-alloy scaffold prototype for entirely-cementless resurfacing arthroplasty endoprostheses-exemplary results of implantation of the Ca-P surface-modified scaffold prototypes in animal model and osteoblast culture evaluation. *Materials* **2016**, *9*, 532.
172. Zhu, Y.; Cao, H.; Qiao, S.; Wang, M.; Gu, Y.; Luo, H.; Meng, F.; Liu, X.; Lai, H. Hierarchical micro/nanostructured titanium with balanced actions to bacterial and mammalian cells for dental implants. *Int. J. Nanomed.* **2015**, *10*, 6659–6674. [CrossRef] [PubMed]
173. Zhao, L.; Wang, H.; Huo, K.; Cui, L.; Zhang, W.; Ni, H.; Zhang, Y.; Wu, Z.; Chu, P.K. Antibacterial nano-structured titania coating incorporated with silver nanoparticles. *Biomaterials* **2011**, *32*, 5706–5716. [CrossRef] [PubMed]
174. De Giglio, E.; Cafagna, D.; Cometa, S.; Allegretta, A.; Pedico, A.; Giannossa, L.C.; Sabbatini, L.; Mattioli-Belmonte, M.; Iatta, R. An innovative, easily fabricated, silver nanoparticle-based titanium implant coating: Development and analytical characterization. *Anal. Bioanal. Chem.* **2013**, *405*, 805–816. [CrossRef] [PubMed]
175. Wu, S.; Liu, X.; Yeung, A.; Yeung, K.W.; Kao, R.Y.; Wu, G.; Hu, T.; Xu, Z.; Chu, P.K. Plasma-modified biomaterials for self-antimicrobial applications. *ACS Appl. Mater. Interfaces* **2011**, *3*, 2851–2860. [CrossRef] [PubMed]
176. Yamaguchi, S.; Nath, S.; Sugawara, Y.; Divakarla, K.; Das, T.; Manos, J.; Chrzanowski, W.; Matsushita, T.; Kokubo, T. Two-in-one biointerfaces-antimicrobial and bioactive nanoporous gallium titanate layers for titanium implants. *Nanomaterials* **2017**, *7*, 229. [CrossRef] [PubMed]
177. Valappil, S.P.; Ready, D.; Abou Neel, E.A.; Pickup, D.M.; O'Dell, L.A.; Chrzanowski, W.; Pratten, J.; Newport, R.J.; Smith, M.E.; Wilson, M.; et al. Controlled delivery of antimicrobial gallium ions from phosphate-based glasses. *Acta Biomater.* **2009**, *5*, 1198–1210. [CrossRef] [PubMed]

178. Cochis, A.; Azzimonti, B.; Della Valle, C.; De Giglio, E.; Bloise, N.; Visai, L.; Cometa, S.; Rimondini, L.; Chiesa, R. The effect of silver or gallium doped titanium against the multidrug resistant acinetobacter baumannii. *Biomaterials* **2016**, *80*, 80–95. [CrossRef] [PubMed]
179. Kaneko, Y.; Thoendel, M.; Olakanmi, O.; Britigan, B.E.; Singh, P.K. The transition metal gallium disrupts pseudomonas aeruginosa iron metabolism and has antimicrobial and antibiofilm activity. *J. Clin. Investig.* **2007**, *117*, 877–888. [CrossRef] [PubMed]
180. Lu, T.; Liu, X.; Qian, S.; Cao, H.; Qiao, Y.; Mei, Y.; Chu, P.K.; Ding, C. Multilevel surface engineering of nanostructured TiO_2 on carbon-fiber-reinforced polyetheretherketone. *Biomaterials* **2014**, *35*, 5731–5740. [CrossRef] [PubMed]
181. Toniatto, T.V.; Rodrigues, B.V.M.; Marsi, T.C.O.; Ricci, R.; Marciano, F.R.; Webster, T.J.; Lobo, A.O. Nanostructured poly (lactic acid) electrospun fiber with high loadings of TiO_2 nanoparticles: Insights into bactericidal activity and cell viability. *Mater. Sci. Eng. C Mater. Biol. Appl.* **2017**, *71*, 381–385. [CrossRef] [PubMed]
182. Nogueira, F.; Karumidze, N.; Kusradze, I.; Goderdzishvili, M.; Teixeira, P.; Gouveia, I.C. Immobilization of bacteriophage in wound-dressing nanostructure. *Nanomedicine* **2017**, *13*, 2475–2484. [CrossRef] [PubMed]
183. Jiang, Y.; Zheng, W.; Kuang, L.; Ma, H.; Liang, H. Hydrophilic phage-mimicking membrane active antimicrobials reveal nanostructure-dependent activity and selectivity. *ACS Infect. Dis.* **2017**, *3*, 676–687. [CrossRef] [PubMed]
184. Tripathy, A.; Sen, P.; Su, B.; Briscoe, W.H. Natural and bioinspired nanostructured bactericidal surfaces. *Adv. Colloid Interface Sci.* **2017**, *248*, 85–104. [CrossRef] [PubMed]
185. Diu, T.; Faruqui, N.; Sjostrom, T.; Lamarre, B.; Jenkinson, H.F.; Su, B.; Ryadnov, M.G. Cicada-inspired cell-instructive nanopatterned arrays. *Sci. Rep.* **2014**, *4*, 7122. [CrossRef] [PubMed]
186. Bhadra, C.M.; Truong, V.K.; Pham, V.T.; Al Kobaisi, M.; Seniutinas, G.; Wang, J.Y.; Juodkazis, S.; Crawford, R.J.; Ivanova, E.P. Antibacterial titanium nano-patterned arrays inspired by dragonfly wings. *Sci. Rep.* **2015**, *5*, 16817. [CrossRef] [PubMed]
187. Hizal, F.; Zhuk, I.; Sukhishvili, S.; Busscher, H.J.; van der Mei, H.C.; Choi, C.H. Impact of 3D hierarchical nanostructures on the antibacterial efficacy of a bacteria-triggered self-defensive antibiotic coating. *ACS Appl. Mater. Interfaces* **2015**, *7*, 20304–20313. [CrossRef] [PubMed]
188. Zhang, X.Y.; Fang, G.; Zhou, J. Additively manufactured scaffolds for bone tissue engineering and the prediction of their mechanical behavior: A review. *Materials* **2017**, *10*, 50. [CrossRef] [PubMed]
189. Wang, X.; Lu, T.; Wen, J.; Xu, L.; Zeng, D.; Wu, Q.; Cao, L.; Lin, S.; Liu, X.; Jiang, X. Selective responses of human gingival fibroblasts and bacteria on carbon fiber reinforced polyetheretherketone with multilevel nanostructured TiO_2. *Biomaterials* **2016**, *83*, 207–218. [CrossRef] [PubMed]
190. Baranowski, A.; Klein, A.; Ritz, U.; Ackermann, A.; Anthonissen, J.; Kaufmann, K.B.; Brendel, C.; Gotz, H.; Rommens, P.M.; Hofmann, A. Surface functionalization of orthopedic titanium implants with bone sialoprotein. *PLoS ONE* **2016**, *11*, e0153978. [CrossRef] [PubMed]
191. Graves, J.L., Jr.; Tajkarimi, M.; Cunningham, Q.; Campbell, A.; Nonga, H.; Harrison, S.H.; Barrick, J.E. Rapid evolution of silver nanoparticle resistance in escherichia coli. *Front. Genet.* **2015**, *6*, 42. [CrossRef] [PubMed]
192. Soto-Quintero, A.; Romo-Uribe, A.; Bermudez-Morales, V.H.; Quijada-Garrido, I.; Guarrotxena, N. 3D-hydrogel based polymeric nanoreactors for silver nano-antimicrobial composites generation. *Nanomaterials* **2017**, *7*, 209. [CrossRef] [PubMed]
193. Li, J.P.; de Wijn, J.R.; van Blitterswijk, C.A.; de Groot, K. Porous Ti6AL4V scaffolds directly fabricated by 3D fibre deposition technique: Effect of nozzle diameter. *J. Mater. Sci. Mater. Med.* **2005**, *16*, 1159–1163. [CrossRef] [PubMed]
194. Murr, L.E.; Esquivel, E.V.; Quinones, S.A.; Gaytan, S.M.; Lopez, M.I.; Martinez, E.Y.; Medina, F.; Hernandez, D.H.; Martinez, E.; Stafford, S.W.; et al. Microstructures and mechanical properties of electron beam-rapid manufactured Ti-6AL-4V biomedical prototypes compared to wrought Ti-6AL-4V. *Mater. Charact.* **2009**, *60*, 96–105. [CrossRef]
195. Mullen, L.; Stamp, R.C.; Brooks, W.K.; Jones, E.; Sutcliffe, C.J. Selective laser melting: A regular unit cell approach for the manufacture of porous, titanium, bone in-growth constructs, suitable for orthopedic applications. *J. Biomed. Mater. Res. B Appl. Biomater.* **2009**, *89*, 325–334. [CrossRef] [PubMed]
196. Vandenbroucke, B.K.; Kruth, J.-P. Selective laser melting of biocompatible metals for rapid manufacturing of medical parts. *Rapid Prototyp. J.* **2007**, *13*, 196–203. [CrossRef]

197. Ryan, G.E.; Pandit, A.S.; Apatsidis, D.P. Porous titanium scaffolds fabricated using a rapid prototyping and powder metallurgy technique. *Biomaterials* **2008**, *29*, 3625–3635. [CrossRef] [PubMed]
198. Alvarez, K.; Nakajima, H. Metallic scaffolds for bone regeneration. *Materials* **2009**, *2*, 790–832. [CrossRef]
199. Hotchkiss, K.M.; Reddy, G.B.; Hyzy, S.L.; Schwartz, Z.; Boyan, B.D.; Olivares-Navarrete, R. Titanium surface characteristics, including topography and wettability, alter macrophage activation. *Acta Biomater.* **2016**, *31*, 425–434. [CrossRef] [PubMed]
200. Shah, F.A.; Stenlund, P.; Martinelli, A.; Thomsen, P.; Palmquist, A. Direct communication between osteocytes and acid-etched titanium implants with a sub-micron topography. *J. Mater. Sci. Mater. Med.* **2016**, *27*, 167. [CrossRef] [PubMed]

3

Modulation of Osteoclast Interactions with Orthopaedic Biomaterials

Chris Steffi, Zhilong Shi, Chee Hoe Kong and Wilson Wang *

Department of Orthopaedic Surgery, Yong Loo Lin School of Medicine, National University of Singapore, NUHS Tower Block, Level 11, 1E Kent Ridge Road, Singapore 119228, Singapore; chrissteffi@u.nus.edu (C.S.); dossz@nus.edu.sg (Z.S.); e0012328@u.nus.edu (C.H.K.)

* Correspondence: doswangw@nus.edu.sg

Abstract: Biomaterial integration in bone depends on bone remodelling at the bone-implant interface. Optimal balance of bone resorption by osteoclasts and bone deposition by osteoblasts is crucial for successful implantation, especially in orthopaedic surgery. Most studies examined osteoblast differentiation on biomaterials, yet few research has been conducted to explore the effect of different orthopaedic implants on osteoclast development. This review covers, in detail, the biology of osteoclasts, in vitro models of osteoclasts, and modulation of osteoclast activity by different implant surfaces, bio-ceramics, and polymers. Studies show that surface topography influence osteoclastogenesis. For instance, metal implants with rough surfaces enhanced osteoclast activity, while smooth surfaces resulted in poor osteoclast differentiation. In addition, surface modification of implants with anti-osteoporotic drug further decreased osteoclast activity. In bioceramics, osteoclast development depended on different chemical compositions. Strontium-incorporated bioceramics decreased osteoclast development, whereas higher concentrations of silica enhanced osteoclast activity. Differences between natural and synthetic polymers also modulated osteoclastogenesis. Physiochemical properties of implants affect osteoclast activity. Hence, understanding osteoclast biology and its response to the natural microarchitecture of bone are indispensable to design suitable implant interfaces and scaffolds, which will stimulate osteoclasts in ways similar to that of native bone.

Keywords: osteoclasts; monocytes; osteoblasts; implants; polymers and scaffolds

---

1. Bone Biology of Osteoclasts

1.1. Bone Remodelling

Bone is a vastly dynamic tissue, which goes through remodelling during the course of life, even if it seems static. Bone constantly adapts itself to various loads. The phenomenon of adaptation of bone structure to various loads, or rather bone remodelling, was explained by Julius Wolff and is known as Wolff's Law [1]. For decades, bone remodelling has been investigated and explained from the macroscopic tissue level to microscopic cellular/molecular level. Bone homeostasis at macroscopic level is termed as bone turn over and the turn-over rate for adult human bone is about 10% per annum [2], whereas, the cellular mechanism causing bone turn-over is called as bone remodelling [2]. Constant bone remodelling, the physiological process of replacing old or damaged bone with new bone tissue, contributes an imperative role in scar-free bone healing and regeneration of damaged bone, while maintaining mineral homeostasis [3–7]. Bone remodelling is performed mainly via the coordinated activities between bone-forming osteoblasts and bone-resorbing osteoclasts. The functional and anatomical site of bone remodelling will contain bone cells, including osteoblasts, osteoclasts, bone-lining cells, and osteocytes, that form a basic multicellular unit (BMU). In addition to these cells, immune cells including macrophages, B-cells, and T-cells are also involved in bone remodelling [8].

Bone remodelling occurs due to the composite interactions of various cells in a closely-regulated environment. This process has five distinct and sequential phases (Figure 1).

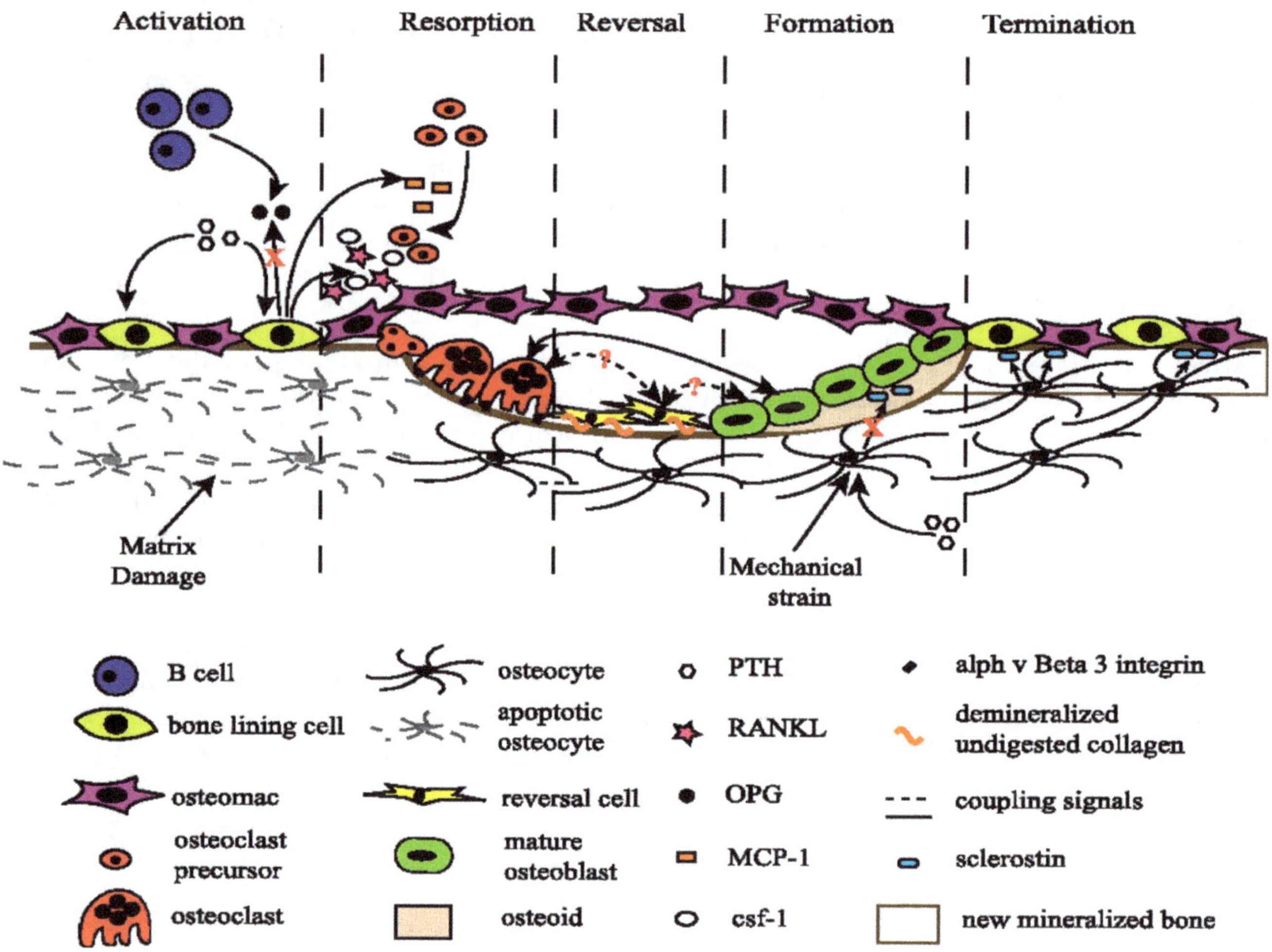

Figure 1. A schematic representation of different stages of bone remodelling. B cells in the marrow of resting bone secrete osteoprotegerin (OPG), which controls osteoclast activation. *Activation phase*: Damaged bone matrix triggers osteocyte apoptosis. Parathyroid (PTH) activates bone cells to recruit osteoclast precursors. *Resorption phase*: monocyte chemoattractant protein-1 (MCP-1) secreted by osteoblasts attracts osteoclast precursors to the damaged site. Osteoblasts also secrete Receptor Activator of NF-κB ligand (RANKL) and colony stimulating factor-1 (CSF-1), which lead to proliferation and differentiation of osteoclast precursors. Functionally-mature osteoclasts attach to the surface, form a sealing zone, and resorb damaged matrix. *Reversal phase*: matrix debris, such as undigested collagen, are removed by reversal cells. Coupling signals generated by reversal cells stimulate bone formation and conclude bone resorption. *Formation phase*: mechanical signals and PTH curb sclerostin expression by osteocytes, resulting in Wnt signalling activation to promote osteoblast differentiation. *Termination phase*: osteocytes secrete sclerostin to terminate bone formation. The newly-formed bone is mineralized. Reprinted from Ref. [9].

1. Activation Phase: This is the first phase that requires a trigger generated either from cytokines released during apoptosis of osteocytes in the impaired bone, the detection of physical forces by osteocytes in the normal bone, or the hormonal (examples are estrogen or parathyroid hormone, PTH) actions on bone cells as a feedback mechanism for the systemic fluctuations due to homeostasis.

2. Resorption Phase: Osteoblasts react on the mechanical or endocrine signals via the engagement of preosteoclastic cells to the remodeling location. Cytokines, secreted by osteoblasts, promote the propagation of these precursor osteoclastic cells along with coordinating the differentiation to

multinucleated mature osteoclasts. They further stimulate resorption of bones and prolong the lifespan for these mature osteoclasts. The mature cells anchor onto the bone surface and create an isolated microenvironment beneath the cells where dissolution of mineralized matrix occurs to create resorption lacunae.

3. Reversal Phase: Following osteoclast-mediated bone resorption, reversal cells remove the matrix debris before receiving or producing signals to initiate the transition from resorption to bone growth in BMUs. Studies have shown that the reversal cells express osteogenic markers, such as Runx 2, which are usually expressed by the cells of the osteoblast lineage [10]. Reversal cells modify or smoothen the bone surface resorbed by osteoclasts making it a suitable osteoblast maturation.

4. Formation Phase: Degraded bone matrix, osteoclasts, and possibly reversal cells create molecular cues to encourage the return of mesenchymal stem cells or premature osteoblast precursors to the resorption lacunae. These cells will then undergo differentiation and eventually mineralization to form new bone.

5. Termination Phase: After a comparable quantity of resorbed bone is restored with new mechanically stronger bone, the remodelling cycle concludes [9]. This bone resorption process occurs for weeks, whereas new bone formation takes months.

In the regular bone remodelling cycle, tight coupling of bone-forming osteoblasts and bone-resorbing osteoclasts occurs consecutively at a constant functional site without alteration in bone shape, bulk, or quality. Dysfunction of bone remodelling can cause the development of several metabolic bone disorders, including osteoporosis, osteopetrosis, and Paget's disease [4].

Postmenopausal osteoporotic fractures have become a global concern. Globally, about 9 million people are affected by osteoporotic fractures per annum [11]. The suboptimal microenvironment of fragile osteoporotic bone hinders new bone formation [12]. The physiological imbalances cause bone resorption to exceed bone formation, which causes delayed fracture healing, hence, leading to post-surgical complications, such as implant loosening, mal-union, and implant failure [13–15]. Moreover, poor bone microarchitecture and low bone mineral density impair the anchorage and osseointegration of orthopaedic implants [16]. Revision surgeries impose huge physiological and economical burdens on elderly patients, not to mention the associated risks and complications. Anti-osteoporotic drugs were administered as an adjunct to surgery to reduce post-surgical complications. Systemic administration of anti-osteoporotic drugs, such as strontium ranelate and parathyroid hormone (PTH), augmented fracture healing in osteoporotic patients [17–20]. Bone-stimulating agents, such as bone morphogenetic protein-2 and -7, were also administered locally to stimulate bone healing and reduce post-surgical complications [21,22]. Additionally, technologies with new implant design, use of bone cements, new implant coatings have been explored to improve implant fixation in osteoporotic bone [23–26]. High bone resorption of osteoporotic bone is not desirable, especially bone resorption at the bone-implant interface may lead to non-union and implant failure. Understanding the physiology of osteoclastic bone resorption and influence of implants on osteoclast development is crucial to determine the success of the implant integration. The biology of osteoclasts and influence of various biomaterials on osteoclast development has been discussed in detail in the subsequent sections of this review.

1.2. Osteoclasts

Osteoclasts are multi-nucleated macrophage-like cells, which originated from hematopoietic stem cells of monocyte-macrophage lineage. These cells are highly migratory and they are the only ones in charge of mineralized bone matrix resorption in remodelling. Osteoclastogenesis consists of several steps, including survival of progenitors from hematopoietic stem cells, differentiation of progenitors to mononuclear preosteoclasts, fusion into multi-nuclear mature osteoclasts, and activation to form bone-resorbing osteoclasts (Figure 2) [27].

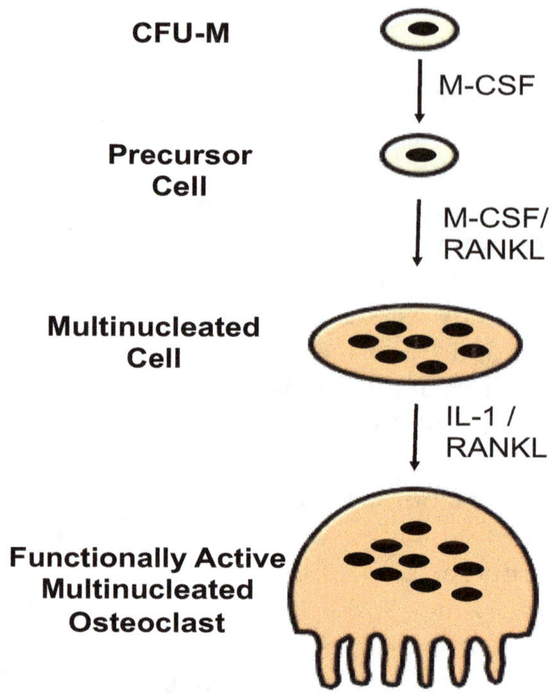

Figure 2. Schematic representation of osteoclast differentiation pathway and various cytokines involved at various stages of differentiation.

Osteoclast differentiation and activation are affected by several cytokines and growth factors. Among them, RANKL and monocyte/macrophage colony–stimulating factor (M-CSF) are two essential factors [28,29]. RANKL is secreted through osteoblasts, osteocytes, and stromal cells, while M-CSF is produced by osteoblasts, stromal cells, and activated immune cells. Both RANKL and M-CSF, combining with receptors found on the monocytic/macrophagic cells, stimulate the undertaking to osteoclast phenotype; an activity restricted by osteoprotegerin (OPG) [27]. Additionally, recent studies have shown that tumour necrosis factor α (TNFα) [30], interleukin 1 (IL-1) [27], and lipopolysaccharides [31] can affect osteoclast development without RANKL-RANK interaction.

During bone remodelling, osteoclasts first attach to bone surfaces through distinctive podosomes, adhesive networks that have actin filaments as the central core. They then undergo profound morphological changes and polarize to activate bone-resorbing cells [32]. Four different membrane domains can be perceived in activated osteoclasts: the sealing zone, the ruffled border, the basolateral domain, and the functional secretory domain [33]. Both the sealing zone and ruffled border are adjacent to the bone, while the basolateral domain and functional secretory domain are not. The sealing zone is a ring-like superstructure formed by rearrangement of podosomes upon activation of osteoclasts. It consists of a highly-ordered filamentous actin bundle that can be easily investigated with confocal microscopy after immunostaining with phalloidin (Figure 3).

This serves as a diffusion barrier. Through the sealing zone, osteoclasts tightly adhere to the bone surface and seal a closed compartment where bone resorption takes place. The ruffled border, which is away from the surrounding tissue due to the presence of sealing zone, forms part of the cell membrane.

The sealing zone and the ruffled border are characteristic structures for bone resorbing-osteoclasts. In the ruffled border, a vacuolar-type H+-ATPase pumps protons to help acidify the resorption lacuna (pH < 4) [34,35]. The mineral phase of bone is dissolved mainly due to the presence of local acidification. At the same time, several matrix metalloproteinases (MMPs), lysosomal proteinases, like cathepsin K [36,37], as well as additional cysteine proteinases are released [38]. These enzymes are responsible for degrading the organic phase of bone, primarily collagen I fibres. Tartrate-resistant acid phosphatase (TRAP) is secreted from the ruffled border [4], which is often used as a characteristic marker of osteoclasts [39]. The degraded products are subsequently endocytosed across the ruffled border and transcytosed in vesicles, and released through the functional secretory domain into the extracellular space. Excluding the sealing zone, ruffled border, and the functional secretory domain, the remaining membrane is known as the basolateral membrane. In the transcytosed vesicles, TRAP with highly-destructive reactive oxygen species can further implicate the degraded products [4,6,33].

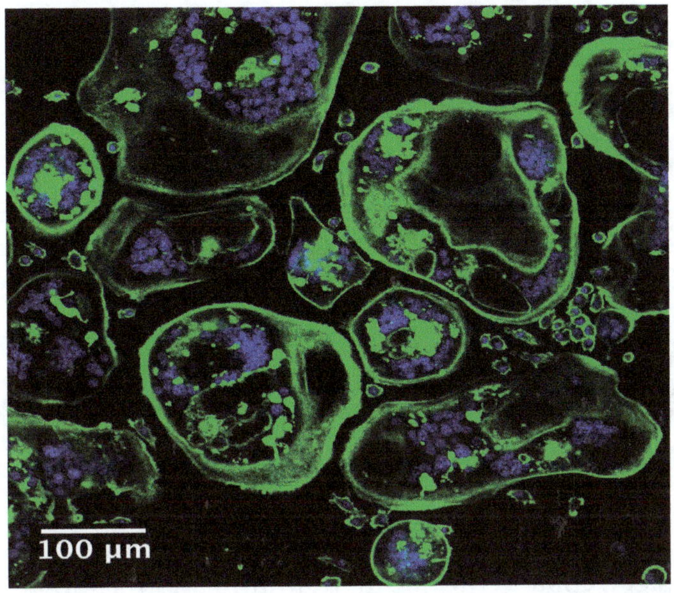

Figure 3. RAW 264.7 cells were cultured in presence of RANKL for five days, to induce osteoclast differentiation. The actin of multinucleated osteoclast cells is stained with phalloidin Alexa fluor 488 (green) and nuclei are stained with DAPI (blue).

1.3. In Vitro Models of Osteoclasts

In vitro experiments are often performed to investigate cell material interactions in the early phases of biomaterial development. Desirable conditions can be easily defined for cost effective screening of the potency in newly-developed biomaterial. The cell source must be identified when using osteoclast cultures. Both primary osteoclast precursor cells [40,41] and cell lines [42,43] are routinely used. Precursor cells are either harvested from bone marrow of animals/humans, or obtained from peripheral blood (mononuclear cells) [44]. One of the advantages in using precursor cells is that they possess high differentiation potency, and cytokines, for example, M-CSF and RANKL, are sufficient to differentiate these cells [45]. Although primary cells have a similar phenotype as cells in the body, they often have a limited lifespan and are genetically diverse if collected from different donors [46]. Additionally, primary osteoclasts are relatively scarce, as well as difficult to culture and study in vitro as compared to primary osteoblasts.

On the other hand, preosteoclasts obtained from cell lines are homogeneous with high differentiation potential [47]. The RAW 264.7 macrophage cell line of murine origin can differentiate into osteoclasts when stimulated with RANKL. It, along with another macrophage-like cell line, the C7 cell line, has been widely utilized for in vitro osteoclastic studies and bone remodelling [42,48]. Currently no human cell lines for osteoclasts have been established.

2. Biomaterials

Biomaterials have been widely used to restore the functions of damaged tissues in the human body. Currently, biomaterials with diverse chemical and physical properties are developed to suit the mechanical requirements and biological function of diverse tissue types, which vary from soft tissues, such as skin, to hard tissues such as bone [49–51]. In this review, the various biomaterials used in bone, such as metals, bioceramics, and polymers, has been reviewed. Each material type has its own advantages and disadvantages, as listed in Table 1. The success of a biomaterial depends on the host response and biological function of the implant. This is mainly dependent on the biomaterials' interaction with the cells when exposed to the tissue environment in the human body. The surface physiochemical properties of the implant affect the cellular responses. The importance of the osteoclast response in the bone-implant interface has been recognized [52]. Yet, the response of osteoclasts on bone implants has not been as widely explored as osteoblasts. Hence, the review mainly focuses on the osteoclast activity on implants and studies of osteoclast response to different types of biomaterial is discussed in subsequent sections.

Table 1. Advantages and disadvantages of orthopaedic biomaterials.

Biomaterials	Advantages	Disadvantages
Metals	High strength, fatigue resistance	Metal ion toxicity, wear
Bioceramics	High bioactivity (bioactive glasses), biodegradability (TCP), low friction coefficient and wear rate (bioinert ceramics)	Brittleness, low fatigue resistance
Polymers	Ease of ease of manufacture and modification	Low strength

3. Metals

3.1. Introduction

Metals, like stainless steel, cobalt-chromium, titanium, and its alloys, have been widely used in fracture fixation and joint replacement for decades [53]. With the aging population and active lifestyle, the demand for metal implants are expected to increase in orthopaedic surgery [54]. Compared to bioceramics and polymeric biomaterials, metals are the first choice in load-bearing orthopaedic usage because of their outstanding mechanical properties. Among the metals, titanium and its alloys are by far the most prevalent, thanks to their exceptional chemical qualities and biocompatibility with human tissues [53].

Despite the prevalent use of metals, clinically, successful integration of metal implants with bone tissue, known as osseointegration, remains a concern. Osseointegration indicates the forming of a direct interface between the implant and bone, short of the soft tissue interfering [55,56]. High mechanical stability of implants in the host tissue can be obtained by having no foreign body response or encapsulation. At the bone-implant interface, constant dynamic remodelling requires close collaboration of osteoclasts and osteoblasts for osseointegration. Although much effort has been devoted to study the effects of different surface characteristics on metals in osteoblast bone formation, little data is presented about the osteoclast interaction with metal surfaces. Surface modification of metal implants is an encouraging advancement to improve osseointegration [56]. Surface topography and chemical modifications are commonly used to modulate cell behaviours on metal surfaces.

3.2. Surface Topography

Surface topography describes the general surface landscape involving undulations, pores, gradients, and small variations in an atomically flat surface to visible grooves and texture. Measuring arithmetical mean roughness (Ra) is one of the widely-used techniques to quantify surface roughness. Sandblasting, acid etching, and grinding are often used to increase surface roughness.

Several groups have studied osteoclast formation and activation on rough surfaces. Sommer et al. used titanium, TiAl6Mo7, CoCr28Mo6, and FeCrNi substrates with polished and sandblasted surfaces to evaluate osteoclastogenesis in vitro [57]. The results showed that TRAP activity and the number of osteoclast were higher on the sandblasted surfaces than that on the polished surfaces, while different metal alloys did not affect osteoclastogenesis significantly. Brinkmann et al. investigated the osteoclastogensis on titianium substrates with smooth (TS), acid-etched (TA), and sandblasted acid-etched (TLA) surfaces and compared it with that on the native bone using RAW 264.7 cell lines [58]. The results revealed that osteoclasts on rough surfaces such as TA and TLA showed similar osteoclastogenesis to those on native bone, whereas impaired osteoclastogenesis was observed on smooth surfaces. Nanotube structures on titanium surfaces by anodization has also been fabricated to investigate its interaction with osteoclasts [59]. Nanotube diameters of 30, 80, and 120 nm were prepared by anodization at 10, 40, and 60 V. The number of osteoclasts, TRAP activity, and the related gene expression on nanotube titanium were decreased compared to the pristine titanium. Osteoclastogenesis decreased with increasing the nanotube diameter.

Titanium surfaces were treated to varying roughness via wet grinding using 2000-, 1200-, 600-, and 180-grit abrasive papers. Molecular analysis of the initial osteoclast differentiation was then conducted [60]. It revealed that osteoclast differentiation markers, like TRAP and cathepsin K, increased in a roughness-dependent manner under RANKL stimulation. The gene expression of RANKL receptor, RANK, and its adapter protein TNF receptor-associated factor 6 (TRAF6) boosted with surface roughness. It was claimed that surface roughness assisted the maturation of osteoclasts by activating the RANK-TRAF6 pathway.

Surface topography can influence the stability and integrity of the sealing zone, which have imperative functions on bone resorption. By ranging the titanium roughness from 1 to 4.5 μm R_a to allow osteoclast bonding, Geblinger et al., investigated the sealing zone dynamics with direct live-cell microscopy [61]. Surface roughness stabilized the sealing zone, but negatively affected its translocation rate. Ridge-like barriers running parallel to the perimeter locally arrested the sealing zone. However, by advancing through less obstructed regions, the barriers could be bypassed. Nonetheless, when the sealing zone was surrounded by steep obstacles, the translocation would eventually stop and stabilize the sealing zone rings.

In general, increased osteoclastogensis are demonstrated on rough surfaces than those on smooth ones. Metal implants with rough surfaces have been shown to establish better osseointegration in clinical use [62]. It is speculated that poor osteoclast differentiation on smooth surfaces could be related to the delayed osseointegration of smooth surfaces compared to that of rough ones [58,63]. However, imbalanced osteoclast-osteoblast ratios due to elevated osteoclastogensis on rough surfaces remains a common concern.

3.3. Surface Chemistry

Surface chemical modification of metals with biomolecules and hydroxyapatite has been investigated for osteoclastogenesis. Makihira et al. covalently immobilized OPG-Fc fusion protein, a competitive inhibitor of RANKL, on titanium surfaces to improve osseointegration by preventing osteoclast formation locally [64]. The results showed that the gene expression for TRAP and cathepsin K of RAW 267.4 cells under RANKL stimulation were significantly reduced on OPG-Fc-immobilized titanium surfaces compared to that of the pristine surfaces. It is still unclear whether the immobilized OPG-Fc blocked RANKL-RANK interactions on the membrane. Moreover, this novel metal implants requires further in vivo animal models.

Decreased periprosthetic bone quality in osteoporotic patients inhibits implants from integrating with the surrounding bone. Surface coating with anti-osteoporotic drugs can impair bone resorption of osteoclasts around host bone tissues, which will benefit osteoporotic patients [65,66]. Bosco et al. developed a hydroxyapatite coating incorporated with bisphosphonate anti-osteoporotic drugs on titanium surfaces [67]. The electrospray deposition technique was used to deposit a hydroxyapatite coating without compromising the drug activity. Another interesting approach was developed by Huang et al. wherein polyelectrolyte multilayer coating techniques were used to immobilize anti-osteoporotic drug, calcitonin, and osteoinductive bone morphogenetic protein 2 (BMP-2) on a titanium surface [66]. Released calcitonin and BMP-2 from the titanium surface were expected to accelerate bone formation with a concomitant inhibition on bone resorption. In vivo results 30 days and 60 days after implantation for osteoporotic rabbits demonstrated that the coating on the implants enhanced bone-implant osseointegration significantly.

4. Bioceramics

4.1. Introduction

Bioceramics refer to biocompatible ceramic materials, such as crystalline and amorphous forms. They can be categorized according to their chemical composition into two groups: calcium phosphates (CaP), and the other constituting silicate-based bioactive glasses and glass-ceramics, like alumina and zirconia [68,69]. CaP ceramics include several materials with different chemical compositions and crystal phases. Among them, the two most studied CaP ceramics are beta-tricalcium phosphate (β-TCP) and hydroxyapatite (HA). Bioactive glasses and glasses-ceramics are made typically from the Na_2O-CaO-MgO-P_2O_5-SiO_2 system of varying composition. Bioactive ceramics, such as HA, β-TCP, and bioactive glasses, have been used as bone graft substitutes or scaffolds. Bioinert ceramics, including alumina and zirconia, have been used as parts in an integrated orthopaedic implant system during surgery. Some physical forms of bioceramics are granules, block, scaffolds, cements, and coating on metal implants.

Bone graft substitutes or scaffolds should be entirely degraded in a suitable time frame for effective bone regeneration. However, an optimal degradation rate is not defined for any biomaterial [7]. It is generally accepted that degradation of bioceramics is established on two distinctive mechanisms: resorption by chemical dissolution, passively, and cell-mediated degradation by osteoclastic resorption. Modulation on osteoclastic resorption of bioceramics is mainly through tuning the material compositions and surface topography.

4.2. Material Composition

β-TCP degrades too fast due to high solubility. On the other hand, HA is essentially insoluble and its degradation is only limited to the surface by osteoclasts since cells are not able to breach the microporous ceramic arrangement. Biphasic calcium phosphate (BCP), a mix of HA and β-TCP with varying ratios, may provide an optimal formulation in terms of bone resorption and final degradation. Yamada et al. investigated using neonatal rabbit bone cells to determine osteoclastic resorption on HA substrates, β-TCP substrates, and two types of BCP substrates in different HA/β-TCP ratios of 25/75 and 75/25 for two days [70]. The results showed that BCP with a HA/β-TCP ratio of 25/75 had the most extensive resorption by osteoclasts, which produced typical track-like resorption lacunae. On β-TCP substrates, smaller discontinuous island-like lacunae can be observed. No resorption lacunae can be found on HA or BCP with a HA/β-TCP ratio of 75/25. At the osteoclast-ceramic interface, it is speculated that free calcium ions in the acidic microenvironment may actually change the resorption pattern. In another study, Mayr et al. evaluated the degradation behaviour of HA, β-TCP, and four BCP with different HA/β-TCP ratios through stimulated osteoclast-like RAW 264.7 cells [71]. The monocytic progenitor cells were found to have matured into osteoclasts on all ceramics. The cell differentiation was the greatest on ceramics with HA/β-TCP ratios of 80/20, 60/40, and 40/60. All but β-TCP ceramic had bone resorption. It is claimed that BCP with HA/beta-TCP ratios of 80/20 and 60/40 revealed the most potential to assist as synthetic bone substitute materials due to their optimized dissolution and resorption properties. HA was resorbed by osteoclasts matured from rat bone marrow cells cultured after eight days and the U-937 human monocyte-like cell line after 21 days [72,73]. The contrast in results may be due to the different osteoclast cells used and culture time in studies.

Metals, like strontium (Sr), zinc (Zn), and magnesium (Mg), have been doped into bioceramics to influence osteoclast behavior [74–76]. Roy et al. assessed the outcomes of 1.0 wt % Sr and 1.0 wt % Mg incorporated into β-TCP on the osteoclast differentiation of RAW 264.7 cells under stimulation of RANKL [76]. Osteoclasts could be observed on β-TCP and Sr-incorporated β-TCP at day 8, but the cells were lacking on Mg-incorporated β-TCP. Zn-doped β-TCP (0.25 wt %) was reported to restrict osteoclast differentiation and a greater resorption pit volume was observed on this substrate after 28 days as in contrast with that of β-TCP [75]. Yamada et al. reported that Zn-doped β-TCP with a Zn content of 0.316 wt % and 0.633 wt % in β-TCP subjugated osteoclastic resorption. This would be attributed to the inhibition of osteoclast resorbing activity, which was demonstrated by fewer actin rings formed on Zn-doped β-TCP than those on β-TCP [77]. Recently, Sr has also been added into CaP cement and bioactive glasses to reduce the resorption [74,78]. Schumacher et al. found that Sr in CaP cement significantly decreased osteoclastic resorption in comparison to the pristine CaP cement, but did not inhibit osteoclastogenesis [78].

Silicon (Si) has also been incorporated into HA and CaP cement [79–82]. Botelho et al. demonstrated higher osteoclastic resorption activity on 1.5 wt % Si-substituted HA compared to that of HA [81]. In another study, osteoclast numbers after 21 days in vitro were comparable on HA, Si-HA (0.5 wt % Si) and Si-HA (1.2 wt % Si), but actin ring sealing zone morphology on Si-HA bore semblance to those found normally on bone. Greater individual pit volumes detected on Si-HA (1.2 wt % Si) may result from the relatively constant sealing zones of osteoclasts and improved lattice solubility [79]. Si increased osteoclast activity in vitro after doped into CaP cement [82]. However, Si released from S53P4 bioactive glass inhibited osteoclastogenesis [83], while another report depicted the presence of resorption lacunae on sol–gel-derived bioactive glasses and glass ceramics [84,85].

4.3. Surface Topography

In addition to material composition, the surface topography can be tailored to affect osteoclast behavior on bioceramics. Costa-Rodrigues assessed the osteoclastogenesis in human peripheral blood mononuclear cells (PBMCs) together with the co-culture of human bone marrow cells (hBMCs) on surface-abraded HA substrates of three different roughnesses (R_a from 0.0437 to 0.582 μm). Characteristic osteoclast properties were seen in PBMCs added with M-CSF and RANKL, or the co-culture with hBMCs. Osteoclastogenesis improved with greater surface roughness in PBMCs added with M-CSF and RANKL, but decreased when in co-culture with hBMCs [86]. HA substrates of three distinct surface roughness (R_a 0.02, 0.18, and 1.45 μm) were also used to investigate osteoclastgenesis with stimulated RAW 264.7 cells [7]. It was shown that the HA surface with a R_a of 0.18 μm demonstrated the greatest osteoclastic differentiation, indicating the positive effect of smaller structures. Conversely, a smoother surface encouraged greater osteoclast formation than one with a rough surface, which could be rationalized by the possibility of optimal cell spreading on the rough surface. Higher resorption activity of human-derived osteoclasts on rough HA thermal spray coating is observed versus those on polished HA coating of metal implants [87]. Another study using neonatal rabbit osteoclasts showed the manifestation of resorption lacunae only on smooth HA coatings, while micro-rough surfaces reduced such lacunae [88]. It can be shown that the differences in differentiation routes of pre-osteoclasts can have a significant effect on osteoclastogenesis for HA surfaces with different roughness.

By modifying surface architecture, it is very probable to regulate the osteoclastic resorption of β-TCP. β-TCP substrates with either submicron- or micron-scale surface topographical structures were used to investigate resorption by human peripheral blood monocyte-derived osteoclasts. On submicrostructured β-TCP, osteoclasts considerably resorbed the substrate, whereas microstructured β-TCP caused the attenuation of osteoclast survival, TRAP activation, and fusion. Effectively, no actin ring and resorption was seen on microstructured β-TCP. This approach presented an advantageous approach in designing resorbable substitutes for bone grafts [89].

5. Polymers

Interaction of polymeric biomaterials with osteoclasts has been investigated limitedly, although polymers, especially biodegradable ones, are often used to fabricate scaffolds in bone tissue engineering and regeneration medicine. Recently, chitosan, a natural polymer from crustaceans, was evaluated for osteoclast formation before and after fibrinogen (Fg) modification with primary human peripheral blood monocytes [90]. Similar cell adhesion patterns were observed in both unmodified and Fg-modified chitosan substrates. By 21 days of culture, Fg-modified chitosan has a significantly higher number of multinucleated osteoclasts (>10 nuclei/cell) than that of the unmodified one.

Quantification of cell-induced material resorption showed that Fg modification resulted in considerably greater resorption by 17 days of culture. Textile chitosan fibre scaffolds with or without collagen I, which is widely used as a scaffold for bone regeneration, were investigated on their interactions with mature osteoclasts derived from human primary monocytes after adding M-CSF and RANKL [91]. The results revealed that both modified and unmodified chitosan fibre scaffolds supported adherence and maturation of monocytes to osteoclasts. The capability of textile chitosan fibre scaffolds to encourage the migration and bonding of human monocytes before merging to form multinucleated osteoclast cells was also exhibited in the study. Interestingly, chitosan had also been added into CaP cement to inhibit the osteoclastic resorption [92]. Collagen coating on polymers can further enhance osteoclastogenesis. When polydimethylsiloxane (PDMS) was coated with collagen, increased osteoclastic activity was reported [93]. Yet, clumps of undifferentiated RAW 264.7 cells were observed at higher surface densities of collagen on PDMS. This suggested that substrate compositions affected the behaviour of monocytes.

Synthetic biodegradable polymer, poly(3-hydroxybutyrate-*co*-3-hydroxyvalerate) (PHBV), reinforced with various phases of calcium phosphate allowed osteoclast attachment although it was unsuccessful in materializing actin rings or resorption pits on every PHBV surfaces [94]. Similar results were observed in another synthetic biodegradable polymer, poly(L-lactic acid) (PLLA) [95].

6. Conclusions and Outlook

Less attention is spent on understanding the influence of orthopaedic biomaterials on osteoclast development than on osteoblasts. The successful clinical use of orthopaedic biomaterials requires the balanced activation of osteoclasts and osteoblasts, as with that in native bone remodelling [96]. Understanding the mechanism of osteoclast interactions with orthopaedic implant would be beneficial to design suitable metal implant surface, and engineer appropriate scaffolds which can then modulate osteoclast development in desirable ways. Research attention in this area is crucial.

Metals are widely used in clinical settings to restore the mechanical strength and function of the damaged bone. The physical and chemical properties of the implant surface can be modified to control the osteoclast development. For instance, surface roughness enhanced osteoclastogenesis, whereas chemical modification of the implant surface with proteins or anti-osteoporotic drugs decreased osteoclast function. Bioceramics researched as bone graft substitutes or scaffolds were shown to influence osteoclast development. The osteoclast development varied with different chemical composition of bioceramics; for instance, Sr incorporation reduced osteoclastic resorptive activity, whereas Si increased osteoclast activity. The surface topography of bioceramics also controlled osteoclast differentiation. Like bioceramics, polymers are used to develop bone scaffolds in bone tissue engineering. Although research of the osteoclast-polymer response is limited, the studies reviewed here depict the influence of different polymers on osteoclast response. This shows that the choice of polymer affects the osteoclast activity and, hence, can be tailored to meet the clinical needs.

Fractured bone at the submicron level has a topographically complex surface, which provides adequate biochemical and biophysical cues to osteoblasts and osteoclasts for their proliferation and differentiation, for forming healthy bone. Understanding the natural surface topography and chemistry of the bone's surface, osteoclast resorption pits and trails could provide valuable information. Simulating such natural surface features on implants via various surface modification techniques would induce osteogenesis in a way comparable to natural bone remodelling. Such biomimetic approaches will help to enhance osseointegration of implants. Additionally, the osteoclast interactions with biodegradable polymers and bioceramics have been reviewed to a small extent, although they are widely used as scaffolds in bone tissue engineering. Detailed investigation of osteoclast-induced bioresorption of scaffolds will help to optimize the design of scaffolds.

Given that the osteoclasts and osteoblasts are in complex crosstalk in the in vivo environment, co-culture of osteoclasts and osteoblasts will provide a more suitable model to investigate the nature of bone remodelling on orthopaedic biomaterials. However, challenges still exist to design optimal culture medium compositions, define the osteoclast/osteoblast ratio, and culture time to stimulate the native bone environment. Nonetheless, separate cultures of osteoblasts and osteoclasts help to understand the independent physiologies of their development, which is one of the advantages of using independent cell cultures over co-cultures.

Acknowledgments: The authors acknowledge the financial support provided by NMRC and Department of Orthopaedic Surgery, NUS. S.C would like to thank NUS Research Scholarship.

References

1. Lee, T.C.; Taylor, D. Bone remodelling: Should we cry wolff? *Ir. J. Med. Sci.* **1999**, *168*, 102. [CrossRef] [PubMed]
2. Väänänen, H.K. Mechanism of bone turnover. *Ann. Med.* **1993**, *25*, 353–359. [CrossRef] [PubMed]
3. Davies, J.E. Bone bonding at natural and biomaterial surfaces. *Biomaterials* **2007**, *28*, 5058–5067. [CrossRef] [PubMed]
4. Boyle, W.J.; Simonet, W.S.; Lacey, D.L. Osteoclast differentiation and activation. *Nature* **2003**, *423*, 337–342. [CrossRef] [PubMed]
5. Ducy, P.; Schinke, T.; Karsenty, G. The osteoblast: A sophisticated fibroblast under central surveillance. *Science* **2000**, *289*, 1501–1504. [CrossRef] [PubMed]
6. Teitelbaum, S.L. Bone resorption by osteoclasts. *Science* **2000**, *289*, 1504–1508. [CrossRef] [PubMed]
7. Detsch, R.; Boccaccini, A.R. The role of osteoclasts in bone tissue engineering. *J. Tissue Eng. Regen. Med.* **2015**, *9*, 1133–1149. [CrossRef] [PubMed]
8. Takayanagi, H. Osteoimmunology and the effects of the immune system on bone. *Nat. Rev. Rheumatol.* **2009**, *5*, 667–676. [CrossRef] [PubMed]
9. Raggatt, L.J.; Partridge, N.C. Cellular and molecular mechanisms of bone remodeling. *J. Biol. Chem.* **2010**, *285*, 25103–25108. [CrossRef] [PubMed]
10. Delaisse, J.-M. The reversal phase of the bone-remodeling cycle: Cellular prerequisites for coupling resorption and formation. *BoneKEy Rep.* **2014**, *3*, 561. [CrossRef] [PubMed]
11. Johnell, O.; Kanis, J.A. An estimate of the worldwide prevalence and disability associated with osteoporotic fractures. *Osteoporos. Int.* **2006**, *17*, 1726–1733. [CrossRef] [PubMed]
12. Kyllönen, L.; D'Este, M.; Alini, M.; Eglin, D. Local drug delivery for enhancing fracture healing in osteoporotic bone. *Acta Biomater.* **2015**, *11*, 412–434. [CrossRef] [PubMed]
13. Stover, M. Distal femoral fractures: Current treatment, results and problems. *Injury* **2001**, *32*, 3–13. [CrossRef]
14. Syed, A.; Agarwal, M.; Giannoudis, P.; Matthews, S.; Smith, R. Distal femoral fractures: Long-term outcome following stabilisation with the LISS. *Injury* **2004**, *35*, 599–607. [CrossRef]
15. Bolhofner, B.R.; Carmen, B.; Clifford, P. The results of open reduction and internal fixation of distal femur fractures using a biologic (indirect) reduction technique. *J. Orthop. Trauma* **1996**, *10*, 372–377. [CrossRef] [PubMed]
16. Sessa, G.; Evola, F.R.; Costarella, L. Osteosynthesis systems in fragility fracture. *Aging Clin. Exp. Res.* **2011**, *23*, 69–70. [PubMed]
17. Negri, A.L.; Spivacow, F.R. Healing of subtrochanteric atypical fractures after strontium ranelate treatment. *Clin. Cases Miner. Bone Metab. Off. J. Ital. Soc. Osteoporos. Miner. Metab. Skelet. Dis.* **2012**, *9*, 166–169.
18. Larsson, S.; Fazzalari, N.L. Anti-osteoporosis therapy and fracture healing. *Arch. Orthop. Trauma Surg.* **2014**, *134*, 291–297. [CrossRef] [PubMed]
19. Koval, K.J.; Meek, R.; Schemitsch, E.; Liporace, F.; Strauss, E.; Zuckerman, J.D. An AOA critical issue. Geriatric trauma: Young ideas. *J. Bone Joint Surg. Am.* **2003**, *85*, 1380–1388. [CrossRef] [PubMed]
20. Liu, J.; Xu, X. Stress shielding and fracture healing. *Zhonghua Yi Xue Za Zhi* **1994**, *74*, 483–485. [PubMed]
21. Govender, S.; Csimma, C.; Genant, H.K.; Valentin-Opran, A.; Amit, Y.; Arbel, R.; Aro, H.; Atar, D.; Bishay, M.; Börner, M.G. Recombinant human bone morphogenetic protein-2 for treatment of open tibial fractures. *J. Bone Joint Surg.* **2002**, *84*, 2123–2134. [CrossRef] [PubMed]
22. Giannoudis, P.V.; Tzioupis, C. Clinical applications of BMP-7: The UK perspective. *Injury* **2005**, *36*, S47–S50. [CrossRef] [PubMed]

23. Tejwani, N.C.; Guerado, E. Improving fixation of the osteoporotic fracture: The role of locked plating. *J. Orthop. Trauma* **2011**, *25* (Suppl. S2), S56–S60. [CrossRef] [PubMed]
24. Wähnert, D.; Hofmann-Fliri, L.; Richards, R.G.; Gueorguiev, B.; Raschke, M.J.; Windolf, M. Implant Augmentation: Adding Bone Cement to Improve the Treatment of Osteoporotic Distal Femur Fractures: A Biomechanical Study Using Human Cadaver Bones. *Medicine* **2014**, *93*, e166. [CrossRef] [PubMed]
25. Agarwal, R.; González-García, C.; Torstrick, B.; Guldberg, R.E.; Salmerón-Sánchez, M.; García, A.J. Simple coating with fibronectin fragment enhances stainless steel screw osseointegration in healthy and osteoporotic rats. *Biomaterials* **2015**, *63*, 137–145. [CrossRef] [PubMed]
26. Li, G.; Zhang, L.; Wang, L.; Yuan, G.; Dai, K.; Pei, J.; Hao, Y. Dual modulation of bone formation and resorption with zoledronic acid-loaded biodegradable magnesium alloy implants improves osteoporotic fracture healing: An in vitro and in vivo study. *Acta Biomater.* **2018**, *65*, 486–500. [CrossRef] [PubMed]
27. Takahashi, N.; Udagawa, N.; Suda, T. A new member of tumor necrosis factor ligand family, ODF/OPGL/TRANCE/RANKL, regulates osteoclast differentiation and function. *Biochem. Biophys. Res. Commun.* **1999**, *256*, 449–455. [CrossRef] [PubMed]
28. Tsurukai, T.; Udagawa, N.; Matsuzaki, K.; Takahashi, N.; Suda, T. Roles of macrophage-colony stimulating factor and osteoclast differentiation factor in osteoclastogenesis. *J. Bone Miner. Metab.* **2000**, *18*, 177–184. [CrossRef] [PubMed]
29. Tanaka, S.; Takahashi, N.; Udagawa, N.; Tamura, T.; Akatsu, T.; Stanley, E.R.; Kurokawa, T.; Suda, T. Macrophage colony-stimulating factor is indispensable for both proliferation and differentiation of osteoclast progenitors. *J. Clin. Investig.* **1993**, *91*, 257–263. [CrossRef] [PubMed]
30. Azuma, Y.; Kaji, K.; Katogi, R.; Takeshita, S.; Kudo, A. Tumor necrosis factor-alpha induces differentiation of and bone resorption by osteoclasts. *J. Biol. Chem.* **2000**, *275*, 4858–4864. [CrossRef] [PubMed]
31. Islam, S.; Hassan, F.; Tumurkhuu, G.; Dagvadorj, J.; Koide, N.; Naiki, Y.; Mori, I.; Yoshida, T.; Yokochi, T. Bacterial lipopolysaccharide induces osteoclast formation in RAW 264.7 macrophage cells. *Biochem. Biophys. Res. Commun.* **2007**, *360*, 346–351. [CrossRef] [PubMed]
32. Lakkakorpi, P.T.; Väänänen, H.K. Cytoskeletal changes in osteoclasts during the resorption cycle. *Microsc. Res. Tech.* **1996**, *33*, 171–181. [CrossRef]
33. Florencio-Silva, R.; Sasso, G.R.; Sasso-Cerri, E.; Simoes, M.J.; Cerri, P.S. Biology of Bone Tissue: Structure, Function, and Factors That Influence Bone Cells. *Biomed. Res. Int.* **2015**, *2015*, 421746. [CrossRef] [PubMed]
34. Blair, H.; Teitelbaum, S.; Ghiselli, R.; Gluck, S. Osteoclastic bone resorption by a polarized vacuolar proton pump. *Science* **1989**, *245*, 855–857. [CrossRef] [PubMed]
35. Silver, I.A.; Murrills, R.J.; Etherington, D.J. Microelectrode studies on the acid microenvironment beneath adherent macrophages and osteoclasts. *Exp. Cell Res.* **1988**, *175*, 266–276. [CrossRef]
36. Yamaza, T.; Goto, T.; Kamiya, T.; Kobayashi, Y.; Sakai, H.; Tanaka, T. Study of immunoelectron microscopic localization of cathepsin K in osteoclasts and other bone cells in the mouse femur. *Bone* **1998**, *23*, 499–509. [CrossRef]
37. Bossard, M.J.; Tomaszek, T.A.; Thompson, S.K.; Amegadzie, B.Y.; Hanning, C.R.; Jones, C.; Kurdyla, J.T.; McNulty, D.E.; Drake, F.H.; Gowen, M.; et al. Proteolytic Activity of Human Osteoclast Cathepsin K: Expression, Purification, Activation, and Substrate Identification. *J. Biol. Chem.* **1996**, *271*, 12517–12524. [CrossRef] [PubMed]
38. Everts, V.; Delaisse, J.M.; Korper, W.; Niehof, A.; Vaes, G.; Beertsen, W. Degradation of collagen in the bone-resorbing compartment underlying the osteoclast involves both cysteine-proteinases and matrix metalloproteinases. *J. Cell. Physiol.* **1992**, *150*, 221–231. [CrossRef] [PubMed]
39. Minkin, C. Bone acid phosphatase: Tartrate-resistant acid phosphatase as a marker of osteoclast function. *Calcif. Tissue Int.* **1982**, *34*, 285–290. [CrossRef] [PubMed]
40. Webster, T.J.; Ergun, C.; Doremus, R.H.; Siegel, R.W.; Bizios, R. Enhanced osteoclast-like cell functions on nanophase ceramics. *Biomaterials* **2001**, *22*, 1327–1333. [CrossRef]
41. Yang, L.; Perez-Amodio, S.; Barrère-de Groot, F.Y.F.; Everts, V.; van Blitterswijk, C.A.; Habibovic, P. The effects of inorganic additives to calcium phosphate on in vitro behavior of osteoblasts and osteoclasts. *Biomaterials* **2010**, *31*, 2976–2989. [CrossRef] [PubMed]
42. Midha, S.; van den Bergh, W.; Kim, T.B.; Lee, P.D.; Jones, J.R.; Mitchell, C.A. Bioactive glass foam scaffolds are remodelled by osteoclasts and support the formation of mineralized matrix and vascular networks in vitro. *Adv. Healthc. Mater.* **2013**, *2*, 490–499. [CrossRef] [PubMed]

43. Hefti, T.; Frischherz, M.; Spencer, N.D.; Hall, H.; Schlottig, F. A comparison of osteoclast resorption pits on bone with titanium and zirconia surfaces. *Biomaterials* **2010**, *31*, 7321–7331. [CrossRef] [PubMed]
44. Kartsogiannis, V.; Ng, K.W. Cell lines and primary cell cultures in the study of bone cell biology. *Mol. Cell. Endocrinol.* **2004**, *228*, 79–102. [CrossRef] [PubMed]
45. Cody, J.J.; Rivera, A.A.; Liu, J.; Liu, J.M.; Douglas, J.T.; Feng, X. A simplified method for the generation of human osteoclasts in vitro. *Int. J. Biochem. Mol. Biol.* **2011**, *2*, 183–189. [PubMed]
46. Hoebertz, A.; Arnett, T.R. Isolated osteoclast cultures. *Methods Mol. Med.* **2003**, *80*, 53–64. [PubMed]
47. Collin-Osdoby, P.; Osdoby, P. RANKL-mediated osteoclast formation from murine RAW 264.7 cells. *Methods Mol. Biol.* **2012**, *816*, 187–202. [PubMed]
48. Miyamoto, A.; Kunisada, T.; Hemmi, H.; Yamane, T.; Yasuda, H.; Miyake, K.; Yamazaki, H.; Hayashi, S.I. Establishment and characterization of an immortal macrophage-like cell line inducible to differentiate to osteoclasts. *Biochem. Biophys. Res. Commun.* **1998**, *242*, 703–709. [CrossRef] [PubMed]
49. Burg, K.J.; Porter, S.; Kellam, J.F. Biomaterial developments for bone tissue engineering. *Biomaterials* **2000**, *21*, 2347–2359. [CrossRef]
50. Currie, L.J.; Sharpe, J.R.; Martin, R. The use of fibrin glue in skin grafts and tissue-engineered skin replacements: A review. *Plast. Reconstr. Surg.* **2001**, *108*, 1713–1726. [CrossRef] [PubMed]
51. Liberski, A.; Ayad, N.; Wojciechowska, D.; Kot, R.; Vo, D.M.P.; Aibibu, D.; Hoffmann, G.; Cherif, C.; Grobelny-Mayer, K.; Snycerski, M.; et al. Weaving for heart valve tissue engineering. *Biotechnol. Adv.* **2017**, *35*, 633–656. [CrossRef] [PubMed]
52. Minkin, C.; Marinho, V.C. Role of the osteoclast at the bone-implant interface. *Adv. Dent. Res.* **1999**, *13*, 49–56. [CrossRef] [PubMed]
53. Geetha, M.; Singh, A.K.; Asokamani, R.; Gogia, A.K. Ti based biomaterials, the ultimate choice for orthopaedic implants—A review. *Prog. Mater. Sci.* **2009**, *54*, 397–425. [CrossRef]
54. Kurtz, S.; Ong, K.; Lau, E.; Mowat, F.; Halpern, M. Projections of primary and revision hip and knee arthroplasty in the United States from 2005 to 2030. *J. Bone Joint Surg. Am.* **2007**, *89*, 780–785. [PubMed]
55. Albrektsson, T.; Brånemark, P.-I.; Hansson, H.-A.; Kasemo, B.; Larsson, K.; Lundström, I.; McQueen, D.H.; Skalak, R. The interface zone of inorganic implantsIn vivo: Titanium implants in bone. *Ann. Biomed. Eng.* **1983**, *11*, 1–27. [CrossRef]
56. Kasemo, B. Biological surface science. *Surf. Sci.* **2002**, *500*, 656–677. [CrossRef]
57. Sommer, B.; Felix, R.; Sprecher, C.; Leunig, M.; Ganz, R.; Hofstetter, W. Wear particles and surface topographies are modulators of osteoclastogenesis in vitro. *J. Biomed. Mater. Res. A* **2005**, *72*, 67–76. [CrossRef] [PubMed]
58. Brinkmann, J.; Hefti, T.; Schlottig, F.; Spencer, N.D.; Hall, H. Response of osteoclasts to titanium surfaces with increasing surface roughness: An in vitro study. *Biointerphases* **2012**, *7*, 34. [CrossRef] [PubMed]
59. Li, Y.; Li, F.; Zhang, C.; Gao, B.; Tan, P.; Mi, B.; Zhang, Y.; Cheng, H.; Liao, H.; Huo, K.; et al. The Dimension of Titania Nanotubes Influences Implant Success for Osteoclastogenesis and Osteogenesis Patients. *J. Nanosci. Nanotechnol.* **2015**, *15*, 4136–4142. [CrossRef] [PubMed]
60. Makihira, S.; Mine, Y.; Kosaka, E.; Nikawa, H. Titanium surface roughness accelerates RANKL-dependent differentiation in the osteoclast precursor cell line, RAW264.7. *Dent. Mater. J.* **2007**, *26*, 739–745. [CrossRef] [PubMed]
61. Geblinger, D.; Zink, C.; Spencer, N.D.; Addadi, L.; Geiger, B. Effects of surface microtopography on the assembly of the osteoclast resorption apparatus. *J. R. Soc. Interface* **2012**, *9*, 1599–1608. [CrossRef] [PubMed]
62. Shalabi, M.M.; Gortemaker, A.; Van't Hof, M.A.; Jansen, J.A.; Creugers, N.H. Implant surface roughness and bone healing: A systematic review. *J. Dent. Res.* **2006**, *85*, 496–500. [CrossRef] [PubMed]
63. Nagasawa, M.; Cooper, L.F.; Ogino, Y.; Mendonca, D.; Liang, R.; Yang, S.; Mendonca, G.; Uoshima, K. Topography Influences Adherent Cell Regulation of Osteoclastogenesis. *J. Dent. Res.* **2016**, *95*, 319–326. [CrossRef] [PubMed]
64. Makihira, S.; Mine, Y.; Nikawa, H.; Shuto, T.; Kosaka, E.; Sugiyama, M.; Hosokawa, R. Immobilized-OPG-Fc on a titanium surface inhibits RANKL-dependent osteoclast differentiation in vitro. *J. Mater. Sci. Mater. Med.* **2010**, *21*, 647–653. [CrossRef] [PubMed]
65. Peter, B.; Gauthier, O.; Laib, S.; Bujoli, B.; Guicheux, J.; Janvier, P.; van Lenthe, G.H.; Muller, R.; Zambelli, P.Y.; Bouler, J.M.; et al. Local delivery of bisphosphonate from coated orthopedic implants increases implants mechanical stability in osteoporotic rats. *J. Biomed. Mater. Res. A* **2006**, *76*, 133–143. [CrossRef] [PubMed]

66. Huang, L.; Luo, Z.; Hu, Y.; Shen, X.; Li, M.; Li, L.; Zhang, Y.; Yang, W.; Liu, P.; Cai, K. Enhancement of local bone remodeling in osteoporotic rabbits by biomimic multilayered structures on Ti6Al4V implants. *J. Biomed. Mater. Res. A* **2016**, *104*, 1437–1451. [CrossRef] [PubMed]
67. Bosco, R.; Iafisco, M.; Tampieri, A.; Jansen, J.A.; Leeuwenburgh, S.C.G.; van den Beucken, J.J.J.P. Hydroxyapatite nanocrystals functionalized with alendronate as bioactive components for bone implant coatings to decrease osteoclastic activity. *Appl. Surf. Sci.* **2015**, *328*, 516–524. [CrossRef]
68. Navarro, M.; Michiardi, A.; Castano, O.; Planell, J.A. Biomaterials in orthopaedics. *J. R. Soc. Interface* **2008**, *5*, 1137–1158. [CrossRef] [PubMed]
69. Hench, L. Bioceramics: From Concept to Clinic. *J. Am. Ceram. Soc.* **1991**, *74*, 1487–1510. [CrossRef]
70. Yamada, S.; Heymann, D.; Bouler, J.M.; Daculsi, G. Osteoclastic resorption of calcium phosphate ceramics with different hydroxyapatite/beta-tricalcium phosphate ratios. *Biomaterials* **1997**, *18*, 1037–1041. [CrossRef]
71. Mayr, H.; Schlufter, S.; Detsch, R.; Ziegler, G. Influence of phase composition on degradation and resorption of biphasic calcium phosphate ceramics. *Key Eng. Mater.* **2008**, *361–363*, 1043–1046. [CrossRef]
72. Gomi, K.; Lowenberg, B.; Shapiro, G.; Davies, J.E. Resorption of sintered synthetic hydroxyapatite by osteoclasts in vitro. *Biomaterials* **1993**, *14*, 91–96. [CrossRef]
73. Detsch, R.; Mayr, H.; Ziegler, G. Formation of osteoclast-like cells on HA and TCP ceramics. *Acta Biomater.* **2008**, *4*, 139–148. [CrossRef] [PubMed]
74. Gentleman, E.; Fredholm, Y.C.; Jell, G.; Lotfibakhshaiesh, N.; O'Donnell, M.D.; Hill, R.G.; Stevens, M.M. The effects of strontium-substituted bioactive glasses on osteoblasts and osteoclasts in vitro. *Biomaterials* **2010**, *31*, 3949–3956. [CrossRef] [PubMed]
75. Roy, M.; Fielding, G.; Bandyopadhyay, A.; Bose, S. Effects of Zinc and Strontium Substitution in Tricalcium Phosphate on Osteoclast Differentiation and Resorption. *Biomater. Sci.* **2013**, *1*, 74–82. [CrossRef] [PubMed]
76. Roy, M.; Bose, S. Osteoclastogenesis and osteoclastic resorption of tricalcium phosphate: Effect of strontium and magnesium doping. *J. Biomed. Mater. Res. A* **2012**, *100*, 2450–2461. [CrossRef] [PubMed]
77. Yamada, Y.; Ito, A.; Kojima, H.; Sakane, M.; Miyakawa, S.; Uemura, T.; LeGeros, R.Z. Inhibitory effect of Zn^{2+} in zinc-containing beta-tricalcium phosphate on resorbing activity of mature osteoclasts. *J. Biomed. Mater. Res. A* **2008**, *84*, 344–352. [CrossRef] [PubMed]
78. Schumacher, M.; Wagner, A.S.; Kokesch-Himmelreich, J.; Bernhardt, A.; Rohnke, M.; Wenisch, S.; Gelinsky, M. Strontium substitution in apatitic CaP cements effectively attenuates osteoclastic resorption but does not inhibit osteoclastogenesis. *Acta Biomater.* **2016**, *37*, 184–194. [CrossRef] [PubMed]
79. Friederichs, R.J.; Brooks, R.A.; Ueda, M.; Best, S.M. In vitro osteoclast formation and resorption of silicon-substituted hydroxyapatite ceramics. *J. Biomed. Mater. Res. A* **2015**, *103*, 3312–3322. [CrossRef] [PubMed]
80. Tortelli, F.; Pujic, N.; Liu, Y.; Laroche, N.; Vico, L.; Cancedda, R. Osteoblast and osteoclast differentiation in an in vitro three-dimensional model of bone. *Tissue Eng. Part A* **2009**, *15*, 2373–2383. [CrossRef] [PubMed]
81. Botelho, C.M.; Brooks, R.A.; Spence, G.; McFarlane, I.; Lopes, M.A.; Best, S.M.; Santos, J.D.; Rushton, N.; Bonfield, W. Differentiation of mononuclear precursors into osteoclasts on the surface of Si-substituted hydroxyapatite. *J. Biomed. Mater. Res. A* **2006**, *78*, 709–720. [CrossRef] [PubMed]
82. Vahabzadeh, S.; Roy, M.; Bose, S. Effects of Silicon on Osteoclast Cell Mediated Degradation, In Vivo Osteogenesis and Vasculogenesis of Brushite Cement. *J. Mater. Chem. B Mater. Biol. Med.* **2015**, *3*, 8973–8982. [CrossRef] [PubMed]
83. Wilson, T.; Parikka, V.; Holmbom, J.; Ylanen, H.; Penttinen, R. Intact surface of bioactive glass S53P4 is resistant to osteoclastic activity. *J. Biomed. Mater. Res. A* **2006**, *77*, 67–74. [CrossRef] [PubMed]
84. Karpov, M.; Laczka, M.; Leboy, P.S.; Osyczka, A.M. Sol-gel bioactive glasses support both osteoblast and osteoclast formation from human bone marrow cells. *J. Biomed. Mater. Res. A* **2008**, *84*, 718–726. [CrossRef] [PubMed]
85. Cacciotti, I.; Lehmann, G.; Camaioni, A.; Bianco, A. AP40 Bioactive Glass Ceramic by Sol-Gel Synthesis: In Vitro Dissolution and Cell-Mediated Bioresorption. *Key Eng. Mater.* **2013**, *541*, 41–50. [CrossRef]
86. Costa-Rodrigues, J.; Fernandes, A.; Lopes, M.A.; Fernandes, M.H. Hydroxyapatite surface roughness: Complex modulation of the osteoclastogenesis of human precursor cells. *Acta Biomater.* **2012**, *8*, 1137–1145. [CrossRef] [PubMed]
87. Gross, K.A.; Muller, D.; Lucas, H.; Haynes, D.R. Osteoclast resorption of thermal spray hydoxyapatite coatings is influenced by surface topography. *Acta Biomater.* **2012**, *8*, 1948–1956. [CrossRef] [PubMed]

88. Costa, D.O.; Prowse, P.D.; Chrones, T.; Sims, S.M.; Hamilton, D.W.; Rizkalla, A.S.; Dixon, S.J. The differential regulation of osteoblast and osteoclast activity by surface topography of hydroxyapatite coatings. *Biomaterials* **2013**, *34*, 7215–7226. [CrossRef] [PubMed]
89. Davison, N.L.; ten Harkel, B.; Schoenmaker, T.; Luo, X.; Yuan, H.; Everts, V.; Barrere-de Groot, F.; de Bruijn, J.D. Osteoclast resorption of beta-tricalcium phosphate controlled by surface architecture. *Biomaterials* **2014**, *35*, 7441–7451. [CrossRef] [PubMed]
90. Torres, A.L.; Santos, S.G.; Oliveira, M.I.; Barbosa, M.A. Fibrinogen promotes resorption of chitosan by human osteoclasts. *Acta Biomater.* **2013**, *9*, 6553–6562. [CrossRef] [PubMed]
91. Heinemann, C.; Heinemann, S.; Bernhardt, A.; Lode, A.; Worch, H.; Hanke, T. In vitro osteoclastogenesis on textile chitosan scaffold. *Eur. Cell Mater.* **2010**, *19*, 96–106. [CrossRef] [PubMed]
92. Rochet, N.; Balaguer, T.; Boukhechba, F.; Laugier, J.P.; Quincey, D.; Goncalves, S.; Carle, G.F. Differentiation and activity of human preosteoclasts on chitosan enriched calcium phosphate cement. *Biomaterials* **2009**, *30*, 4260–4267. [CrossRef] [PubMed]
93. Shafieyan, Y.; Tiedemann, K.; Goulet, A.; Komarova, S.; Quinn, T.M. Monocyte proliferation and differentiation to osteoclasts is affected by density of collagen covalently bound to a poly(dimethyl siloxane) culture surface. *J. Biomed. Mater. Res. A* **2012**, *100*, 1573–1581. [CrossRef] [PubMed]
94. Cool, S.M.; Kenny, B.; Wu, A.; Nurcombe, V.; Trau, M.; Cassady, A.I.; Grondahl, L. Poly(3-hydroxybutyrate-co-3-hydroxyvalerate) composite biomaterials for bone tissue regeneration: In vitro performance assessed by osteoblast proliferation, osteoclast adhesion and resorption, and macrophage proinflammatory response. *J. Biomed. Mater. Res. A* **2007**, *82*, 599–610. [CrossRef] [PubMed]
95. Jones, G.L.; Motta, A.; Marshall, M.J.; El Haj, A.J.; Cartmell, S.H. Osteoblast: Osteoclast co-cultures on silk fibroin, chitosan and PLLA films. *Biomaterials* **2009**, *30*, 5376–5384. [CrossRef] [PubMed]
96. Jeon, O.H.; Panicker, L.M.; Lu, Q.; Chae, J.J.; Feldman, R.A.; Elisseeff, J.H. Human iPSC-derived osteoblasts and osteoclasts together promote bone regeneration in 3D biomaterials. *Sci. Rep.* **2016**, *6*, 26761. [CrossRef] [PubMed]

4

Experimentally Achievable Accuracy Using a Digital Image Correlation Technique in measuring Small-Magnitude (<0.1%) Homogeneous Strain Fields

Alice Acciaioli, Giacomo Lionello and Massimiliano Baleani *

IRCCS—Istituto Ortopedico Rizzoli, Laboratorio di Tecnologia Medica, 40136 Bologna, Italy; alice.acciaioli@ior.it (A.A.); giacomo.lionello@ior.it (G.L.)

* Correspondence: baleani@tecno.ior.it

Abstract: Measuring small-magnitude strain fields using a digital image correlation (DIC) technique is challenging, due to the noise-signal ratio in strain maps. Here, we determined the level of accuracy achievable in measuring small-magnitude (<0.1%) homogeneous strain fields. We investigated different sets of parameters for image processing and imaging pre-selection, based on single-image noise level. The trueness of DIC was assessed by comparison of Young's modulus (E) and Poisson's ratio (ν) with values obtained from strain gauge measurements. Repeatability was improved, on average, by 20–25% with experimentally-determined optimal parameters and image pre-selection. Despite this, the intra- and inter-specimen repeatability of strain gauge measurements was 5 and 2.5 times better than DIC, respectively. Moreover, although trueness was also improved, on average, by 30–45%, DIC consistently overestimated the two material parameters by 1.8% and 3.2% for E and ν, respectively. DIC is a suitable option to measure small-magnitude homogeneous strain fields, bearing in mind the limitations in achievable accuracy.

Keywords: digital image correlation; homogeneous strain; small deformation level; accuracy; precision; calcium phosphate cements

---

1. Introduction

Calcium phosphate cements (CPCs) are bone substitute materials used for tissue defects filling [1]. Although they should mimic the mechanical behavior of bone tissue, their mechanical properties are still far from optimal. In fact, CPCs are brittle [2–4], and the limited data available in the literature suggests that this material can only withstand small strain levels (range 0.1–0.2%) before failure [5,6]. Therefore, new CPC formulations are still under development [7].

CPC testing is performed on small specimens (typically up to 20 mm in their largest dimension) [8–10]. Accurately measuring strain values the material undergoes to during testing is useful to compare different formulations of CPCs regarding elastic response and toughness enhancement. However, due to CPC characteristics, this is a challenge. In fact, contact-type extensometers cannot be used, because the knife edges would damage the specimen surface. Conversely, strain gauge installation may affect CPC response because of the unavoidable penetration of cyanoacrylate adhesive into the pores, which are always present in the cement matrix [8,11,12]. Therefore, the alternatives are non-contact techniques, i.e., optical methods based on interferometric techniques, or digital image correlation (DIC).

Interferometric techniques may be highly accurate, but are not practical for large sample size studies. They also may be too sensitive to environmental conditions, or could be limited to measurements on quasi-static loading scenarios [13–18]. Conversely, the DIC technique can be easily implemented, as demonstrated by its wide range of applications [19–23]. Video extensometry, initially based on feature-based image registration techniques that is evolving into a real-time DIC [24], can measure high strain level with small errors. However, strain errors increases if the specimen's dimensions decrease [25]. Moving on to DIC, experimental studies have defined effective procedures to calibrate DIC systems and/or to process the acquired images [26–29], thereby improving measurement accuracy. Unfortunately, although DIC has been demonstrated to be accurate in measuring medium-large strain levels [30–36], non negligible errors have been found when measuring small (<0.1% or 1000 microstrain) strain values [37–40], i.e., of the same order of magnitude of strain that CPCs can withstand before fracture. To the authors' knowledge, there is only one report showing that the DIC technique has the potential to provide an accuracy level comparable to the strain gauge in measuring small strain values [41]. However, that study was carried out analyzing artificial images, i.e., in absence of experimental errors. Conversely, studies based on experimentally-acquired images suggest that the measurement of small strain values may be affected by errors with an order of magnitude of up to 10% [28,38,39,42–44].

The present study investigated the suitability of DIC for measuring small-magnitude, homogeneous strain field, by experimentally determining the accuracy achievable using DIC to measure Young's modulus (E) and the Poisson's ratio (ν) of a specimen subjected to strain levels smaller than 0.1%.

2. Materials and Methods

The strain gauge (SG) technique was chosen as a reference technique to determine the error in measuring E and ν using the DIC technique. Aluminum was used instead of CPCs, to avoid any problems related to the SG application (described in the introduction section), i.e., an undesired reinforcing effect on the porous brittle material. Five parallelepiped specimens (10 mm square cross section, 20 mm height) were machined from an AA1050 (maximum grain size 80 μm) square bar, in order to ensure material uniformity. Each specimen underwent two series of uniaxial compression tests.

In the first series, a DIC system (Aramis 5M, GOM mbH, Braunschweig, Germany) was used to measure surface strain fields. Two digital cameras (2050 × 2448 pixels, TXG50i, Baumer Optronic GmbH, Radeberg, Germany), equipped with 2.8 FL/50 mm Titanar lenses and polarization filters (Schneider-Kreuznach, Bad Kreuznach, Germany) simultaneously monitored two opposite sides of the specimen at 15 Hz (Figure 1a).

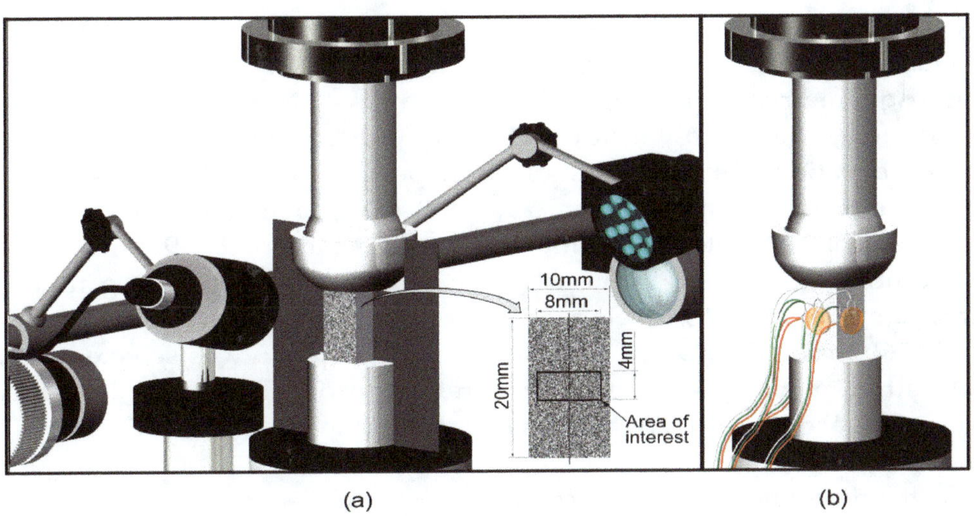

Figure 1. Scheme of the experimental setup used to measure surface strain. (**a**) Arrangement of the DIC system. The area of interest on the specimen surface is also shown. (**b**) Specimen instrumented with triaxial rosettes.

Both cameras were mounted onto a rigid support integrated into the testing machine frame and oriented in order to have the specimen surface centered in the view, while assuring a perpendicularity error smaller than 0.5 degrees. The camera-specimen distance was adjusted to the minimum focusing distance—about 150 mm from the polarizing filter placed in front of the camera lens to the specimen surface—obtaining a 12.6 × 15.0 mm measuring window. The resulting pixel size was 0.006 mm. A smaller pixel size, experimentally achievable with higher focal length lens, would have required a smaller dot size—determining the need to replace the airbrushing procedure (see below)—and would have reduced the subset dimension into millimeters (see below), thus introducing potential noise, due to the local strain gradient that occurs across grain boundaries. Speckle patterns (black dots on a white background) were previously created on two opposite surfaces of the specimen using an airbrush (Iwata HP-CH, 0.3 mm nozzle, Anest Iwata Europe S.r.l., Torino, Italy). Airbrush settings (air pressure = 3 bar; paint reduction by volume = 40%; airflow at the nozzle = 2 screw turns; needle travel length = 3 screw turns; spraying distance about 15 cm) were chosen using an internal airbrush-specific algorithm [45], in order to achieve an optimal speckle size of 3–5 pixels [46,47]. A trained operator (A.A.) created all patterns trying to achieve a coverage factor falling within the range of 42–50%, in order to minimise strain noise [48]. Average speckle size and coverage factor, calculated using the technique proposed by Lecompte et al. [49] and Shih [50], were 4.3 pixels (mean value range: 4.1–4.5 pixels) and 49% (range 47–50%) respectively. Images were acquired under the best achievable experimental conditions, i.e., at the smallest lens aperture (1/16, to get a sufficient depth of field), using the maximum exposure time (56 ms, due to the frame rate set to 15 Hz), while maximizing uniform lighting conditions over the entire area of interest (a white-light led was placed at about 80 mm from the specimen surface, the minimum allowable distance without interference of the 9W-led body with the field of view while maintaining the lamp heat-sink above and behind the camera lens). 2D calibration of each camera was carried out before each test-session by using a cubic-shaped 15 × 12 mm panel, following the manufacturer's recommendations [28].

An 8 by 4 mm rectangular area in the center of the specimen surface (Figure 1a) was selected as the area of interest, to exclude a local effect due to end effects. Preliminarily, the interaction between the subset size, step size, and strain window was investigated to select optimal parameters for image processing. The theoretically-set optimal subset size was calculated as three times the sum of the mean of the speckle size and distance (calculated values fell in the range 25 × 25–28 × 28 pixels), rounded to the nearest multiple of ten. Therefore, a subset size of 30 × 30 pixels was chosen. The step size was set at 1, 3, 8 and 15 pixels.

Image processing was carried out using a dedicated software (Aramis V 6.3.0, GOM mbH, Braunschweig, Germany). Surface strain in a measurement point, i.e., the center of a subset, was calculated using a square grid containing the center points of N × N neighboring subsets [51,52], hereinafter referred to as the strain window. The 2D deformation gradient tensor was calculated solving the system of equation, based on a first-order shape function, by the least square method [53,54]. The strain window was increased, starting from 3 × 3 subset, i.e., a field of center points of 3 × 3 subset, and increasing in steps of 2 subsets, up the maximum dimension of 9 × 9. Since increasing the step size decreased the noise in zero-strain maps (Figure 2), and the processing time without losing independent data, a step size of 15 pixels was chosen, i.e., an overlap ratio between neighboring subsets of 50% [55,56]. Similarly, a 9 × 9 strain window dimension was selected, because the noise decreased in zero-strain maps by increasing the strain window (Figure 2) [57]. Therefore the first image processing was carried out using a subset size of 30 × 30 pixels, a 50% overlap ratio and a 9 × 9 strain window.

A second image processing was carried out using the same parameters, except for the subset size, which was set at 60 × 60 pixels. This size was experimentally determined starting from the previous (30 × 30 pixels), and increasing it in steps of 10 pixels. The selection of the experimentally-determined optimal subset size to be used for image processing was based on the values of the coefficient of variation (CV, i.e., the ratio of the standard deviation to the mean, expressed in percent) of the principal strain values calculated for pooled data obtained from each couple of images. Indeed, CV values, which should theoretically be zero, are affected by both experimental and processing errors; the latter decreases by increasing the subset size. Since no further significant reduction was found when passing from pixel sizes 60 × 60 to 70 × 70, the 60 × 60 dimension was selected as the experimentally determined optimal subset size, as mentioned above (Figure 3, see also Supplementary Materials, Figure S1).

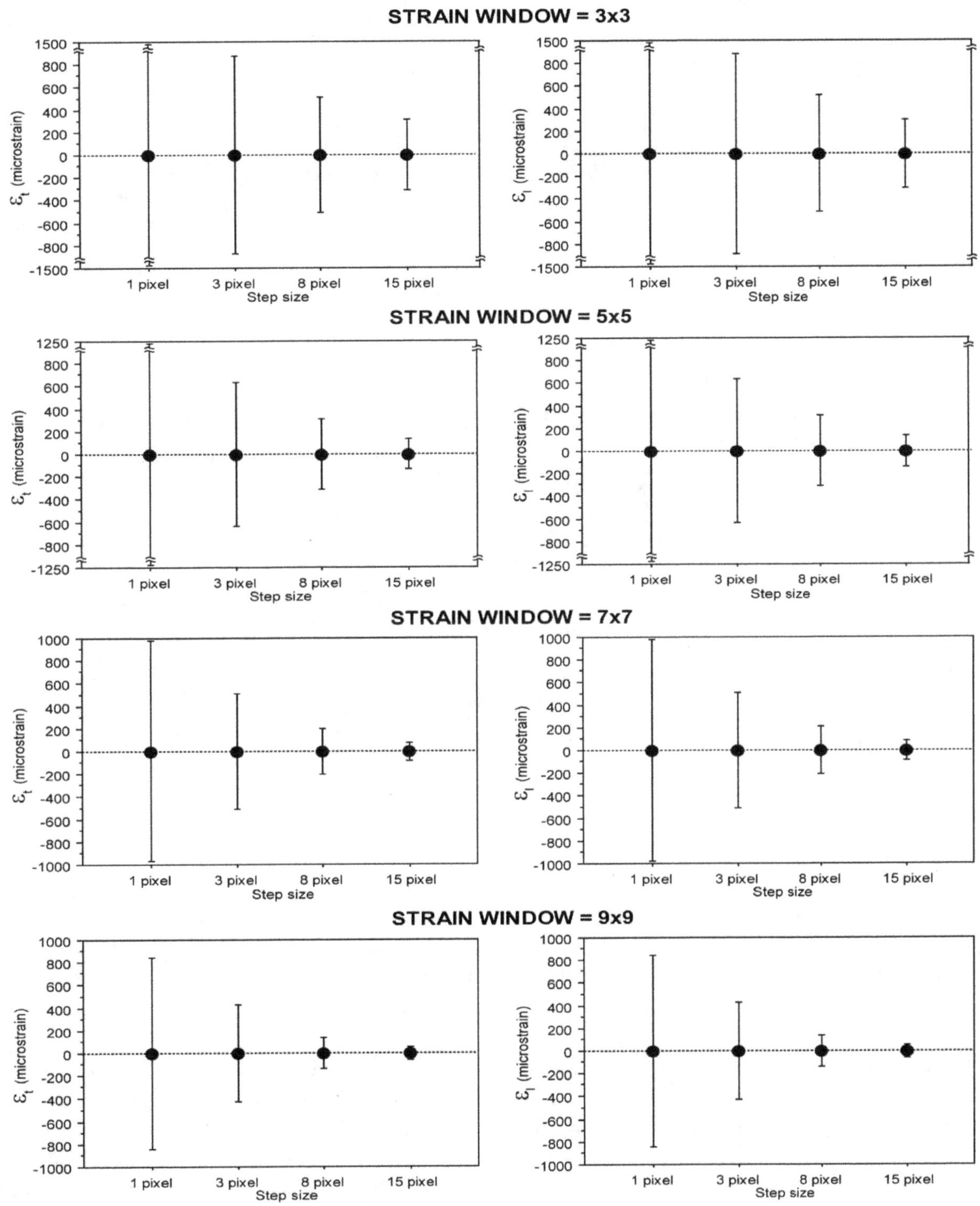

Figure 2. Errors in a zero-strain map achieved using a subset size of 30 × 30 pixels with different overlap values and strain window dimensions (error bar = standard deviation).

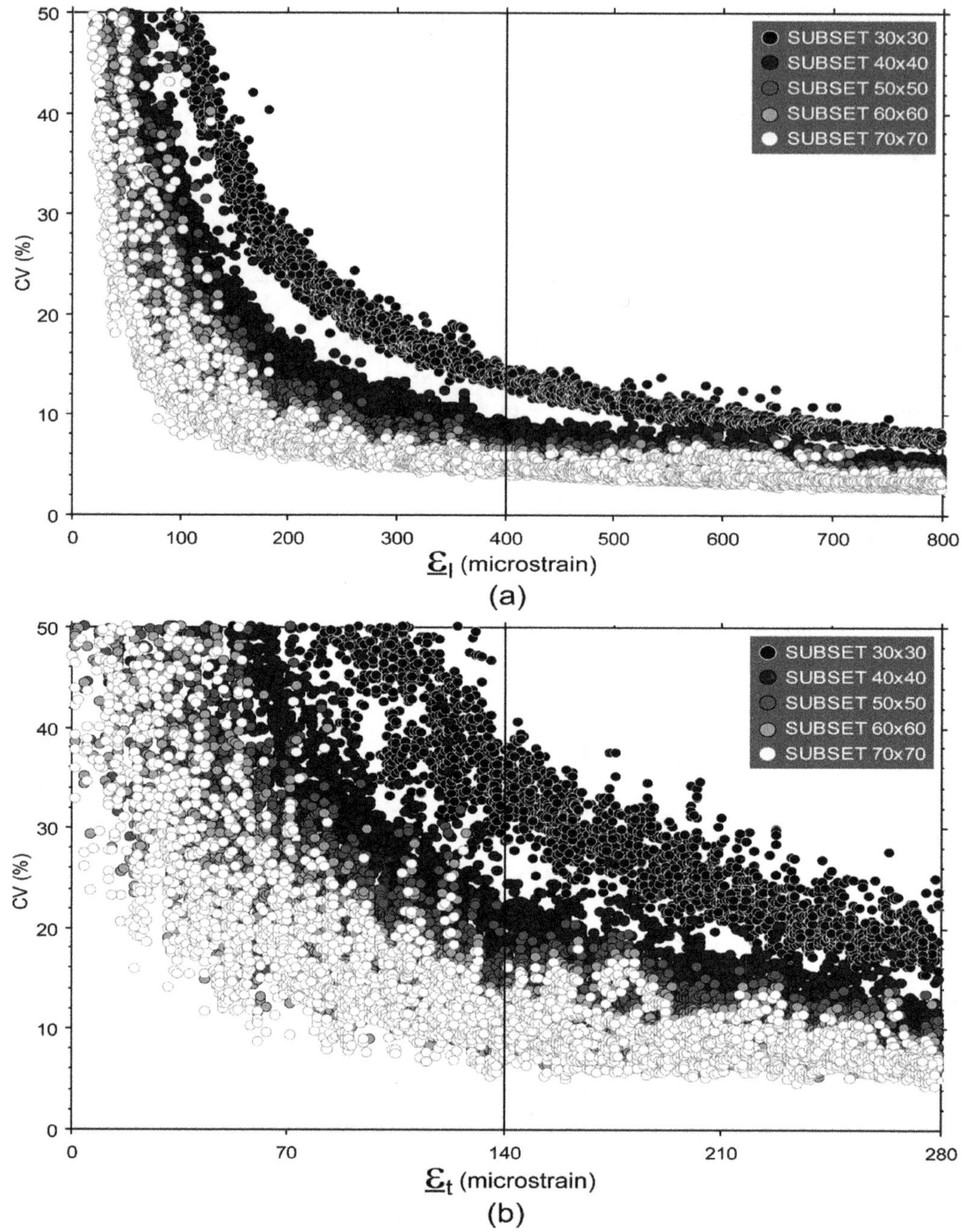

Figure 3. Representation of CV values calculated on the same image datasets changing the subset size from 30 × 30 to 70 × 70 pixels. (**a**) ε_l values; (**b**) ε_t values. Note: Each circle represents the CV of all strain values (ε) measured on the area of interest of a couple of images simultaneously acquired on both sides of the specimen.

A third image processing step was carried out using the previous parameters and an image pre-selection. Since noise on the strain map determines angle fluctuation of principal compressive (or longitudinal strain ε_l) and tensile strain (or transverse strain ε_t) direction, image pre-selection was based on the distribution of angle fluctuation: an image, and the image simultaneously acquired on the opposite surface of the specimen, was automatically discarded when three times the standard deviation of θ values ($3SD_\theta$) was greater than 0.1 rad, where θ was the angle between local ε_t and the horizontal direction (Figure 4).

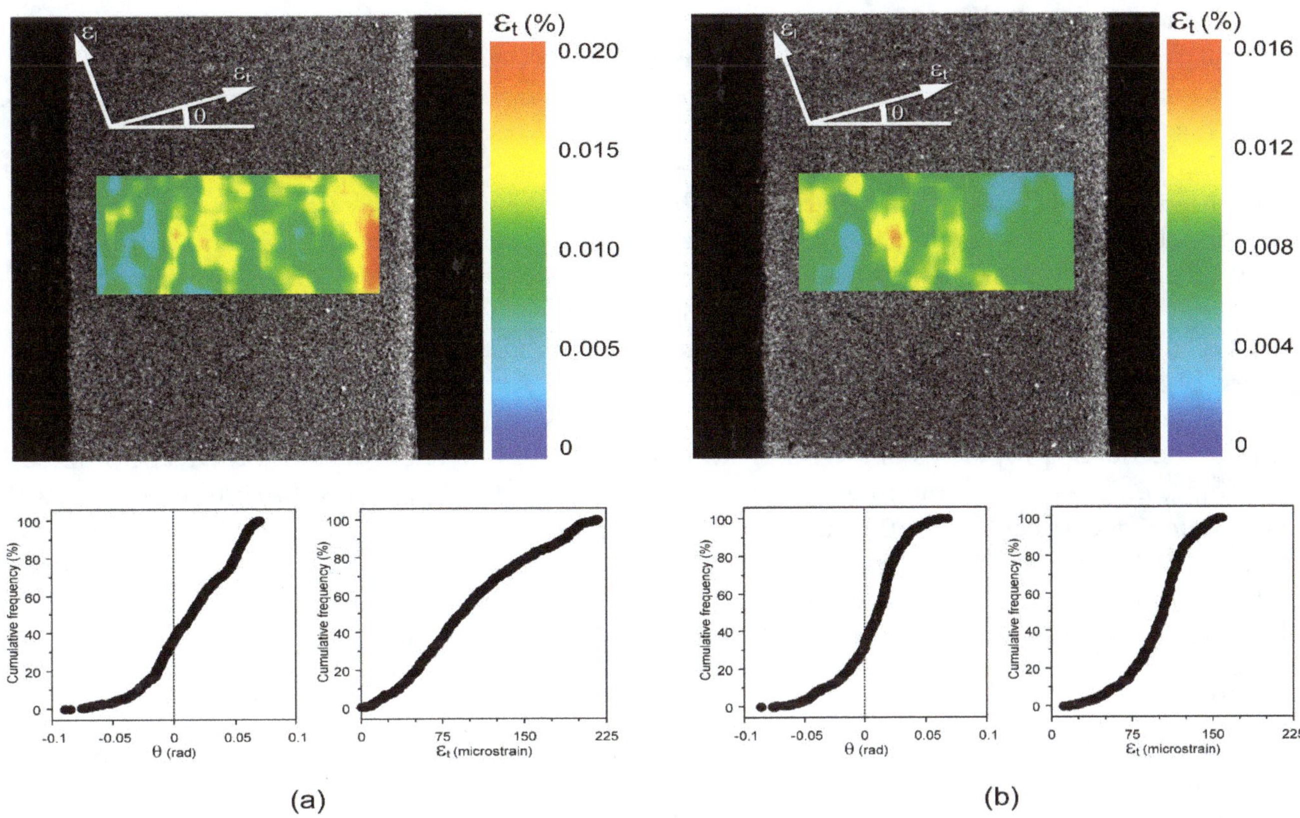

Figure 4. Two strain maps, with a cumulative distribution of θ and ε_t values, calculated for the same ε_l value (ε_l = 280 microstrain) on the same specimen surface during two different test-sessions. (**a**) $3SD_\theta > 0.1$ rad: this image, and the image simultaneously acquired on the opposite surface of the specimen, must be discarded; (**b**) $3SD_\theta \leq 0.1$ rad: this image is accepted if θ distribution determined for the image simultaneously acquired on the opposite surface of the specimen fulfils the same requirement.

For all the three image processing, the average values (indicated as $\underline{\varepsilon}$) of ε_l and ε_t were calculated over the two areas of interest which were simultaneously acquired by the two cameras.

In the second series, triaxial rosettes with pre-attached lead wire (UFRA-3-350, Tokyo Sokki Kenkyuio Co, Tokyo, Japan) were used to measure strain reference values; this was necessary to determine the accuracy of the DIC technique (Figure 1b). After having carefully prepared the surface (Vishay Precision Group, 2014), a rosette was attached in the center of all four sides of the specimen surface (Figure 1b). Strain data were acquired at 100 Hz, using a multichannel data logger (System 6000, Vishay Precision Group, Raileigh, NC, USA), and processed to determine the principal directions and principal strains using a dedicated software (StrainSmart V4.31, Vishay Precision Group, Raileigh, NC, USA). The average values ($\underline{\varepsilon}$) of ε_l and ε_t simultaneously acquired by the four rosettes were calculated.

Both test series were performed at a constant displacement rate of 0.1 mm/min. Specimens were mounted onto a fixed platen placed onto a 10 kN load cell and loaded through an unlocked spherical seat platen fixed to the actuator of the testing machine (Mod.8502, Instron, Norwood, MA, USA), allowing alignment to the specimen end surface. A customized jig was used in order to align the specimen to the spherical seat, while maintaining the two patterned surfaces orthogonal to the DIC cameras. An initial preload (about 20 N) was applied to maintain the position of the specimen before removing the customized jig. All tests were limited to −5.6 kN, in order to reach a maximum compressive strain value just above a target value of 800 microstrain (i.e., 0.08%). The minimum compressive strain value was chosen considering the image processing errors. Indeed, referring to the experimentally-determined optimal subset size 60 × 60, CV values started to increase exponentially for $\underline{\varepsilon}_t$ values falling below 140 microstrain (Figure 3). Therefore this value, which corresponds to 400 microstrain in term of $\underline{\varepsilon}_l$, was set as minimum strain value in calculating E and ν.

Each test-session of five specimens was repeated five times after dismounting and remounting the whole setup. For each test repetition, E and ν were calculated using $\underline{\varepsilon}_l$ and $\underline{\varepsilon}_t$, measured as described above using both techniques. $\underline{\varepsilon}_l$ values were limited to a range of 400–800 microstrain for the aforementioned reasons. The E value was determined as the slope of the stress-$\underline{\varepsilon}_l$ curve. The ν value was calculated as the mean value of all the absolute ratios of $\underline{\varepsilon}_t$ to $\underline{\varepsilon}_l$. Inter- and intra-specimen repeatability was expressed as CV, calculated for five repetitions carried out on the same specimen and for each set of five specimens respectively. DIC trueness was assessed by analyzing differences between E and ν mean values, which were determined using DIC and SG techniques on each specimen, by means of a paired t-test.

Finally, on the basis of the achieved results (see below), the third image processing was used to determine the elastic properties of a CPC prototype formulation. The formulation was optimized for 3D plotting, i.e., the paste allowed extrusion from a thin needle and assured printed shape stability. Ten parallelepiped specimens (10 mm square cross section, 20 mm height) were printed in air and immersed in deionized water for two weeks to achieve full setting. CPC specimens underwent monotonic compressive tests performed at a constant displacement rate of 0.1 mm/min. E and ν were calculated limiting $\underline{\varepsilon}_l$ to the range of 400–800 microstrain for the aforementioned reasons.

3. Results

Noise in zero strain readings was negligible for SG; in all cases, measured values were smaller than 4 microstrain. Conversely, although $\underline{\varepsilon}_t$ and $\underline{\varepsilon}_l$ values calculated using DIC technique were smaller than 10 microstrain, ε standard deviation was 10–20 microstrain, with peak values up to 70 microstrain.

Approximately, 360 images were captured by each camera during a test against about 2400 triplets of data acquired from each rosette. Image pre-selection was used in the third processing procedure for DIC data. This process discarded, on average, 12% of images (range 0–35%). Discarded images were generally acquired in the first part of the test, i.e., where $\underline{\varepsilon}_t$ values calculated using DIC fell into the lower part of $\underline{\varepsilon}_t$ range. An example of the effect of image pre-selection on collected data is show in Figures 5 and 6.

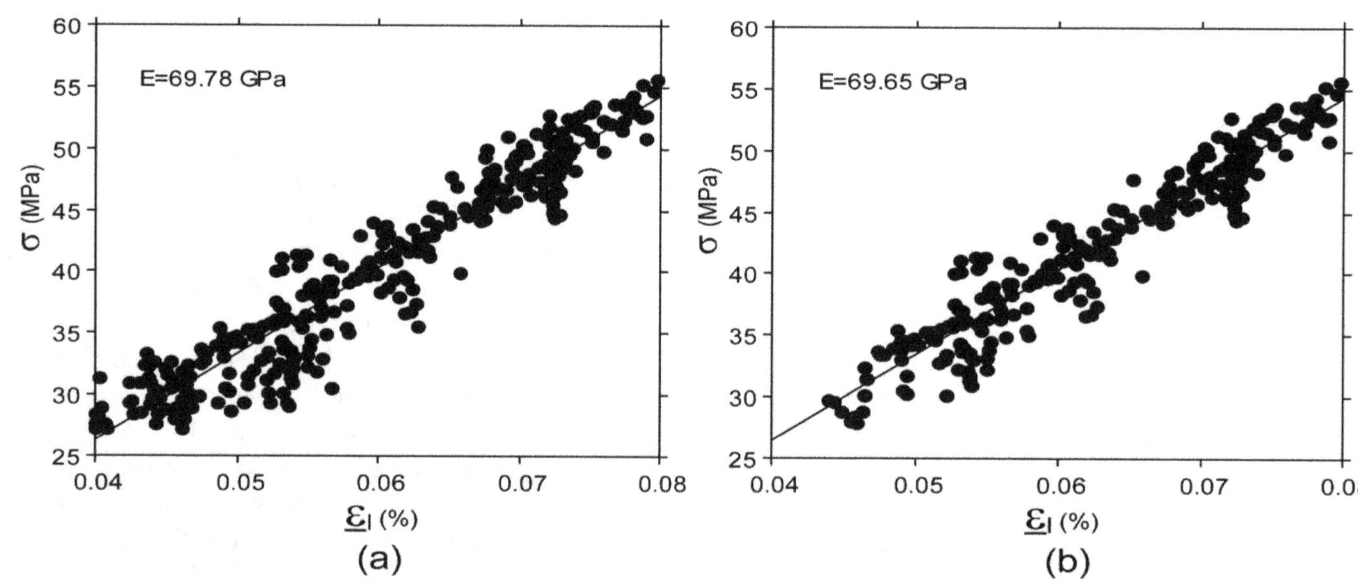

Figure 5. E value determined for one specimen. (**a**) Regression slope obtained using a subset size of 60 × 60 pixels. (**b**) Regression slope obtained using a subset size of 60 × 60 pixels and image pre-selection.

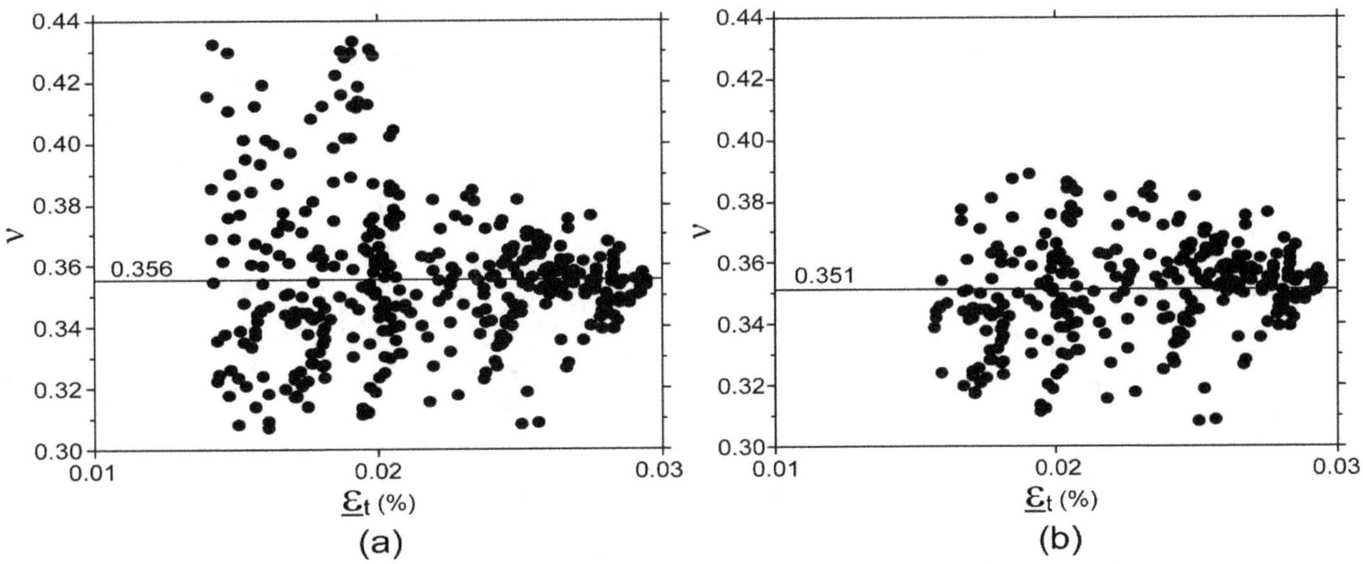

Figure 6. ν mean value determined for one specimen. (**a**) Data obtained using a subset size of 60 × 60 pixels. (**b**) Data obtained using a subset size of 60 × 60 pixels and image pre-selection. Note 1: The 140 microstrain threshold to ε_t had already been applied before calculating ν values reported in this graph. Note 2: Interchanging ε_l to ε_t in x-axis would: (i) scale the x-axis by a factor of 1/0.35 (ii) cause a small horizontal drift of each point, the entity and direction of which would depend on the difference between the current value and 0.35; no changes would occur in ν mean values.

Intra- and inter-specimen repeatability values, calculated for the two techniques, are summarized in Tables 1 and 2 for E and ν values respectively. The three CV values reported for DIC technique refer to the three different image processing procedures. Intra- and inter-specimen repeatability of DIC were comparable. Conversely, inter-specimen repeatability of SG was double that of intra-specimen. In general, both techniques were more precise for determining E values. However, regardless of the measured parameter, the intra- and inter-specimen repeatability of SG measurements was better than DIC by about 5 and 2.5 times respectively. An improvement in DIC repeatability was found by increasing the subset size, and by adding image pre-selection. This improvement was more noticeable when looking at the worst CV values calculated for ν values.

Table 1. Intra- and inter-specimen repeatability for E values. The mean and the worst (maximum) CV values are reported.

Young's Modulus (E)	Strain Gauge Mean (Worst)	DIC Subset 30 × 30 Mean (Worst)	DIC Subset 60 × 60 Mean (Worst)	DIC Subset 60 × 60 + Image pre-Selec. Mean (Worst)
Intra-specimen repeatability	0.4% (0.7%)	2.2% (2.4%)	1.9% (2.2%)	1.8% (2.0%)
Inter-specimen repeatability	0.8% (1.0%)	2.3% (2.9%)	2.0% (2.7%)	1.9% (2.4%)

Table 2. Intra- and inter-specimen repeatability for ν values. The mean and the worst (maximum) CV values are reported.

Poisson's Ratio (ν)	Strain Gauge Mean (Worst)	DIC Subset 30 × 30 Mean (Worst)	DIC Subset 60 × 60 Mean (Worst)	DIC Subset 60 × 60 + Image Pre-Selec. Mean (Worst)
Intra-specimen repeatability	0.8% (1.2%)	4.4% (6.4%)	3.8% (5.4%)	3.3% (4.4%)
Inter-specimen repeatability	1.6% (2.2%)	4.3% (6.3%)	3.8% (5.5%)	3.5% (4.9%)

The trueness of DIC is shown in Figure 7, where values experimentally determined using SGs were used as reference. Although the bias decreased by increasing the subset size and adding image pre-selection, the difference was statistically significant in all three comparisons.

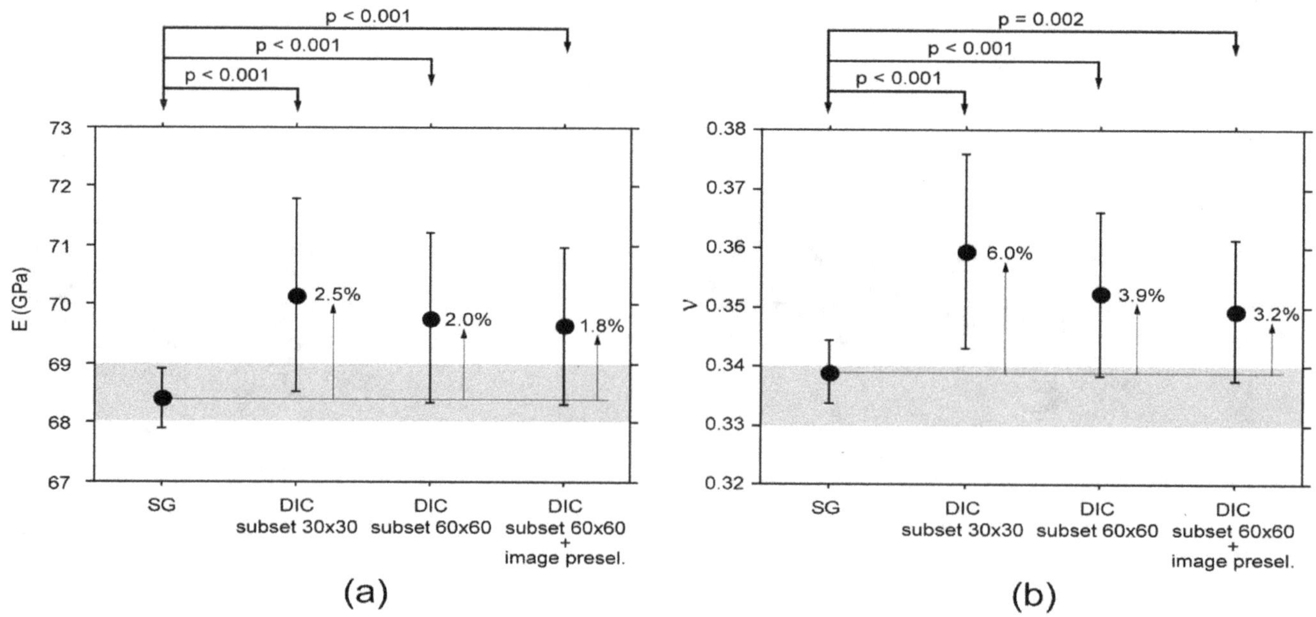

Figure 7. (**a**) E and (**b**) ν mean values, and relative standard deviations, determined using SG and DIC technique. The grey bands represent the range of E and ν values for AA1050, as reported in the literature. Note: The total sample size is 25, with 5 repeated measurements taken on the same specimen.

The pilot study on a CPC prototype formulation was successfully carried-out using the described experimental procedure. Indeed, elastic mechanical properties were determined for all ten tested specimens. E and ν were 9.0 ± 1.2 GPa and 0.22 ± 0.04 respectively.

4. Discussion

This study shows that DIC can measure small-magnitude (<0.1%) homogeneous strain fields with satisfactory accuracy, as demonstrated by the good agreement between E and ν values determined using SG (reference values) and DIC technique.

Although the DIC technique is extensively used to investigate material response to loads, these results were not foreseeable because, in general, published studies measured surface strain values with magnitudes of 1% or greater, both at macro and microscopic scales, [23,25,35,36,42,58–60] and reported error values of the same order of magnitude of the strain range as those investigated in the present study [28,39,42–44,61]. Indeed, the above-mentioned accuracy was achieved by minimizing the noise level, by (i) measuring each strain value (ε) on a 60 × 60 pixels subset, using a 50% overlap ratio (step size 30 pixel) and a 9 × 9 strain window, meaning that each strain value was calculated on a squared area of 300 × 300 pixels, i.e., 1.8 × 1.8 mm, and (ii) averaging all the strain values measured over an area of 64 mm^2 to calculate the $\underline{\varepsilon}_l$ and $\underline{\varepsilon}_t$ value for each couple of images simultaneously acquired, i.e., averaging about 900 ε values. Despite all this, some level of noise in $\underline{\varepsilon}_l$ and $\underline{\varepsilon}_t$ values, of up to 40 microstrain (in agreement with previous findings [62]), still remains, as shown by the dispersion of ν values in Figure 6. It has been widely demonstrated that the overlap ratio (or step size), subset size, and strain window dimension (or computation size) in image processing impact the DIC accuracy. These parameters were optimized in the present study for the described setup. Indeed, the chosen overlap ratio fell into the optimal range recommended in the literature, i.e., 50–75% [52,63,64]. A greater overlap ratio, i.e., smaller step size, would produce oversampled data, and increase noise on the strain field [48,65]. Similarly, a subset size greater than 60 × 60 pixels would not further reduce the residual error. It is acknowledged that increasing the subset size will increase the accuracy with which displacements are determined [49,66,67]. Indeed, CVs of ε values decrease as the subset size increases from 30 × 30 to 60 × 60, as shown in Figure 3. However, beyond a 60 × 60 pixel size, no further improvement was found; this is in agreement with previous studies showing that there is a plateau in noise reduction [25,42,66,67]. It must be acknowledged that subset sizes used in the literature are generally smaller than 60 $\times$ 60 pixels [30,31,68,69]. However, those studies investigated strain levels greater than 1%. Indeed, trends observed in Figure 3 suggest that subset size smaller than 60 $\times$ 60 become appropriate for measuring strain levels greater than 0.08%, thus increasing the ability of DIC to capture strain gradients. However when strain levels smaller that 0.1% are investigated, the optimal subset size increases [41,70]. It is noteworthy that CV values do not converge to zero. It seems unlikely that this noise is due to strain localization across grain boundaries, since the subset dimension, in millimeters, was at least one order of magnitude greater than the grain dimension. In other words, we assumed that the aluminum surface deformation appeared homogeneous at subset scale level. Noise in DIC measurements contributes to a residual trend. However, the actual strain distribution was non-uniform over the cross section, due to undesired off-axis loading on the specimen. In fact, although specimen alignment was performed carefully, a misalignment error of up to 0.1 mm may have occurred, which contributes up to 6.5% to residual CV value. The DIC setup (i.e., two cameras monitoring simultaneously two opposite side of the specimen), as well as the four-rosette configuration, was chosen in order to compensate for the misalignment error, and to determine accurate E value. Referring to the strain window dimension, a large value (9 $\times$ 9) was used, i.e., each ε value was calculated over a quite large area, as explained above. This choice decreases the ability of DIC to capture strain gradients, and therefore to accurately monitor what happens in proximity of any nucleating crack, which is irrelevant in the homogeneous strain field. Greater strain window dimensions might further lightly smooth ε values, but would not change the $\underline{\varepsilon}$ value calculated over the entire area of interest, and ultimately, would not change the results.

Other known sources of error are due to inaccuracies in preparing the specimen surface (speckle pattern), or in setting up the experimental model (loading condition, lens alignment, lighting, etc.). Special attention was paid in the specimen preparation. The speckle pattern was created by spraying black dots on the specimen surface following a previously developed procedure [45]. This involved the use of an airbrush-specific algorithm, which allows a trained operator to achieve the desired dot size of 3–5 pixels, and a coverage factor closer to 50%. On the basis of the data available in the literature [42,47,48,65,71], the achieved pattern should minimize the correlation error. In addition, the experimental model was set up attempting to achieve the best operating conditions. Additionally, the experimental setup minimized the error of perpendicularity between camera and specimen surface, decreasing the out-of-plane motion. Indeed, residual errors in calculating Poisson's ratio determined using the DIC technique, are comparable to those reported in the literature using the DIC 3D setup [72], which is unaffected by out-of-plane motion, without the need to manipulate DIC data. Finally, another source of error was deleted by simultaneously monitoring two opposite sides, in order to compensate for the problem of a non-axial-load applied on the specimen due to small misalignment between specimen axis and spherical seat. However, other errors are operator dependent (e.g., focusing camera lenses, lighting homogeneously both specimen surfaces). Despite the fact that the same trained operator carried out all test-sessions, the repeatability in achieving the experimental optimal conditions for the investigated strain range appeared to be a problem. However, it must be acknowledged that other sources of errors, such as thermal noise or CCD sensor noise [73] may have affected strain measurements. Whatever the cause, when experimental "sub-optimal" conditions occurred, image pre-selection played a role in reducing error and slightly improving DIC accuracy. In fact, image pre-selection discarded several images in all but one test session. The image pre-selection criterion is based on a priori knowledge of strain directions. It deletes all and only images that are noisy, which is more effective than data filtering, slightly improving both DIC trueness and precision in determining E and ν values (although a residual bias and a quite large dispersion still exists). Dispersion values can be ascribed to specimen inhomogeneity only for a small part. Indeed, apart from the fact that specimens were machined from the same bar, in order to minimize material inhomogeneity due to processing route, the inter-specimen repeatability achieved using SG was excellent. It could be argued that the E and ν values determined using SG are not true values, and therefore, that it is not possible to conclude that DIC overestimates the two mechanical parameters. However, although SG data are affected by some degree of uncertainty, the E and ν values determined using SG are in agreement with those reported in the literature for AA1050. This observation indirectly supports the aforementioned conclusion.

Other known sources of error are the quality of DIC hardware [28,74,75], and the correlation algorithm [34,37,54,74,76,77]. However, it was out of the scope of this study to compare different hardware or algorithms. Therefore, one commercial system was used to carry out the experimental series; this is a major limitation of this work. In fact, it cannot be excluded that different hardware components or different sub-pixel registration algorithms might have further improved the accuracy and precision achieved in the present study. However, the described procedure appeared suitable to determine CPC elastic mechanical properties, whose accuracy is a key for the reliability of numerical models of CPC 3D structures.

5. Conclusions

DIC can be practical and effective in measuring small-magnitude (<0.1%) homogeneous strain fields. The experimentally-determined optimal parameters for image processing, including the identification of the optimal subset size for the actual speckle pattern, and image pre-selection based on strain direction, can minimize the noise level. Under these conditions, a trueness better than 2% and 4% in measuring E and ν can be achieved, keeping in mind that both parameters are overestimated. However, DIC repeatability must be taken into account when calculating the sample size.

Author Contributions: M.B. conceived and designed the experiments; A.A. and G.L. performed the experiments; A.A. and G.L. analyzed the data; A.A. and M.B. wrote the paper, with the help of G.L.

Acknowledgments: The authors wish to thank Luigi Lena for the artworks and Lucia Mancini for her help in revising the manuscript.

References

1. Zhang, J.; Liu, W.; Schnitzler, V.; Tancret, F.; Bouler, J.-M. Calcium phosphate cements for bone substitution: Chemistry, handling and mechanical properties. *Acta Biomater.* **2014**, *10*, 1035–1049. [CrossRef] [PubMed]
2. Ajaxon, I.; Öhman, C.; Persson, C. Long-Term In Vitro Degradation of a High-Strength Brushite Cement in Water, PBS, and Serum Solution. *BioMed Res. Int.* **2015**, *2015*, 575079. [CrossRef] [PubMed]
3. Ambard, A.J.; Mueninghoff, L. Calcium phosphate cement: Review of mechanical and biological properties. *J. Prosthodont.* **2006**, *15*, 321–328. [CrossRef] [PubMed]
4. Chow, L. Next generation calcium phosphate-based biomaterials. *Dent. Mater. J.* **2009**, *28*, 1–10. [CrossRef] [PubMed]
5. Charrière, E.; Terrazzoni, S.; Pittet, C.; Mordasini, P.; Dutoit, M.; Lemaìtre, J.; Zysset, P. Mechanical characterization of brushite and hydroxyapatite cements. *Biomaterials* **2001**, *22*, 2937–2945. [CrossRef]
6. Ajaxon, I.; Acciaioli, A.; Lionello, G.; Ginebra, M.P.; Öhman-Mägi, C.; Baleani, M.; Persson, C. Elastic properties and strain-to-crack-initiation of calcium phosphate bone cements: Revelations of a high-resolution measurement technique. *J. Mech. Behav. Biomed. Mater.* **2017**, *74*, 428–437. [CrossRef] [PubMed]
7. Geffers, M.; Groll, J.; Gbureck, U. Reinforcement Strategies for Load-Bearing Calcium Phosphate Biocements. *Materials* **2015**, *8*, 2700–2717. [CrossRef]
8. Engstrand, J.; Persson, C.; Engqvist, H. The effect of composition on mechanical properties of brushite cements. *J. Mech. Behav. Biomed. Mater.* **2014**, *29*, 81–90. [CrossRef] [PubMed]

9. Ginebra, M.P.; Driessens, F.C.M.; Planell, J.A. Effect of the particle size on the micro and nanostructural features of a calcium phosphate cement: A kinetic analysis. *Biomaterials* **2004**, *25*, 3453–3462. [CrossRef] [PubMed]
10. Luo, J.; Ajaxon, I.; Ginebra, M.P.; Engqvist, H.; Persson, C. Compressive, diametral tensile and biaxial flexural strength of cutting-edge calcium phosphate cements. *J. Mech. Behav. Biomed. Mater.* **2016**, *60*, 617–627. [CrossRef] [PubMed]
11. Grover, L. In vitro ageing of brushite calcium phosphate cement. *Biomaterials* **2003**, *24*, 4133–4141. [CrossRef]
12. Hofmann, M.; Mohammed, A.; Perrie, Y.; Gbureck, U.; Barralet, J. High-strength resorbable brushite bone cement with controlled drug-releasing capabilities. *Acta Biomater.* **2009**, *5*, 43–49. [CrossRef] [PubMed]
13. Davidson, R.J. *A Comparison of Moirè Interferometry and Digital Image Correlation*; Air force Institute of Technology: Dayton, OH, USA, 2008.
14. Erne, O.K.; Chu, Y.E.; Mohr, M.; Miller, J.R.; Bottlang, M. Full-field strain measurement on cortical bone. In Proceedings of the 48th Annual Meeting of the Orthopaedic Research Society, Dallas, TX, USA, 10–13 February 2002.
15. Jacquot, P. Speckle Interferometry: A Review of the Principal Methods in Use for Experimental Mechanics Applications. *Strain* **2008**, *44*, 57–69. [CrossRef]
16. Ohlson, N.G. Classical optical interferometry for strain measurement. In *Imaging Methods for Novel Materials and Challenging Applications*; Jin, H., Sciammarella, C., Furlong, C., Yoshida, S., Eds.; Springer: New York, NY, USA, 2013; Volume 3, pp. 127–132.
17. Post, D.H.B. Moiré Interfe. In *Handbook of Experimental Solid Mechanics*; Sharpe, N.W., Jr., Ed.; Springer: New York, NY, USA, 2008; pp. 1–26.
18. Yang, L.; Xie, X.; Zhu, L.; Wu, S.; Wang, Y. Review of electronic speckle pattern interferometry (ESPI) for three dimensional displacement measurement. *Chin. J. Mech. Eng.* **2014**, *27*, 1–13. [CrossRef]
19. Chevalier, L.; Calloch, S.; Hild, F.; Marco, Y. Digital image correlation used to analyze the multiaxial behavior of rubber-like materials. *Eur. J. Mech.-A/Solids* **2001**, *20*, 169–187. [CrossRef]
20. Sánchez-Arévalo, F.M.; Pulos, G. Use of digital image correlation to determine the mechanical behavior of materials. *Mater. Charact.* **2008**, *59*, 1572–1579. [CrossRef]
21. Tarigopula, V.; Hopperstad, O.S.; Langseth, M.; Clausen, A.H.; Hild, F. A study of localisation in dual-phase high-strength steels under dynamic loading using digital image correlation and FE analysis. *Int. J. Solids Struct.* **2008**, *45*, 601–619. [CrossRef]
22. Zhou, J.; Liu, D.; Shao, L.; Wang, Z. Application of digital image correlation to measurement of packaging material mechanical properties. *Math. Prob. Eng.* **2013**, *2013*, 204875. [CrossRef]
23. Lionello, G.; Fognani, R.; Baleani, M.; Sudanese, A.; Toni, A. Suturing the myotendinous junction in total hip arthroplasty: A biomechanical comparison of different stitching techniques. *Clin. Biomech.* **2015**, *30*, 1077–1082. [CrossRef] [PubMed]
24. Wu, R.; Kong, C.; Li, K.; Zhang, D. Real-Time Digital Image Correlation for Dynamic Strain Measurement. *Exp. Mech.* **2016**, *56*, 1–11. [CrossRef]
25. Pan, B.; Tian, L. Advanced video extensometer for non-contact, real-time, high-accuracy strain measurement. *Opt. Express* **2016**, *24*, 19082–19093. [CrossRef] [PubMed]
26. Hack, E.; Lin, X.; Patterson, E.A.; Sebastian, C.M. A reference material for establishing uncertainties in full-field displacement measurements. *Meas. Sci. Technol.* **2015**, *26*, 75004. [CrossRef]
27. Wang, D.; Diazdelao, F.A.; Wang, W.; Lin, X.; Patterson, E.A.; Mottershead, J.E. Uncertainty quantification in DIC with Kriging regression. *Opt. Lasers Eng.* **2016**, *78*, 182–195. [CrossRef]
28. Lava, P.; Van Paepegem, W.; Coppieters, S.; De Baere, I.; Wang, Y.; Debruyne, D. Impact of lens distortions on strain measurements obtained with 2D digital image correlation. *Opt. Lasers Eng.* **2013**, *51*, 576–584. [CrossRef]
29. Becker, T.; Splitthof, K.; Siebert, T.; Kletting, P. Error estimations of 3D digital image correlation measurements. *SPIE Proc.* **2006**, *6341*, 63410F.
30. Grytten, F.; Daiyan, H.; Polanco-Loria, M.; Dumoulin, S. Use of digital image correlation to measure large-strain tensile properties of ductile thermoplastics. *Polym. Test.* **2009**, *28*, 653–660. [CrossRef]
31. Jerabek, M.; Major, Z.; Lang, R.W. Strain determination of polymeric materials using digital image correlation. *Polym. Test.* **2010**, *29*, 407–416. [CrossRef]
32. Lagattu, F.; Bridier, F.; Villechaise, P.; Brillaud, J. In-plane strain measurements on a microscopic scale by coupling digital image correlation and an in situ SEM technique. *Mater. Charact.* **2006**, *56*, 10–18. [CrossRef]

33. Pritchard, R.H.; Lava, P.; Debruyne, D.; Terentjev, E.M. Precise determination of the Poisson ratio in soft materials with 2D digital image correlation. *Soft Matter* **2013**, *9*, 6037. [CrossRef]
34. Wang, Y.H.; Jiang, J.H.; Wanintrudal, C.; Du, C.; Zhou, D.; Smith, L.M.; Yang, L.X. Whole field sheet-metal tensile test using digital image correlation. *Exp. Tech.* **2010**, *34*, 54–59. [CrossRef]
35. Fuentes, C.A.; Willekens, P.; Hendrikx, N.; Lemmens, B.; Claeys, J.; Croughs, J.; Dupont-Gillain, C.; Seveno, D.; Van Vuure, A. Microstructure and mechanical properties of hemp technical fibres for composite applications by micro computed tomography and digital image correlation. In Proceedings of the 17th European Conference on Composite Materials (ECCM 2016), Munich, Germany, 26–30 June 2016; pp. 26–30.
36. Berfield, T.A.; Patel, J.K.; Shimmin, R.G.; Braun, P.V.; Lambros, J.; Sottos, N.R. Micro- and Nanoscale Deformation Measurement of Surface and Internal Planes via Digital Image Correlation. *Exp. Mech.* **2007**, *47*, 51–62. [CrossRef]
37. Chu, T.C.; Ranson, W.F.; Sutton, M.A. Applications of digital-image-correlation techniques to experimental mechanics. *Exp. Mech.* **1985**, *25*, 232–244. [CrossRef]
38. Hung, P.-C.; Voloshin, A.S. In-plane strain measurement by digital image correlation. *J. Braz. Soc. Mech. Sci. Eng.* **2003**, *25*, 215–221. [CrossRef]
39. Périé, J.-N.; Calloch, S.; Cluzel, C.; Hild, F. Analysis of a multiaxial test on a C/C composite by using digital image correlation and a damage model. *Exp. Mech.* **2002**, *42*, 318–328. [CrossRef]
40. Siebert, T.; Becker, T.; Spiltthof, K.; Neumann, I.; Krupka, R. Error Estimations in Digital Image Correlation Technique. *Appl. Mech. Mater.* **2007**, *7–8*, 265–270. [CrossRef]
41. Lee, C.; Take, W.A.; Hoult, N.A. Optimum Accuracy of Two-Dimensional Strain Measurements Using Digital Image Correlation. *J. Comput. Civ. Eng.* **2012**, *26*, 795–803. [CrossRef]
42. Rajan, V.P.; Rossol, M.N.; Zok, F.W. Optimization of Digital Image Correlation for High-Resolution Strain Mapping of Ceramic Composites. *Exp. Mech.* **2012**, *52*, 1407–1421. [CrossRef]
43. Begonia, M.T.; Dallas, M.; Vizcarra, B.; Liu, Y.; Johnson, M.L.; Thiagarajan, G. Non-contact strain measurement in the mouse forearm loading model using digital image correlation (DIC). *Bone* **2015**, *81*, 593–601. [CrossRef] [PubMed]
44. Robert, L.; Nazaret, F.; Cutard, T.; Orteu, J.-J. Use of 3-D Digital Image Correlation to Characterize the Mechanical Behavior of a Fiber Reinforced Refractory Castable. *Exp. Mech.* **2007**, *47*, 761–773. [CrossRef]
45. Lionello, G.; Cristofolini, L. A practical approach to optimizing the preparation of speckle patterns for digital-image correlation. *Meas. Sci. Technol.* **2014**, *25*, 107001. [CrossRef]
46. Schreier, H.; Orteu, J.-J.; Sutton, M.A. *Image Correlation for Shape, Motion and Deformation Measurements*; Springer: New York, NY, USA, 2009.
47. Zhou, P. Subpixel displacement and deformation gradient measurement using digital image/speckle correlation (DISC). *Opt. Eng.* **2001**, *40*, 1613. [CrossRef]
48. Carter, J.L.W.; Uchic, M.D.; Mills, M.J. Impact of Speckle Pattern Parameters on DIC Strain Resolution Calculated from In-situ SEM Experiments. *Fract. Fatigue Fail. Damage Evol.* **2015**, *5*, 119–126.
49. Lecompte, D.; Sol, H.; Vantomme, J.; Habraken, A. Analysis of speckle patterns for deformation measurements by digital image correlation. *Proc. SPIE* **2006**, *6341*. [CrossRef]
50. Shih, F.Y. *Image Processing and Mathematical Morphology*; CRC Press: New York, NY, USA, 2009.
51. Wang, Y.; Lava, P.; Reu, P.; Debruyne, D. Theoretical analysis on the measurement errors of local 2D DIC: Part II assessment of strain errors of the local smoothing method-Approaching an answer to the overlap question. *Strain* **2016**, *52*, 129–147. [CrossRef]
52. Eriksen, R.; Berggreen, C.; Boyd, S.W.; Dulieu-Barton, J.M. Towards high velocity deformation characterisation of metals and composites using Digital Image Correlation. *EPJ Web Conf.* **2010**, *6*, 31013. [CrossRef]
53. Schreier, H.W.; Sutton, M.A. Systematic errors in Digital Image Correlation due to unermatched subset shape functions. *Exp. Mech.* **2002**, *42*, 303–310. [CrossRef]
54. Pan, B.; Asundi, A.; Xie, H.; Gao, J. Digital image correlation using iterative least squares and pointwise least squares for displacement field and strain field measurements. *Opt. Lasers Eng.* **2009**, *47*, 865–874. [CrossRef]
55. Gu, X.; Pierron, F. Towards the design of a new standard for composite stiffness identification. *Compos. Part A Appl. Sci. Manuf.* **2016**, *91*, 448–460. [CrossRef]
56. Rossi, M.; Lava, P.; Pierron, F.; Debruyne, D.; Sasso, M. Effect of DIC Spatial Resolution, Noise and Interpolation Error on Identification Results with the VFM. *Strain* **2015**, *51*, 206–222. [CrossRef]

57. Lava, P.; Cooreman, S.; Coppieters, S.; De Strycker, M.; Debruyne, D. Assessment of measuring errors in DIC using deformation fields generated by plastic FEA. *Opt. Lasers Eng.* **2009**, *47*, 747–753. [CrossRef]
58. Joo, S.-H.; Lee, J.K.; Koo, J.-M.; Lee, S.; Suh, D.-W.; Kim, H.S. Method for measuring nanoscale local strain in a dual phase steel using digital image correlation with nanodot patterns. *Scr. Mater.* **2013**, *68*, 245–248. [CrossRef]
59. Kang, J.; Ososkov, Y.; Embury, J.; Wilkinson, D. Digital image correlation studies for microscopic strain distribution and damage in dual phase steels. *Scr. Mater.* **2007**, *56*, 999–1002. [CrossRef]
60. Ravindran, S.; Koohbor, B.; Kidane, A. On the Meso-Macro Scale Deformation of Low Carbon Steel. In *Advancement of Optical Methods in Experimental Mechanics*; Jin, H., Ed.; The Society for Experimental Mechanics: Bethel, CT, USA, 2015; pp. 409–414.
61. Pan, B. Bias error reduction of digital image correlation using Gaussian pre-filtering. *Opt. Lasers Eng.* **2013**, *51*, 1161–1167. [CrossRef]
62. Fayolle, X.; Calloch, S.; Hild, F. Controlling testing machines with digital image correlation. *Exp. Tech.* **2007**, *31*, 57–63. [CrossRef]
63. Koohbor, B.; Ravindran, S.; Kidane, A. Experimental determination of Representative Volume Element (RVE) size in woven composites. *Opt. Lasers Eng.* **2017**, *90*, 59–71. [CrossRef]
64. Leprince, S.; Barbot, S.; Ayoub, F.; Avouac, J.-P. Automatic and Precise Orthorectification, Coregistration, and Subpixel Correlation of Satellite Images, Application to Ground Deformation Measurements. *IEEE Trans. Geosci. Remote Sens.* **2007**, *45*, 1529–1558. [CrossRef]
65. Gu, J.; Cooreman, S.; Smits, A.; Bossuyt, S.; Sol, H.; Lecompte, D.; Vantomme, J. Full-field optical measurement for material parameter identification with inverse methods. *WIT Trans. Built Environ.* **2006**, *85*. [CrossRef]
66. Pan, B.; Xie, H.; Wang, Z.; Qian, K.; Wang, Z. Study on subset size selection in digital image correlation for speckle patterns. *Top. Appl. Phys. Opt. Express* **2008**, *16*, 7037–7048. [CrossRef]
67. Yaofeng, S.; Pang, J.H.L. Study of optimal subset size in digital image correlation of speckle pattern images. *Opt. Lasers Eng.* **2007**, *45*, 967–974. [CrossRef]
68. Carriero, A.; Abela, L.; Pitsillides, A.A.; Shefelbine, S.J. Ex vivo determination of bone tissue strains for an in vivo mouse tibial loading model. *J. Biomech.* **2014**, *47*, 2490–2497. [CrossRef] [PubMed]
69. Zhu, F.; Bai, P.; Zhang, J.; Lei, D.; He, X. Measurement of true stress–strain curves and evolution of plastic zone of low carbon steel under uniaxial tension using digital image correlation. *Opt. Lasers Eng.* **2015**, *65*, 81–88. [CrossRef]
70. Li, G.; Mubashar Hassan, G.; Dyskin, A.; MacNish, C. Study of Natural Patterns on Digital Image Correlation Using Simulation Method. *Int. J. Comput. Electr. Autom. Control Inf. Eng.* **2015**, *9*, 414–421.
71. Wang, Y.Q.; Sutton, M.A.; Bruck, H.A.; Schreier, H.W. Quantitative Error Assessment in Pattern Matching: Effects of Intensity Pattern Noise, Interpolation, Strain and Image Contrast on Motion Measurements. *Strain* **2009**, *45*, 160–178. [CrossRef]
72. Wittevrongel, L.; Badaloni, M.; Balcaen, R.; Lava, P.; Debruyne, D. Evaluation of Methodologies for Compensation of Out of Plane Motions in a 2D Digital Image Correlation Setup. *Strain* **2015**, *51*, 357–369. [CrossRef]
73. Haddadi, H.; Belhabib, S. Use of rigid-body motion for the investigation and estimation of the measurement errors related to digital image correlation technique. *Opt. Lasers Eng.* **2008**, *46*, 185–196. [CrossRef]
74. Barranger, Y.; Doumalin, P.; Dupré, J.C.; Germaneau, A. Digital Image Correlation accuracy: Influence of kind of speckle and recording setup. *EPJ Web Conf.* **2010**, *6*, 31002. [CrossRef]
75. Crammond, G.; Boyd, S.W.; Dulieu-Barton, J.M. Speckle pattern quality assessment for digital image correlation. *Opt. Lasers Eng.* **2013**, *51*, 1368–1378. [CrossRef]
76. Jiang, Z.; Kemao, Q.; Miao, H.; Yang, J.; Tang, L. Path-independent digital image correlation with high accuracy, speed and robustness. *Opt. Lasers Eng.* **2015**, *65*, 93–102. [CrossRef]
77. Tong, W. An Evaluation of Digital Image Correlation Criteria for Strain Mapping Applications. *Strain* **2005**, *41*, 167–175. [CrossRef]

5

The Mechanical Properties and In Vitro Biocompatibility of PM-Fabricated Ti-28Nb-35.4Zr Alloy for Orthopedic Implant Applications

Wei Xu [1,†], Ming Li [1,†], Cuie Wen [2], Shaomin Lv [1], Chengcheng Liu [1], Xin Lu [1,3,4,*] and Xuanhui Qu [1,3,4,*]

1 Institute for Advanced Materials and Technology, University of Science and Technology Beijing, Beijing 100083, China; xuweicool@126.com (W.X.); g20159107@xs.ustb.edu.cn (M.L.); lsmleon@163.com (S.L.); liucc1988@163.com (C.L.)
2 School of Engineering, RMIT University, 3083 Melbourne, Australia; cuie.wen@rmit.edu.au
3 Beijing Key Laboratory for Advanced Powder Metallurgy and Particulate Materials, University of Science and Technology Beijing, Beijing 100083, China
4 Beijing Laboratory of Metallic Materials and Processing for Modern Transportation, University of Science and Technology Beijing, Beijing 100083, China
* Correspondence: luxin@ustb.edu.cn (X.L.); quxh@ustb.edu.cn (X.Q.)
† These authors contributed equally to this work.

Abstract: A biocompatible Ti-28Nb-35.4Zr alloy used as bone implant was fabricated through the powder metallurgy process. The effects of mechanical milling and sintering temperatures on the microstructure and mechanical properties were investigated systematically, before in vitro biocompatibility of full dense Ti-28Nb-35.4Zr alloy was evaluated by cytotoxicity tests. The results show that the mechanical milling and sintering temperatures have significantly effects on the density and mechanical properties of the alloys. The relative density of the alloy fabricated by the atomized powders at 1500 °C is only 83 $\pm$ 1.8%, while the relative density of the alloy fabricated by the ball-milled powders can rapidly reach at 96.4 $\pm$ 1.3% at 1500 °C. When the temperature was increased to 1550 °C, the alloy fabricated by ball-milled powders achieve full density (relative density is 98.1 $\pm$ 1.2%). The PM-fabricated Ti-28Nb-35.4Zr alloy by ball-milled powders at 1550 °C can achieve a wide range of mechanical properties, with a compressive yield strength of 1058 $\pm$ 35.1 MPa, elastic modulus of 50.8 $\pm$ 3.9 GPa, and hardness of 65.8 $\pm$ 1.5 HRA. The in vitro cytotoxicity test suggests that the PM-fabricated Ti-28Nb-35.4Zr alloy by ball-milled powders at 1550 °C has no adverse effects on MC3T3-E1 cells with cytotoxicity ranking of 0 grade, which is nearly close to ELI Ti-6Al-4V or CP Ti. These properties and the net-shape manufacturability makes PM-fabricated Ti-28Nb-35.4Zr alloy a low-cost, highly-biocompatible, Ti-based biomedical alloy.

Keywords: Ti-28Nb-35.4 alloy; powder metallurgy; ball milling; mechanical properties; biocompatibility

---

1. Introduction

Metallic biomaterials, which are the materials of choice for orthopedic implants, are fundamental for improve the quality of life and longevity of human beings [1,2]. Many different metallic materials have been used in a variety of applications in the medical field. Specifically, they are used for internal support and biological tissue replacements such as joint replacement, dental roots, orthopedic fixation and stents [3]. The common metals and alloys that are being utilized for biomedical applications include: stainless steels, Co-based alloys, and Ti-based alloys. Ti-based alloys have dominated in the human hard tissue repair and dentistry fields due to high strength, low elastic modulus, and excellent in vivo corrosion and biocompatibility [4]. However, despite their attractive performance, there are still challenges facing their application in artificial joints [5]. These concerns are mainly related to bio-toxicity, the need for lower elastic modulus and better mechanical strength. For instance, Al elements in extra-low interstitial (ELI) Ti-6Al-4V (hereafter all compositions are given in wt %), Ti-5Al-2.5Fe and Ti-6Al-7Nb [6–8], which is the most widely applied Ti alloy, are considered to be related to some health-related problems, including Alzheimer disease and neuropathy [9,10]. In addition, the elastic modulus (~110 GPa) of these alloys is still considerably higher than those of the cortical bones (~30 GPa), which results in severe 'stress shielding' for implantation failures [11,12]. Hence, considerable amount of effort has been exeerted to develop Al- and V-free lower-modulus β-Ti alloys.

Notable examples include the United States Food and Drug Administration (FDA)-approved proprietary alloys of Ti-13Nb-13Zr and Ti-12Mo-6Zr-2Fe and the non-proprietary alloy of Ti-15Mo. In particular, Ti-Nb-Zr alloys have received significant attention due to their excellent mechanical compatibility and biocompatibility [13–16]. The addition of Nb to Ti can stabilize the β phase and results in improved mechanical properties, which also results in improved wear resistance and corrosion resistance [17,18]. Furthermore, the addition of Zr helps in obtaining the solid solution required for achieving the hardness [19,20]. In addition, as reported by references [21,22], the elastic modulus in Ti-Nb and Ti-Zr alloys decreases with an increase in the content of the Nb and Zr within certain limits. Based on these results, Wen et al. [23] designed the new Ti-Nb-Zr alloys using the d-electron design method combined with the molybdenum equivalence (Mo_{eq}) and electron-to-atom ratio (e/a) approaches. The results show that the alloys have an excellent combination of mechanical properties and biocompatibility. However, at present these alloys are manufactured by the conventional route (i.e., ingot metallurgy in addition to wrought processing and machining with up to 90% being scrapped), which leads to a high manufacturing cost. Hence, in order to reduce costs and enhance the utilization rate of materials, the powder metallurgy (PM) technique is introduced. PM is an advanced net-shape technique which particularly suits to large volume production and can reduce processing steps, hence reducing cost [24–27]. It has already been used to synthesize Ti-based alloys by many researchers. For example, Sharma et al. [28] used a powder metallurgy route consisting of mechanical alloys (MA) of the TiH_2-Nb powder mixture and spark plasma sintering (SPS) to produce Ti-40 mass% Nb alloys. Jia et al. [29] successfully obtained the Ti-22Al-25Nb alloy by PM. Mendes et al. [30] produced the alloy Ti-27Nb-13Zr with low Young's modulus by PM using powders produced by the hydride-dehydride (HDH) process.

In this study, the Ti-28Nb-35.4Zr alloy is fabricated by PM in order to obtain Ti-based alloy with excellent mechanical compatibility and biocompatibility in addition to further reducing the manufacturing cost. The effects of sintering temperatures and mechanical milling on density, microstructure and mechanical properties are investigated systematically, before the in vitro biocompatibility of the full dense Ti-28Nb-35.4Zr is evaluated preliminarily. We aimed to establish a necessary understanding of the low-cost PM-fabricated Ti-28Nb-35.4Zr alloy for orthopedic implant applications.

2. Experimental and Methods

2.1. Materials and Sample Preparation

Atomized Ti-28Nb-35.4Zr powders (purity $\geq$ 99.9%, 75 $\leq$ particle size $\leq$ 150 μm) was supplied by the Wen group (RMIT University, Melbourne, Australia), who fabricated the powders using continuous inert gas atomization without the crucible method. The atomized Ti-28Nb-35.4Zr powders were subjected to ball milling for 30 min using a three-dimensional vibration ball milling machine (HSVM, Nanjing Chishun Science and Technology Co., Ltd., Nanjing, China). The frequency of the vibration ball milling machine was 1400 r/min, while the ball-to-powder weight ratio was 3:1.

The materials of the balls and jars were stainless steel and GCr15 bearing steel, respectively. The milling process was carried out in a high-purity argon atmosphere, with 2 wt % stearate used as the process control agent (PCA). Atomized powder (AP) and ball-milled powder (BMP) were cold-pressed into cylindrical compacts under 450 MPa. Then isothermal sintering was carried out in the argon (Ar) protection environment and implemented in two steps. Specimens were initially heated to 1000 °C for 2 h at 5 °C/min, before being heated at 2 °C/min to six different temperatures between 1200 °C and 1550 °C for 2 h. This was followed by furnace cooling to room temperature to obtain samples.

2.2. Materials Characterization

The density was measured by the Archimedes method and the relative density was calculated by the following formula:

$$\text{Relative density} = \text{the density}/\text{the theoretical density} \tag{1}$$

where the theoretical density is 6.36 g/cm^3. The hardness was carried out using the HDI-1875 Rockwell hardness tester. Five points were measured, before the average value was calculated. X-ray diffraction (XRD) was performed using a Dmax-RB X-ray diffractometer (Cu Kα, λ = 0.15406 nm, Rigaku, Tokyo, Japan). A JSM-6510V (JEOL, Tokyo, Japan) scanning electron microscope (SEM) was used to analyze the powder morphology of the received atomized powders and ball-milled powders and sintered microstructure. Compression specimens with a gauge size (φ) of 3 mm × 5 mm were fabricated by electric discharge machining and the specimen surface was polished with SiC papers. The compression test was performed on an Instron machine (Instron, Boston, MA, USA) at the strain rate of 2×10^{-3} s^{-1} at room temperature. The compressive yield strength and elastic modulus were calculated from the engineering stress strain curves.

2.3. In Vitro Biocompatibility Testing

Cytotoxicity tests were carried out with murine osteoblast cells (MC3T3-E1) to examine the in vitro biocompatibility of the Ti-28Nb-35.4Zr alloy. For comparison, the cast ELI Ti-6Al-4V and CP-Ti were studied simultaneously. The cells were cultured in Dulbecco's modified Eagle's medium (DMEM, Shanghai solarbio Bioscience and Technology Co., Ltd., Shanghai, China) containing 10% fetal bovine serum (FBS), 100 U/mL penicillin, and 100 μg/mL streptomycin at 37 °C under a humidified atmosphere of air containing 5% CO_2. The metal samples were cut into discs of 10 mm in diameter and 1 mm in thickness via electric discharge machining, before the surface was polished with SiC papers (grit 400 down to 5000). After this, the samples were cleaned ultrasonically and sterilized for further use.

In the cytotoxicity test, the extracts were obtained based on the international standard ISO 10993-5 [31]. The cells were incubated by an extraction medium in 96-well plates at the density of 5000 cells per 100 μL. At the desired times (day 1, day 2 and day 3), cells were observed by the optical microscope (LEXT OLS4000, Olympus, Tokyo, Japan), while the 10 μL MTT solution (Shanghai solarbio Bioscience and Technology Co., Ltd., Shanghai, China) was added to each well and were incubated for 4 h. After this, 100 μL of dimethyl sulfoxide (DMSO, Shanghai solarbio Bioscience and Technology Co., Ltd., Shanghai, China) was added to each well, before being incubated for a further 5 min. The absorbance was recorded by a multimode detector on a Synergy HT (BioTek, Winooski, VT, USA) at a wavelength of 570 nm. The cell viability ratio (CVR) was calculated by the formula as follows:

$$CVR = (OD_{570nm} \text{ in experimental extract}/OD_{570nm} \text{ in control extract}) \times 100\% \tag{2}$$

Based on the international standard ISO 10993-5 [31], the cytotoxic level was divided into six groups: 0: ≥100%; I: 75–99%; II: 50–74%; III: 25–49%; IV: 1–24%; V: ≤1%. Cell viability ratio were analyzed using one-way analysis of variance (ANOVA, $P < 0.05$) followed by the Tukey honestly significant difference (HSD) post-hoc test. $P < 0.05$ was considered to be statistically significant.

3. Results and Discussion

3.1. Raw Powder Characterization

Figure 1 depicts the representative SEM micrographs of atomized and ball-milled powders. It can be seen that the atomized powders (Figure 1a) have a typical spherical shape. The particle size of the powders varies from 30.2 to 160.5 μm with an average particles size of approximately 80.5 μm. The morphology of the Ti-Nb-Zr particles after 30 min of ball milling is shown in Figure 1b. The particle size of the ball-milled powders varies from 5.1 to 30.5 μm with an average particle size of approximately 15.2 μm. The shape of the powders becomes irregular, which makes further powder treatment easier (green compaction) as irregular powder particles have higher compressibility and green strength [32].

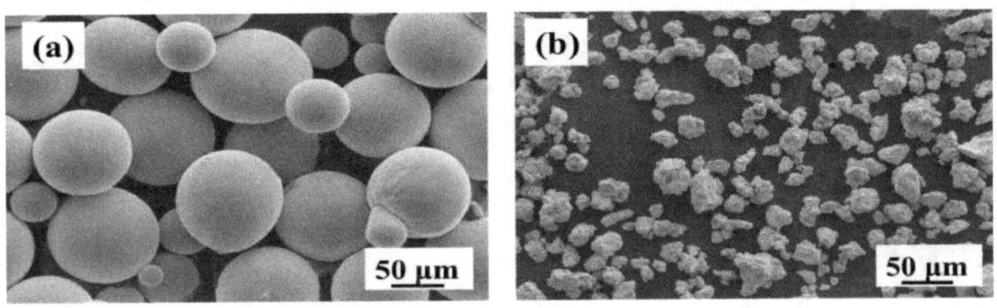

Figure 1. SEM images (800×) of the powders: (**a**) Atomized powders; and (**b**) Ball-milled powders.

Figure 2 shows the XRD patterns of atomized and ball-milled powders. It can be seen that atomized powders consist of a single β-Ti, while the ball-milled powders consist of β-Ti and TiO_2. TiO_2 mainly emerges because there is some oxygen introduced during the process of ball milling. In addition, compared with the atomized powders, the diffraction spectrums of the ball-milled powders shows an obvious broadening and moves to low angle, which is associated with the reduction in grain size, increase in lattice distortion and instrumental effects [33].

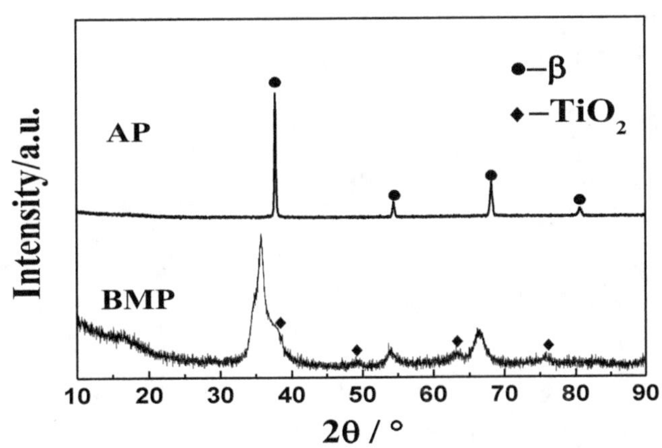

Figure 2. XRD patterns of atomized and ball-milled powders.

3.2. As-Sintered Density

Figure 3 shows the variation in relative density of samples with respect to sintering temperatures and powders. The relative density strongly depends on both sintering temperatures and powders. For the atomized powder, with an increase in the sintering temperature the relative density of the alloys increases gradually, but it is difficult to achieve a high relative density. The relative density of the alloy sintered at 1500 °C is only 83.1 ± 1.8%. Compared to the samples fabricated by atomized powder, the relative density of the samples fabricated by milled powder at 1500 °C rapidly increases to 96.4 ± 1.3%. When the sintering temperature increases to 1550 °C, the relative density of the alloy reaches 98.1 ± 1.2%.

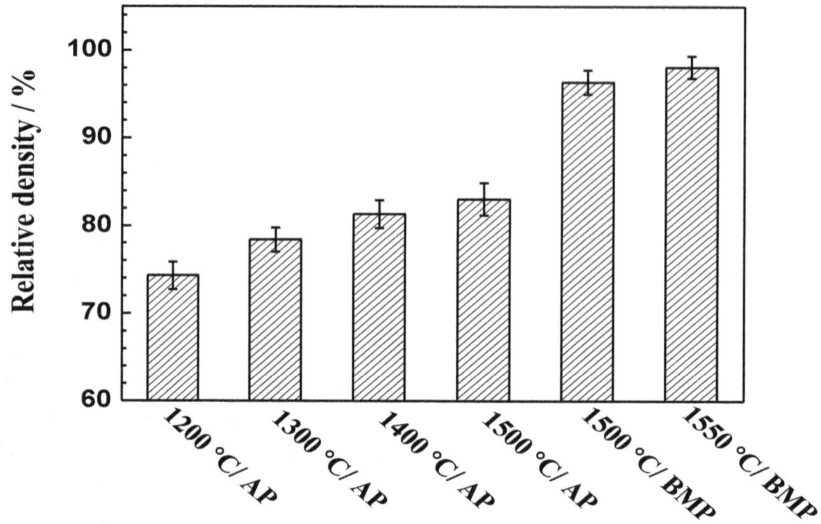

Figure 3. Relative density of Ti-28Nb-35.4Zr alloy prepared with different sintering temperatures and powders.

Figure 4 shows the optional images of Ti-28Nb-35.4Zr prepared with different sintering temperatures and powders. As shown in Figure 4a–d, the porosity of the samples fabricated by atomized powders decreases gradually with an increase in the sintering temperature. However, there are many pores on the surface of the samples even when they are sintered at 1500 °C. As shown by Figure 4e,f, the porosity of alloy prepared by milled powder reduces significantly, while the alloy becomes close to full density when sintered at 1550 °C. This is mainly associated with the sintering process of powder particles. After milling, the average particle sizes of the powders become smaller and hence, the powders have a high interface energy, which makes the sintering neck form more easily. Therefore, compared with the samples fabricated by atomized powder, the alloys prepared by milled powders have a higher density and therefore higher relative density.

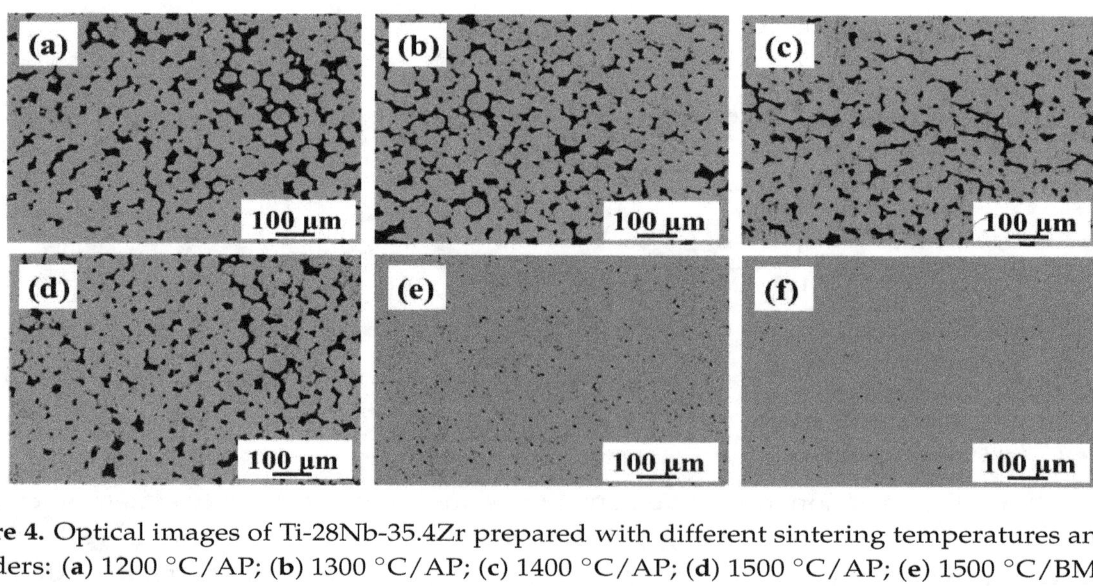

Figure 4. Optical images of Ti-28Nb-35.4Zr prepared with different sintering temperatures and raw powders: (**a**) 1200 °C/AP; (**b**) 1300 °C/AP; (**c**) 1400 °C/AP; (**d**) 1500 °C/AP; (**e**) 1500 °C/BMP and (**f**) 1550 °C/BMP.

3.3. As-Sintered Microstructure

Figure 5 shows the XRD patterns of Ti-28Nb-35.4Zr alloy fabricated by different powders at different sintering temperature. It can be seen that there is no significant difference of XRD patterns of Ti-28Nb-35.4Zr alloy fabricated by different powders and sintering temperatures. The clear diffraction peaks suggest that the samples all have similar phase compositions and mainly consist of single β phases.

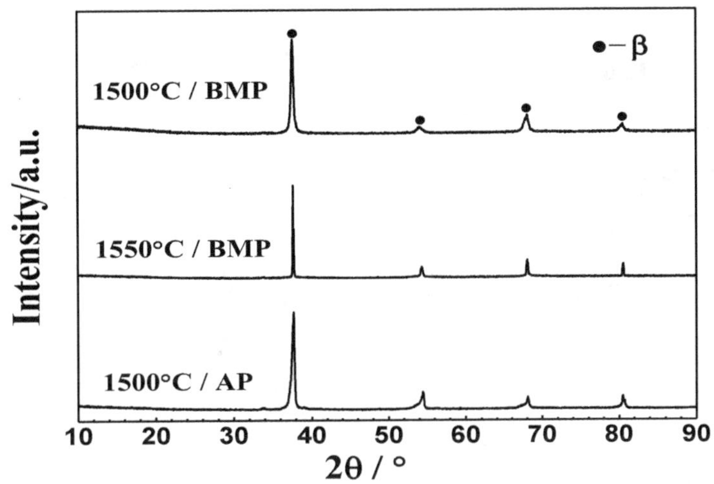

Figure 5. XRD patterns of Ti-28Nb-35.4Zr alloy prepared with different temperatures and powders.

Figure 6 displays the SEM micrographs of Ti-28Nb-35.4Zr alloy samples sintered at different temperatures with different powders, which was taken under 800× magnification. It can be seen that some pores exist in the alloy fabricated by the atomized powder at 1500 °C and the original powder particle boundaries can be observed clearly. However, the alloy prepared by milled powder at 1500 °C has a few pores, while the alloy becomes nearly fully dense with no obvious pores when the sintering temperature increases to 1550 °C. In addition, as shown in Figure 6b,c, the samples fabricated by the milled powder show a similar microstructure, which is consistent with the XRD results. Both samples consist of a single β phase and the average grain size is about 100 ± 10 μm.

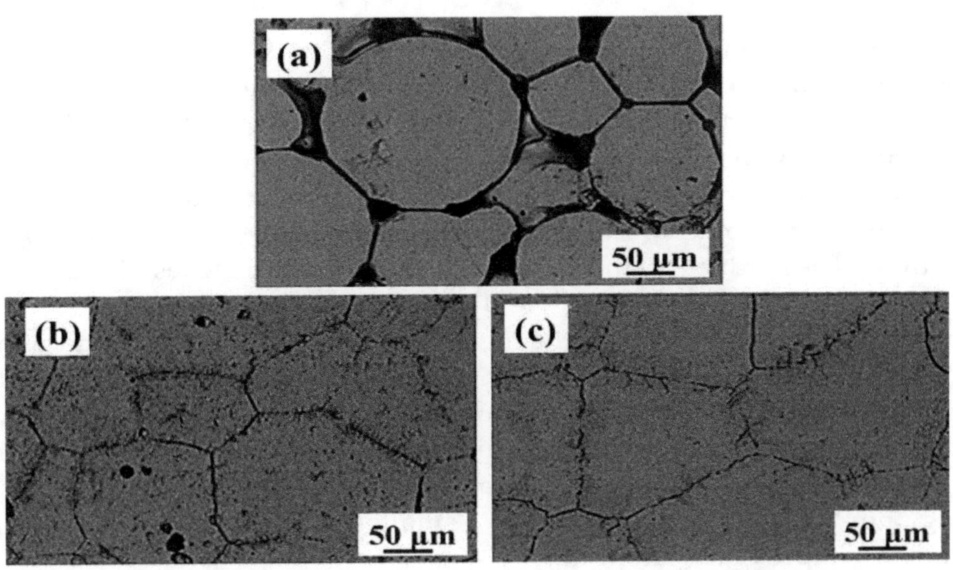

Figure 6. SEM images (800×) of Ti-28Nb-35.4Zr alloy prepared with different sintering temperatures and powders: (**a**) 1500 °C/AP; (**b**) 1500 °C/BMP and (**c**) 1550 °C/BMP.

3.4. Room-Temperature Mechanical Properties

Figure 7 shows compressive engineering stress-strain curves of the Ti-28Nb-35.4Zr alloy fabricated by different powders at different sintering temperatures. As shown in Figure 7, the alloys exhibit similar stress–strain behavior and no fracture was observed during their compression process, demonstrating that the alloys exhibit considerable elastic–plastic deformation ability. Compression tests were stopped after reaching a strain value of about 50%.

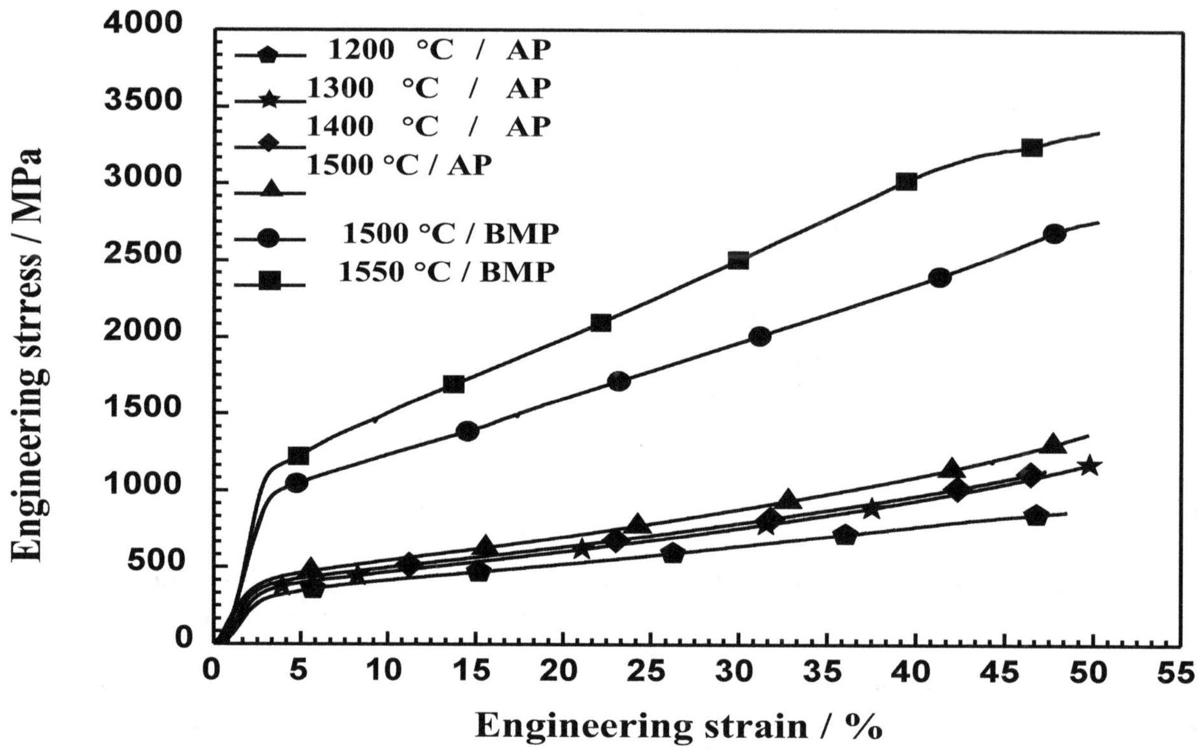

Figure 7. Compressive stress–strain curves of Ti-28Nb-35.4Zr alloy prepared with different sintering temperatures and powders.

The compressive yield strength, elastic modulus and hardness of Ti-28Nb-35.4Zr alloy fabricated by different powders at different sintering temperatures are shown in Figure 8. The hardness, compressive yield strength and elastic modulus of the Ti-28Nb-35.4Zr alloy fabricated atomized powder generally increase with an increase in the sintering temperature, which were in the range of 27.3–39.2 HRA, 273–332 MPa and 15.6–24.0 GPa, respectively. Compared with the alloy fabricated by the atomized powder, the mechanical properties of the alloy prepared by milled powder are significantly improved. The hardness of the alloy sintered at 1550 °C reaches 65.8 $\pm$ 1.5 HRA (Figure 8a) while the elastic modulus and compressive yield strength is 50.8 $\pm$ 3.9 GPa and 1058 $\pm$ 35.1 MPa (Figure 8b), respectively. This is superior to the mechanical properties fabricated by the cold-crucible levitation melting (compressive yield strength of 730 MPa [23]). The improvement in the compressive yield strength of the BMP sintered samples stems from two reasons. The first reason is that there is some oxygen introduced during the process of ball milling, which can also can be seen from the powders XRD results for the powders. In addition, compared with the samples fabricated by cold-crucible levitation melting, the PM-fabricated samples have smaller grains, uniform microstructure and less defects, which can also improve the strength.

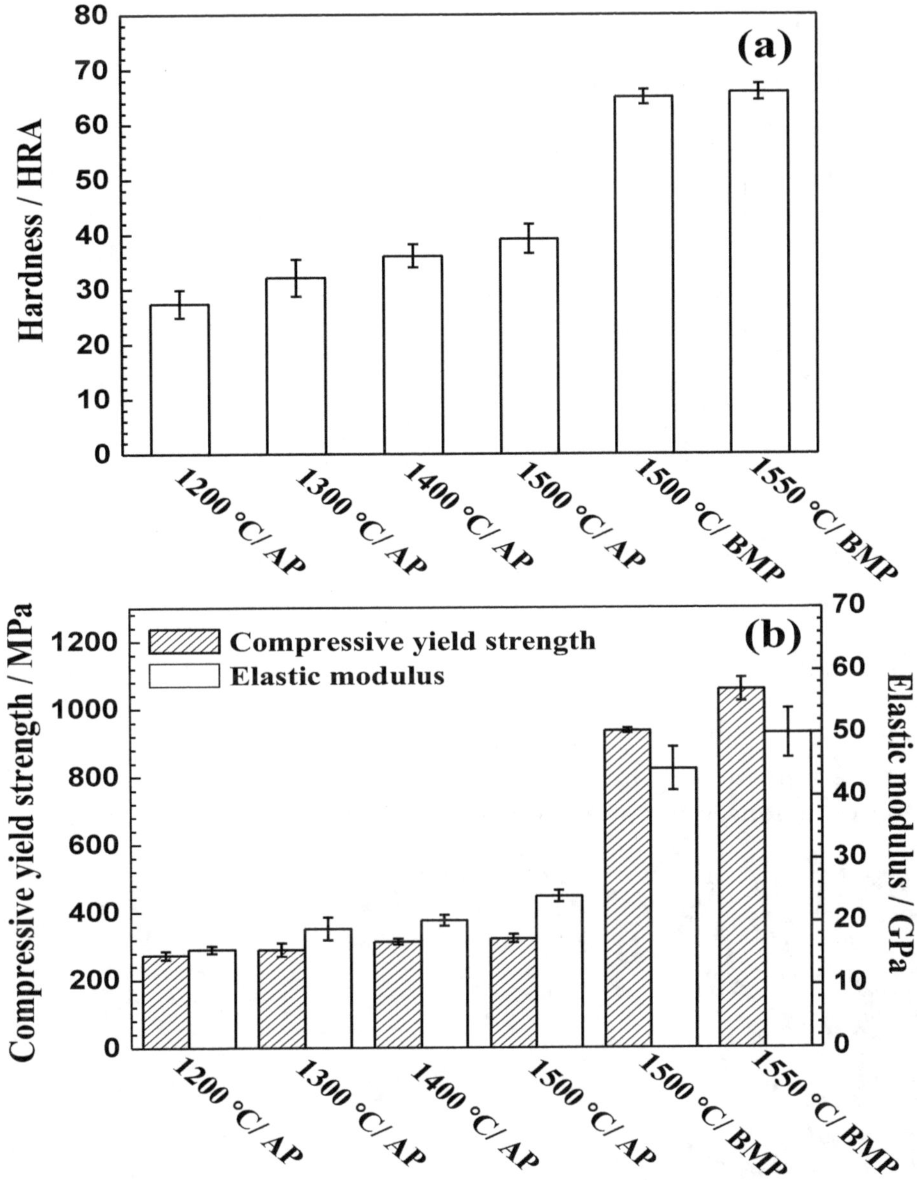

Figure 8. Mechanical properties of Ti-28Nb-34.5Zr alloy prepared with different sintering temperatures and powders: (**a**) Hardness; (**b**) Compressive elastic modulus and yield strength.

3.5. In Vitro Biocompatibility

In vitro biocompatibility of the Ti-28Nb-35.4Zr alloy sintered at 1550 °C by the milled powder was evaluated by cell tests. The CVR was calculated by Equation (2). The control group has a CVR of 100%, which is accepted as a reference for determining the cell viability radio of samples [34]. Figure 9 shows the results of CVR using MC3T3-E1 cells grown in Ti-28Nb-35.4Zr alloy, ELI Ti-6Al-4V and CP-Ti extracts for 1, 2 and 3 days. It can be seen that the average CVR value of all the experimental alloys was above 99%. The Ti-28Nb-35.4Zr alloy exhibits a slightly higher average CVR value than ELI Ti-6Al-4V while was similar to CP Ti. However there were no statistically significant differences among them ($P > 0.05$). According to ISO 10993-5 [31], the cytotoxicity grade of Ti-28Nb-35.4Zr alloy and CP Ti is 0–I grade while that of ELI Ti-6Al-4V is 0–I grade. Consequently, the PM-fabricated Ti-28Nb-35.4Zr alloy shows good in vitro biocompatibility to MC3T3-E1 cells.

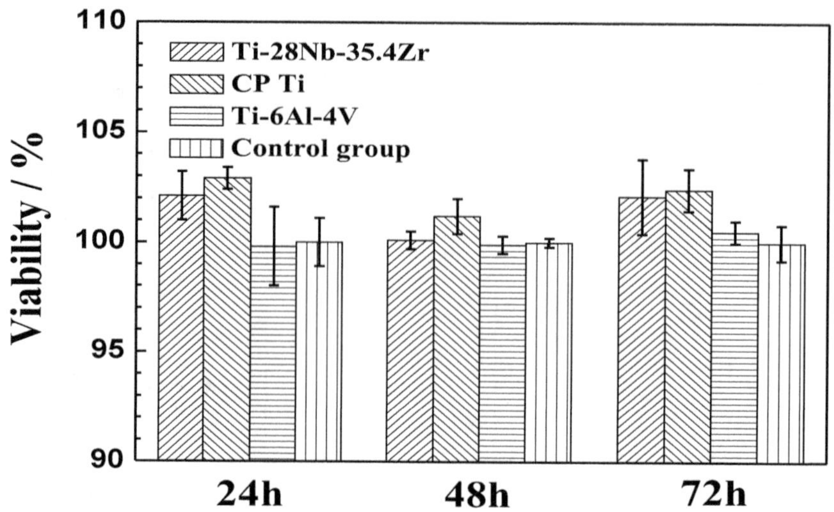

Figure 9. MTT result of MC3T3-E1 cells cultured with extracts of Ti-28Nb-35.4Zr, CP Ti and ELI Ti-6Al-4V.

Figure 10 displays the number and morphology of MC3T3-E1 cells cultured with extracts of Ti-28Nb-35.4Zr ELI Ti-6Al-4V and CP-Ti for different periods (1 day, 2 days and 3 days). It can be seen that the morphologies of all cells are similar for different periods. After a 1-day culture, cells are basically adhered to the well and the shape is spindle. With a prolonged culture time, cells cultured by different Ti alloys become denser and stretched, although there are no significantly changes in MTT.

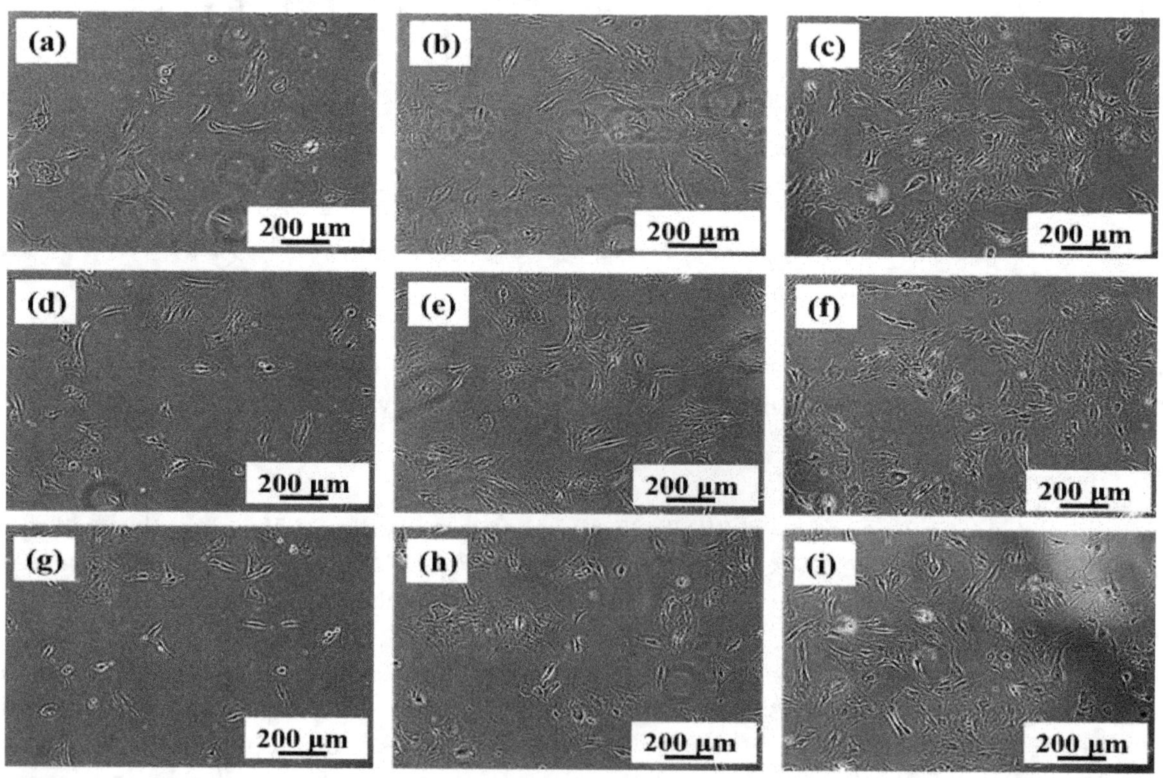

Figure 10. The number and morphology of MC3T3-E1 cells cultured with extracts of Ti-28Nb-35.4Zr ((**a**): 24 h; (**b**): 48 h; (**c**): 72 h), CP Ti ((**d**): 24 h; (**e**): 48 h; (**f**): 72 h) and ELI Ti-6Al-4V ((**g**): 24 h; (**h**): 48 h; (**i**): 72 h).

The in vitro biocompatibility of an implant lies not only in the toxicity of its alloys elements, but also in its corrosion resistance. Ti-Nb-Zr alloys are formed by the solid solutions of pure Ti, Nb and Zr, and maintain a high corrosion resistance and low toxicity [35]. Further, the corrosion resistance of Ti-Nb-Zr alloys is superior to that of CP Ti and ELI Ti-6Al-4V [36]. Spontaneously formed oxides, made up of TiO_2, Nb_2O_3 and Zr_2O_3, will provide a bio-inert layer in aggressive body fluids [37]. The enrichment of TiO_2, Nb_2O_3 and Zr_2O_3 on the surface suppressed the dissolution of Ti, Zr and Nb as ions. Hence, the Ti-28Nb-35.4Zr alloys show high cell viability during the MTT assays. Coupled with the low elastic modulus, high compressive yield strength and net-shape manufacturability, it thus suggests that PM-fabricated Ti-28Nb-35.4Zr alloy may hold promise for the development of next class of low-cost, highly-biocompatible, Ti-based biomedical alloys.

4. Conclusions

(1) Ti-28Nb-35.4Zr alloy with a high relative density and uniform microstructure can be obtained from milled powder via PM. After milling, the average particle sizes of powders was 15.2 μm, and when sintered at 1550 °C, the relative density reaches 98.1 ± 1.2%. The alloy fabricated by milled powders at 1550 °C is characterized by the single β phase.

(2) The alloys fabricated by the ball-milled powder at 1550 °C can achieve a high mechanical properties with the compressive yield strength of 1058 ± 35.1 MPa, the elastic modulus of 50.8 ± 3.9 GP, and the hardness of 65.8 ± 1.5 HRA. This is superior to the mechanical properties fabricated by the cold-crucible levitation melting technique.

(3) From in vitro cytotoxicity tests, the Ti-28Nb-35.4Zr alloy fabricated by milled powder at 1550 °C has no adverse effects on cell proliferation, and the cytotoxicity level is ranked as 0 grade, which is similar to the existing biomedical materials of CP Ti or ELI Ti-6Al-4V.

(4) Based on its demonstrated net-shape manufacturability by PM, high compressive yield strength, low elastic modulus and excellent in vitro biocompatibility, the PM-fabricated Ti-28Nb-35.4Zr can be considered as an attractive orthopedic implant alloy.

Acknowledgments: This research work is supported by Fundamental Research Funds for the Central Universities (FRF-GF-17-B39).

Author Contributions: Wei Xu, Ming Li and Xin Lu conceived and designed the experiments; Wei Xu and Ming Li performed the experiments; Wei Xu and Ming Li analyzed the data and wrote the paper; Chengcheng Liu, Shaomin Lv, Cuie Wen, Xin Lu and Xuanhui Qu revised the manuscript; all authors discussed and approved the final manuscript.

References

1. Okulov, I.V.; Volegov, A.S.; Attar, H.; Bönisch, M.; Ehtemam-Haghighi, S.; Calin, M.; Eckert, J. Composition optimization of low modulus and high-strength TiNb-based alloys for biomedical applications. *J. Mech. Behav. Biomed.* **2016**, *65*, 866–871. [CrossRef] [PubMed]
2. Attar, H.; Bönisch, M.; Calin, M.; Zhang, L.C.; Scudino, S.; Eckert, J. Selective laser melting of in situ titanium-titanium boride composites: Processing, microstructure and mechanical properties. *Acta Mater.* **2014**, *76*, 13–22. [CrossRef]
3. Dai, N.W.; Zhang, J.X.; Chen, C.; Zhang, L.C. Heat treatment degrading the corrosion resistance of selective laser melted Ti-6Al-4V alloy. *J. Electrochem. Soc.* **2017**, *164*, C428–C434. [CrossRef]
4. Biesiekierski, A.; Lin, J.; Li, Y.; Ping, D.H.; Yamabe-Mitarai, Y.; Wen, C.E. Investigations into Ti-(Nb,Ta)-Fe alloys for biomedical applications. *Acta Biomater.* **2016**, *32*, 336–347. [CrossRef] [PubMed]
5. Ehtemam-Haghighi, S.; Prashanth, K.G.; Attar, H.; Chaubey, A.K.; Cao, G.H.; Zhang, L.C. Evaluation of mechanical and wear properties of Ti-xNb-7Fe alloys designed for biomedical applications. *Mater. Des.* **2016**, *111*, 592–599. [CrossRef]
6. Lu, S.L.; Qian, M.; Tang, H.P.; Yan, M.; Wang, J.; StJohn, D.H. Massive transformation in Ti-6Al-4V additively manufactured by selective electron beam melting. *Acta Mater.* **2016**, *104*, 303–311. [CrossRef]

7. Siqueira, R.P.; Sandim, H.R.Z.; Hayama, A.O.F.; Henriques, V.A.R. Microstructural evolution during sintering of the blended elemental Ti-5Al-2.5Fe alloy. *J. Alloys Compd.* **2009**, *476*, 130–137. [CrossRef]
8. Polyakova, V.V.; Semenova, I.P.; Polyakov, A.V.; Magomedova, D.K.; Huang, Y.; Langdon, T.G. Influence of grain boundary misorientations on the mechanical behavior of a near-αTi-6Al-7Nb alloy processed by ECAP. *Mater. Lett.* **2017**, *190*, 256–259. [CrossRef]
9. Flaten, T.P. Aluminium as a risk factor in Alzheimer's disease, with emphasis on drinking water. *Brain Res. Bull.* **2001**, *55*, 187–196. [CrossRef]
10. Lima, P.D.; Vasconcellos, M.C.; Montenegro, R.C.; Bahia, M.O.; Costa, E.T.; Antunes, L.M.; Burbano, R.R. Genotoxic effects of aluminum, iron and manganese in human cells and experimental systems: A review of the literature. *Hum. Exp. Toxicol.* **2011**, *30*, 1435–1444. [CrossRef] [PubMed]
11. Wang, X.J.; Xu, S.Q.; Zhou, S.W.; Xu, W.; Leary, M.; Choong, P.; Qian, M.; Brandt, M.; Xie, Y.M. Topological design and additive manufacturing of porous metals for bone scaffolds and orthopaedic implants: A review. *Biomaterials* **2016**, *83*, 127–141. [CrossRef] [PubMed]
12. Xu, W.; Lu, X.; Zhang, B.; Liu, C.C.; Lv, S.M.; Yang, S.D.; Qu, X.H. Effects of Porosity on Mechanical Properties and Corrosion Resistances of PM-Fabricated Porous Ti-10Mo Alloy. *Metals* **2018**, *8*, 188. [CrossRef]
13. Lee, T.; Park, K.T.; Dong, J.L.; Jeong, J.; Sang, H.O.; Kim, H.S.; Park, C.H.; Lee, C.S. Microstructural evolution and strain-hardening behavior of multi-pass caliber-rolled Ti-13Nb-13Zr. *Mater. Sci. Eng. A* **2015**, *648*, 359–366. [CrossRef]
14. Niinomi, M. Fatigue performance and cyto-toxicity of low rigidity titanium alloy, Ti-29Nb-13Ta-4.6Zr. *Biomaterials* **2003**, *24*, 2673–2683. [CrossRef]
15. Zhang, L.C.; Klemm, D.; Eckert, J.; Hao, Y.L.; Sercombe, T.B. Manufacture by selective laser melting and mechanical behavior of a biomedical Ti-24Nb-4Zr-8Sn alloy. *Scr. Mater.* **2011**, *65*, 21–24. [CrossRef]
16. Niinomi, M.; Nakai, M.; Hieda, J. Development of new metallic alloys for biomedical applications. *Acta Biomater.* **2012**, *8*, 3888–3903. [CrossRef] [PubMed]
17. Zhou, F.Y.; Wang, B.L.; Qiu, K.J.; Lin, W.J.; Li, L.; Wang, Y.B.; Nie, F.L.; Zheng, Y.F. Microstructure, corrosion behavior and cytotoxicity of Zr-Nb alloys for biomedical application. *Mater. Sci. Eng. C* **2012**, *32*, 851–857. [CrossRef]
18. Li, S.J.; Yang, R.; Li, S.; Hao, Y.L.; Cui, Y.Y.; Niinomi, M.; Guo, Z.X. Wear characteristics of Ti-Nb-Ta-Zr and Ti-6Al-4V alloys for biomedical applications. *Wear* **2004**, *257*, 869–876. [CrossRef]
19. Kobayashi, E.; Ando, M.; Tsutsumi, Y.; Doi, H.; Yoneyama, T.; Kobayashi, M.; Hanawa, T. Inhibition effect of zirconium coating on calcium phosphate precipitation of titanium to avoid assimilation with bone. *Mater. Trans.* **2007**, *48*, 301–306. [CrossRef]
20. Hanawa, T.; Okuno, O.; Hamanaka, H. Compositional change in surface of Ti-Zr alloys in artificial bioliquid. *J. Jpn. Inst. Met. Mater.* **1992**, *56*, 1168–1173. [CrossRef]
21. Lee, C.M.; Ju, C.P.; Lin, J.H.C. Structure-property relationship of cast Ti-Nb alloys. *J. Oral Rehabil.* **2002**, *29*, 314–322. [CrossRef] [PubMed]
22. Ho, W.F.; Chen, W.K.; Wu, S.C.; Hsu, H.C. Structure, mechanical properties, and grindability of dental Ti-Zr alloys. *J. Mater. Sci.* **2008**, *19*, 3179–3186. [CrossRef]
23. Ozan, S.; Lin, J.X.; Li, Y.C.; Ipek, R.; Wen, C.E. Development of Ti-Nb-Zr alloys with high elastic admissible strain for temporary orthopedic devices. *Acta Biomater.* **2015**, *20*, 176–187. [CrossRef] [PubMed]
24. Pattanayak, D.K.; Matsushita, T.; Doi, K.; Takadama, H.; Nakamura, T.; Kokubo, T. Effects of oxygen content of porous titanium metal on its apatite-forming ability and compressive strength. *Mater. Sci. Eng. C* **2009**, *29*, 1974–1978. [CrossRef]
25. Niu, W.J.; Bai, C.G.; Qiu, G.B.; Wang, Q. Processing and properties of porous titanium using space holder technique. *Mater. Sci. Eng. C* **2009**, *506*, 148–151. [CrossRef]
26. Liu, Y.; Chen, L.F.; Tang, H.P.; Liu, C.T.; Liu, B.; Huang, B.Y. Design of powder metallurgy titanium alloys and composites. *Mater. Sci. Eng. A* **2006**, *418*, 25–35. [CrossRef]
27. Kipouros, G.J.; Caley, W.F.; Bishop, D.P. On the advantages of using powder metallurgy in new light metal alloy design. *Metall. Mater. Trans. A* **2006**, *37*, 3429–3436. [CrossRef]
28. Sharma, B.; Vaipai, S.K.; Ameyama, K. Microstructure and properties of beta Ti-Nb alloy prepared by powder metallurgy route using titanium hydride powder. *J. Alloys Compd.* **2012**, *656*, 978–986. [CrossRef]
29. Jia, J.; Zhang, K.; Liu, L.; Wu, F.Y. Hot deformation behavior and processing map of a powder metallurgy Ti-22Al-25Nb alloy. *J. Alloys Compd.* **2014**, *600*, 215–221. [CrossRef]

30. Mendes, M.W.D.; Ágreda, C.G.; Bressiani, A.H.; Bressiani, J.C. A new titanium based alloy Ti-27Nb-13Zr produced by powder metallurgy with biomimetic coating for use as a biomaterial. *Mater. Sci. Eng. C* **2016**, *63*, 671–677. [CrossRef] [PubMed]
31. ISO 10993-5. *Biological Evaluation of Medical Devices—Part 5: Tests for Cytotoxicity: In Vitro Methods*; American National Standards Institute: Arlington, VA, USA, 1999.
32. Samal, C.P.; Parihar, J.S.; Chaira, D. The effect of milling and sintering techniques on mechanical properties of Cu-graphite metal matrix composite prepared by powder metallurgy route. *J. Alloys Compd.* **2013**, *569*, 95–110. [CrossRef]
33. Wen, M.; Wen, C.E.; Hodgson, P.; Li, Y.C. Fabrication of Ti-Nb-Ag alloy via powder metallurgy for biomedical applications. *Mater. Des.* **2014**, *56*, 629–634. [CrossRef]
34. Li, Y.; Wen, C.W.; Mushahary, D.; Sravanthi, R.; Harishankar, N.; Pande, G.; Hodgson, P. Mg-Zr-Sr alloys as biodegradable implant materials. *Acta Biomater.* **2012**, *8*, 3177–3188. [CrossRef] [PubMed]
35. Wang, B.L.; Li, L.; Zheng, Y.F. In vitro cytotoxicity and hemocompatibility studies of Ti-Nb, Ti-Nb-Zr and Ti-Nb-Hf biomedical shape memory alloys. *Biomed. Mater.* **2010**, *5*, 044102. [CrossRef] [PubMed]
36. Robin, A.; Carvalho, O.A.S.; Schneider, S.G.; Schneider, S. Corrosion behavior of Ti-xNb-13Zr alloys in Ringer's solution. *Mater. Corros.* **2015**, *59*, 929–933. [CrossRef]
37. Robin, A.; Carvalho, O.A.S. Influence of pH and Fluoride Species on the Corrosion Behavior of Ti-xNb-13Zr Alloys in Ringer's Solution. *Adv. Mater. Sci. Eng.* **2013**, *1*, 1–10. [CrossRef]

6

Effect of Laser Energy Density, Internal Porosity and Heat Treatment on Mechanical Behavior of Biomedical Ti6Al4V Alloy Obtained with DMLS Technology

Żaneta Anna Mierzejewska

Faculty of Mechanical Engineering, Bialystok University of Technology, Wiejska 45c Street, 15-351 Białystok, Poland; a.mierzejewska@pb.edu.pl

Abstract: The purpose of this paper was to determine the influence of selected parameters of Direct Metal Laser Sintering and various heat treatment temperatures on the mechanical properties of Ti6Al4V samples oriented vertically (V, ZX) and horizontally (H, XZ). The performed micro-CT scans of as-build samples revealed that the change in laser energy density significantly influences the change in porosity of the material, which the parameters (130–210 W; 300–1300 mm/s), from 9.31% (130 W, 1300 mm/s) to 0.16% (190 W, 500 mm/s) are given. The mechanical properties, ultimate tensile strength (UTS, Rm) and yield strength (YS, Re) of the DMLS as-build samples, were higher than the ASTM F 1472 standard suggestion (UTS = 1100.13 ± 126.17 MPa, YS = 1065.46 ± 127.91 MPa), and simultaneously, the elongation at break was lower than required for biomedical implants (A = 4.23 ± 1.24%). The low ductility and high UTS were caused by a specific microstructure made of α' martensite and columnar prior β grains. X-Ray Diffraction (XRD) analysis revealed that heat treatment at 850 °C for 2 h caused the change of the microstructure intothe $\alpha + \beta$ combination, affecting the change of strength parameters—a reduction of UTS and YS with the simultaneous increase in elongation (A). Thus, properties similar to those indicated by the standard were obtained (UTS = 908.63 ± 119.49 MPa, YS = 795.9 ± 159.32 MPa, A = 8.72 ± 2.51%), while the porosity remained almost unchanged. Moreover, the heat treatment at 850 °C resulted in the disappearance of anisotropic material properties caused by the layered structure (UTS_{ZX} = 908.36 ± 122.79 MPa, UTS_{XZ} = 908.97 ± 118.198 MPa, YS_{ZX} = 807.83 ± 124.05 MPa, YS_{XZ} = 810.56 ± 124.05 MPa, A_{ZX} = 8.75 ± 2.65%, and A_{XZ} = 8.68 ± 2.41%).

Keywords: Selective Laser Melting; Direct Metal Laser Sintering; porosity; titanium alloys; yield strength; ultimate tensile strength; X-Ray Diffraction

---

1. Introduction

Direct Metal Laser Sintering (DMLS) is predicted to revolutionize the implants manufacturing. However, it is crucial to understand the possibilities and limitations of the process for the Ti6Al4V alloy, which is still the subject of extensive research. Phase transitions, as a result of heat treatment, have a considerable influence on the mechanical properties of the material [1,2], as well as α lath thickness [3]. Hrabe and Quinn [4] conducted a series of experiments to determine the effect of a microstructure on the properties of the samples in order to compare the mechanical properties of the Ti6Al4V alloy. Their work revealed that the orientation of the base plane in relation to the load direction is of great importance. The yield strength was the highest when the direction of the load was perpendicular to the base plane and the lowest in the orientation of an angle of 45°, resulting in a maximum shear stress at the basic plane. They have also proved that the texture has almost no effect on the ductility.

In numerous research papers, it has been proved that the Ti6Al4V alloy's microstructure created with a laser beam has some unique features that are characteristic of DMLS [5]. Tests of Ti6Al4V samples made with the use of Nd: YAG lasers presented that columnar grains are a common feature of microstructures made with additive techniques [6–9]. These grains grow along the boundaries of the original β grains, along with the build direction, as a result of repeated cycles above the β-transus and solidification temperatures, which start at a temperature of about 1660 °C. When passing through the liquidus line, the grain growth of the primary β phase occurs very quickly, making the grains orientation vertical, according to the build direction [10,11]. The laser beam creates a pool of molten material, from which the heat is transferred to the environment and to the already solidified layers. As the material below the top layer is again partially melted, the grains grow epitaxially from the layer below [12–14]. Some researchers suggested that the presence of columnar grains in DMLS samples may result in anisotropic mechanical properties of as-build samples (immediately after sintering) [15,16]. Regarding mechanical properties, it has been shown that cracks tend to spread along columnar grains [17,18]. Depending on the direction of tensile forces and the orientation of the columnar grains, there were differences in the ductility of samples built in a vertical or horizontal direction [7,19,20]. While the tensile strength was approx. 1060 MPa in both directions, the elongation was 11% and 14% for samples build in vertical and horizontal orientation, respectively.

The microstructure of the Ti6Al4V alloy produced by SLM technology is entirely made of the martensitic α′phase [10,21]. This is a result of high rates of heating and cooling of the solidified powder, which are neglected in the DMLS process [22]. Fine martensitic structure α′determines a high yield point and ultimate tensile strength (UTS) of more than 1 GPa, but also has a low elongation value, not exceeding 10%, and therefore lower than forged and casted materials [6,7,10,23]. Vranckenet al. analyzed the effect of various heat treatments on the microstructure of samples manufactured with SLM technology, taking into account different times, temperatures, and cooling rates [24]. The original α′structure has been transformed into a α + β plate mixture with heating below β-transus, while the features of the original microstructure (columnar grains) were preserved. After the heat treatment above the β-transus temperature, a clear change in the microstructure was observed—the columnar β grains were transformed into equiaxed grains.

The presence of defects in the microstructure, which are the source of initiation and propagation of cracks, as well as their random distribution, influences the reduction of fracture strength and fatigue strength due to significant stress peaks [25–28]. The morphology, number, size, and location of defects also affect the durability of samples created with the use of SLM technology. Qui et al., Liu et al., Gong et al., and Zhang et al. proved that spherical defects had less impact on durability if their volume did not exceed 1% [7,26,29,30]. The fracture toughness was significantly lowered, while spherical defects created over 5% of material porosity. Irregular defects in the volume of up to 1% turned out to be much more harmful for the samples tested in terms of mechanical strength. Kasperovich et al. tested samples that were subjected to various types of post-treatment—their aim was crack elimination, which occur in the structure, to improve fatigue strength [31]. Their research indicated that the heat treatment process only affected the change of the microstructure, however, it did not eliminate its defects, and therefore the improvement of fatigue life was negligible. As it is difficult to control the type, quantity, and location of defects in DMLS parts, fatigue strength can be different, even when the manufacturing process is carried out using regular parameters. Therefore, the fatigue strength of components manufactured by SLM technology still raises doubts and requires further research to be improved.

A number of studies conducted by Leuders et al., Qui et al., and Simonelli et al. have shown that it is possible to obtain a density of more than 99.5% for Ti6Al4V samples produced with the use of a laser beam [6,7,10]. Some researchers suggest that, due to the apparent density of the powder (50–60%), small amounts of gas may be entrapped in the material after solidification, resulting in the pores formation, which can be defined as small and empty spaces inside the solid material [3,32]. Gas pores are detrimental to mechanical properties because they act as stress concentrators in components under load, reducing fatigue life and elongation [7,25,33,34]. For this reason, one of the objectives of this work was to analyze the effect of porosity on the mechanical properties of samples obtained with DMLS technology.

The unique properties of titanium in medical applications were discovered relatively recently in the mid-1970s.Pioneering research, which was conducted in 1983, presented that this material promotes bone build-up on its surface (contact osteogenesis), causing a slight inflammatory reaction of tissues to foreign bodies [35]. One of the alloys meeting the requirements for biomaterials is a two-phase alloy Ti6Al4V (Titanium Grade 5/UNS R56400/WNR 3.7165), consisting of aluminum (6%) and vanadium (4%). This alloy is used in many industries, but mainly in biomedical engineering [36].

Concern about the validity of the titanium alloy in biomedical applications arouse the presence of aluminum and vanadium, and its toxicity to living organisms have been well documented [37]. However, specialists in the field of materials and medicine ensure that the occurrence of complications associated with the release of corrosion products to the tissues surrounding the implant is negligible, as titanium and its alloys undergo spontaneous surface passivation [38]. This process is related to the spontaneous formation of a tight and stable TiO_2 layer, formed on the surface, protecting the implant from the aggressive tissue environment and corrosion processes [39]. The unique properties of the Ti6Al4V alloy such as high corrosion resistance, so-called relative strength, low modulus of elasticity, high biocompatibility, excellent osseointegration, or low density, allow for the comprehensive use of its potential [40]. On the basis of ASTM F 1472 specifications for a forged Ti6Al4V alloy used as a medical material, the YS and UTS should not be lower than YS = 868 MPa and UTS = 930 MPa, respectively, and the elongation at the moment of break should be no less than 10%. Obtaining such properties with additive technologies requires a precise selection of DMLS parameters and additional heat treatment, due to which the stresses in the material will be eliminated, and the single-phase martensitic structure will decompose into a two-phase structure suitable for implantable biomaterials.

While the technology of selective laser melting is standardized, each commercial DMLS system presented in the published studies shows a separate characteristic in terms of materials and basic process characteristics (powder delivery to the working field, platform temperature, optical system, and laser) that affect the obtained results [41,42]. Literature analysis indicates a lack of a systematic approach to the study of laser–metal interactions, which would be beneficial for the further development of DMLS. To determine the optimal process parameters, extensive and comprehensive research on the relation of process conditions and product properties are required. Therefore, the key to this study was to investigate how the orientation affects the strength of the material and whether the heat treatment temperature can affect the reduction of the anisotropy of the material obtained with DMLS technology

2. Materials and Methods

The verification of the chemical composition of the analyzed powder was carried out using Thermo ARL Quantris spectrometer Spectrometer (Thermo Fisher Scientific, Waltham, MA, USA). Detailed results of the powder analysis are presented in Table 1. The content of Al and V was within the range specified in ASTMF 2924-14 (Standard Specification for Additive Manufacturing Titanium-6 Aluminum-4 Vanadium with Powder Bed Fusion).

Table 1. Chemical composition and material characteristics of used powder.

Element	Al	V	O	N	H	Fe	C	Ti
wt.%	5.97	4.04	0.195	0.036	0.010	0.24	0.061	Bal.
ASTM F 2924-14	5.5–6.75	3.5–4.5	<0.2	<0.05	<0.015	<0.3	<0.08	Bal.

Powder particle size measurements were performed using the ANALYSETTE 22 Micro Tec plus particle analyzer from FRITSCH GmbH Milling and Sizing (Idar-Oberstein, Germany). According to the powder producer (EOS company, Krailling, Germany), the average particle size is around 30 μm.

However, laboratory analyzes revealed that the particle size was in the range of 10 to 100 μm. The average particle size obtained for three subsequent measurements of the particle distribution was equal to 39.81 μm, with about 94.2% of the particles investigated ranging from 20 to 80 μm (0–30 μm, 18.12%; 30–80 μm, 80.82%, 80–100 μm, and 1.10%). The grains observed under the microscope were spherical and smooth, with numerous satellites, which correspond to the morphology of gas sprayed powder. The advantage of spherical morphology and wide particle size distribution has high fluidity and high packing density.

Thirty groups of test samples were used in experimental research. In each group, different laser powers (130 W, 150 W, 170 W, 190 W, and 210 W) and different beam speeds (300 mm/s, 500 mm/s, 700 mm/s, 900 mm/s, 1100 mm/s, and 1300 mm/s) were used. In all samples, a cross–scan pattern was used and the same distance of scanning vectors was maintained, as well as layer thickness (0.03 mm), spot size (0.1 mm), and hatch distance (0.1 mm). The process parameters used in the present study have been presented in Table 2.

Table 2. Processing parameters.

Scanning Velocity (mm/s)	Laser Power [W]				
	130	150	170	190	210
	Energy Density (J/mm³)				
300	144	166	188	211	233
500	87	100	113	127	140
700	62	71	81	90	100
900	48	56	63	70	74
1100	40	45	52	58	64
1300	33	38	44	49	54

The energy density (E) was calculated based on laser power (P), the distance between the laser scan line (h), scanning speed (v), and layer thickness (t), which is presented in Equation (1) [13].

$$E = \frac{P}{vht}\ [J/mm^3] \quad (1)$$

DMLS samples were divided into five groups—four of them were heat treated and one remained in the as-build state. Samples were heated for 2 h at 650 °C, 750 °C, 850 °C, and 950 °C. Heat treatment was carried out in a vertical furnace, heating at a rate of about 10 °C/ min, under argon atmosphere (to prevent oxidation of the titanium surface). The samples were cooled with the furnace to 500 °C at a rate of about 0.04 °C/s, and then cooled in the air. After heat treatment, the samples were grinded with abrasive paper with gradations of 200, 500, and 800, purified in 70% ethanol, rinsed with deionized water, and then electropolished in a bath solution using a perchloric acid, glacial acetic acid, and distilled water mixture in a volume ratio of 1:10:1.2 [43]. The current density was equal to 0.3 A/cm^2. The samples were treated with fresh solution at room temperature (25 °C) for 15 min. The Bruker Sky Scan 1172 (Brucker, Billerica, MA, USA) scanner with set parameters: Number of rows—2664, number of columns—4000, Au + CU filter, sample rotation—0.2500, and pixel size—4.28 μm was used for microtomographic optical analysis. Scanned images of samples were reconstructed with the use of software dedicated to micro-CT image analysis—NRecon, Data Viewer, CTvox, and CTAn. Tensile properties were studied using a Hegewald and Peschke INSPEKT (Meß—und Prüftechnik GmbH, Nossen, Germany) test machine with a maximum breaking strength of 5 kN. Displacements were measured by using an extensometer with a 25 mm gauge length. Yield stress and Young's modulus were determined according to ASTM E 111. XRD X–ray phase analysis was performed using a Bruker D8 Advance Eco-ray diffractometer (Brucker, Billerica, MA, USA), equipped with a Cu Kα1 X-ray tube = 1.5406 Å and an SSD160 detector (Brucker, Billerica, MA, USA) adapted for ultra–fast XRD diffraction detection.

3. Results and Discussion

All samples were produced on one mounting plate. Due to the specificity of the process, changes in the dimensional accuracy of the samples with respect to nominal dimensions (Figure 1a) were expected. The dimensional accuracy was affected by the intensive degreasing of samples in an ultrasonic washer and resulted in the rinsing out of loose, unmelted powder grains, and consequently, changes in the dimensions of the samples. Thirty randomly selected samples were subjected to detailed measurements in strictly defined places—fourteen points, marked A through M, presented in Figure 1b.

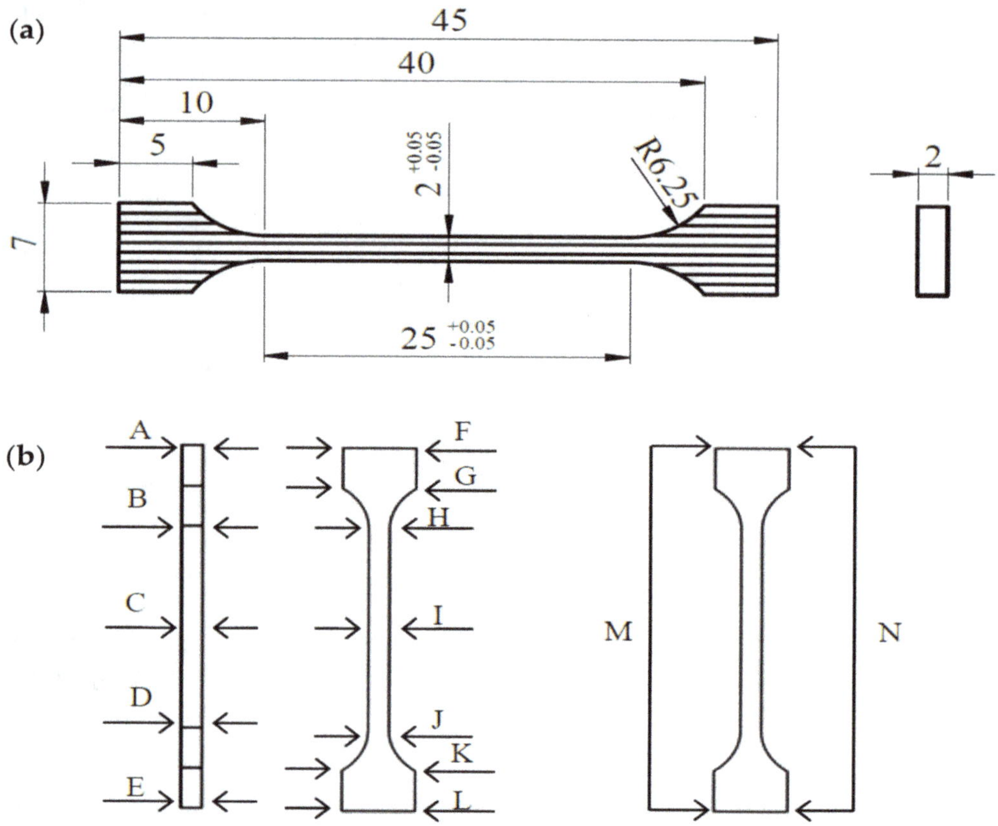

Figure 1. Nominal dimensions of a single sample (**a**) and measurement points (**b**).

The dimensions of each sample were measured with a digital caliper to an accuracy of 0.01 mm. The list of measurements is presented in Table 3.

Table 3. Dimensional accuracy of samples for testing mechanical properties.

Dimension	Thickness A–E [mm]	Necking H/I/J [mm]	Width F/G/K/L [mm]	Length M–N [mm]
Nominal	2	2	7	45
Min	2.48	2.07	6.97	45.55
Max	2.55	2.17	7.16	45.65
Average	2.51	2.12	7.07	45.58
Standard deviation	0.01	0.02	0.06	0.03

3.1. Porosity

Polished and etched surfaces of cylindrical samples were subjected to microscopic observations. The effect can be seen in Figure 2. It was concluded that the change in scanning speed as well as the change in laser power significantly affected the shape and the number of pores.

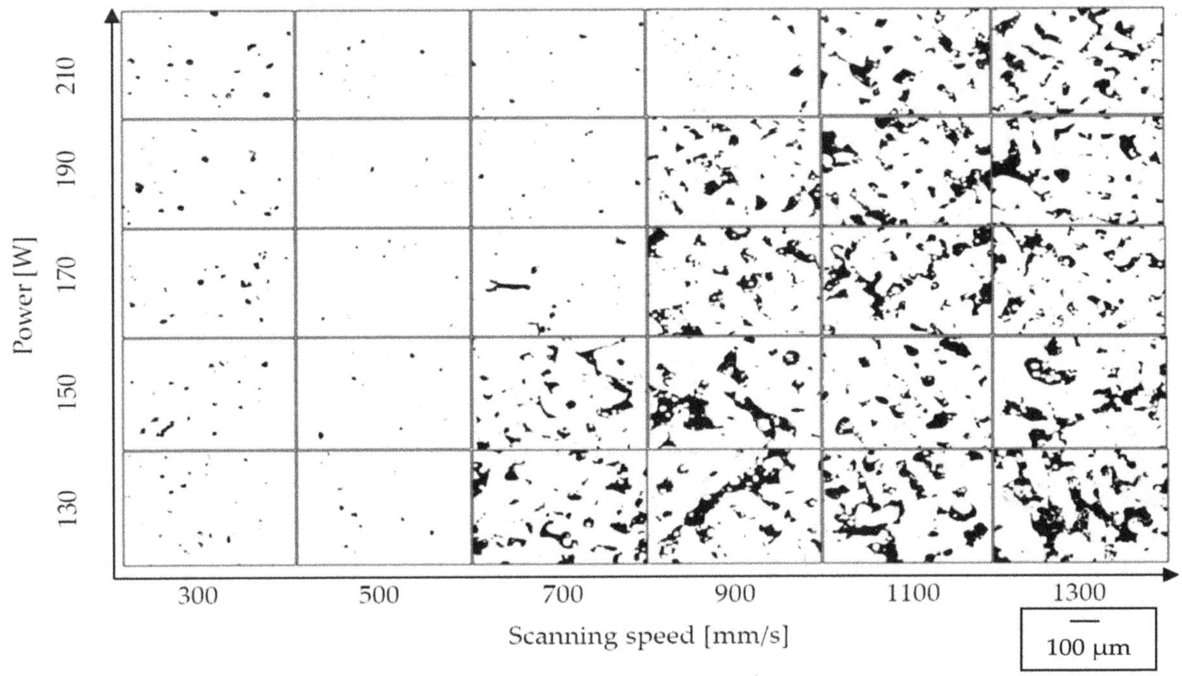

Figure 2. Graphical representation of the variable pore morphology in vertical samples manufactured with Direct Metal Laser Sintering (DMLS) technology, perpendicular to the build direction; 100×.

The quantitative analyzes allowed for a precise assessment of the samples porosity by means of non-destructive microtomographic examination. The correlation between the decreasing value of the melting energy density and the increasing porosity is highly noticeable (Figure 3). However, porosity increases significantly with the increase of scanning speed. This regularity was observed in each group of samples. For samples melted with a laser power of 130 W and a scanning speed of 500 mm/s, the material density was almost 99%. The porosity in the range of 0.72% indicates the presence of internal defects in the structure. An increase is observed below and above 500 mm/s in porosity—from 1.27% at a speed of 300 mm/s to 9.31% at a speed of 1300 mm/s (Figure 3a). Samples melted with a power of 150 W and 300 mm/s were characterized by a porosity of 1.5%. Above 500 mm/s, an increase in porosity was observed—from 3.37% at a speed of 700 mm/s to 8.43% at a speed of 1300 mm/s. The minimum value porosity of 0.46% was observed at a laser speed of 500 mm/s. In comparison to samples manufactured at 130 W with the same speed, the porosity was lower by 0.26%. The difference between the maximum porosity values obtained for the highest laser speed was less than 1% (Figure 3b). For samples melted with a laser power of 170 W at scanning speeds from 300 to 700 mm/s, the porosity of the material varies from 1.69% to 0.8%. Above 700 mm/s, an increase in porosity is observed—from 5.29% at a speed of 900 mm/s to 7.29% at a speed of 1300 mm/s. Samples melted with a power of 170 W achieved a density of more than 99% for two scanning speeds—500 and 700 mm/s. The highest density, 99.73%, was obtained for samples scanned with 700 mm/s (Figure 3c). Additionally, for samples melted with a laser power of 190 W and scanning speed of 500 mm/s and 700 mm/s, porosity did not exceed 1%. The lowest value of porosity was observed for samples melted with 500 mm/s—0.16%. At a scanning speed of 300 mm/s, microstructure defects in the analyzed samples were slightly below 2%, while a further increase in scanning speed above 500 mm/s resulted in higher porosity—from 0.68% for 700 mm/s to 6.57% for 1300 mm/s (Figure 3d). Similar characteristics were found for samples melted with a power of 210 W. The porosity obtained at 300 mm/s exceeded 2% and a decreasing tendency was observed along with the increase of sintering speed to 700 mm/s. After exceeding 700 mm/s, the porosity increased again, reaching a maximum value of 6.16% at a sintering speed of 1300 mm/s. The lowest porosity was obtained at 700 mm/s and was 0.45% (Figure 3e).

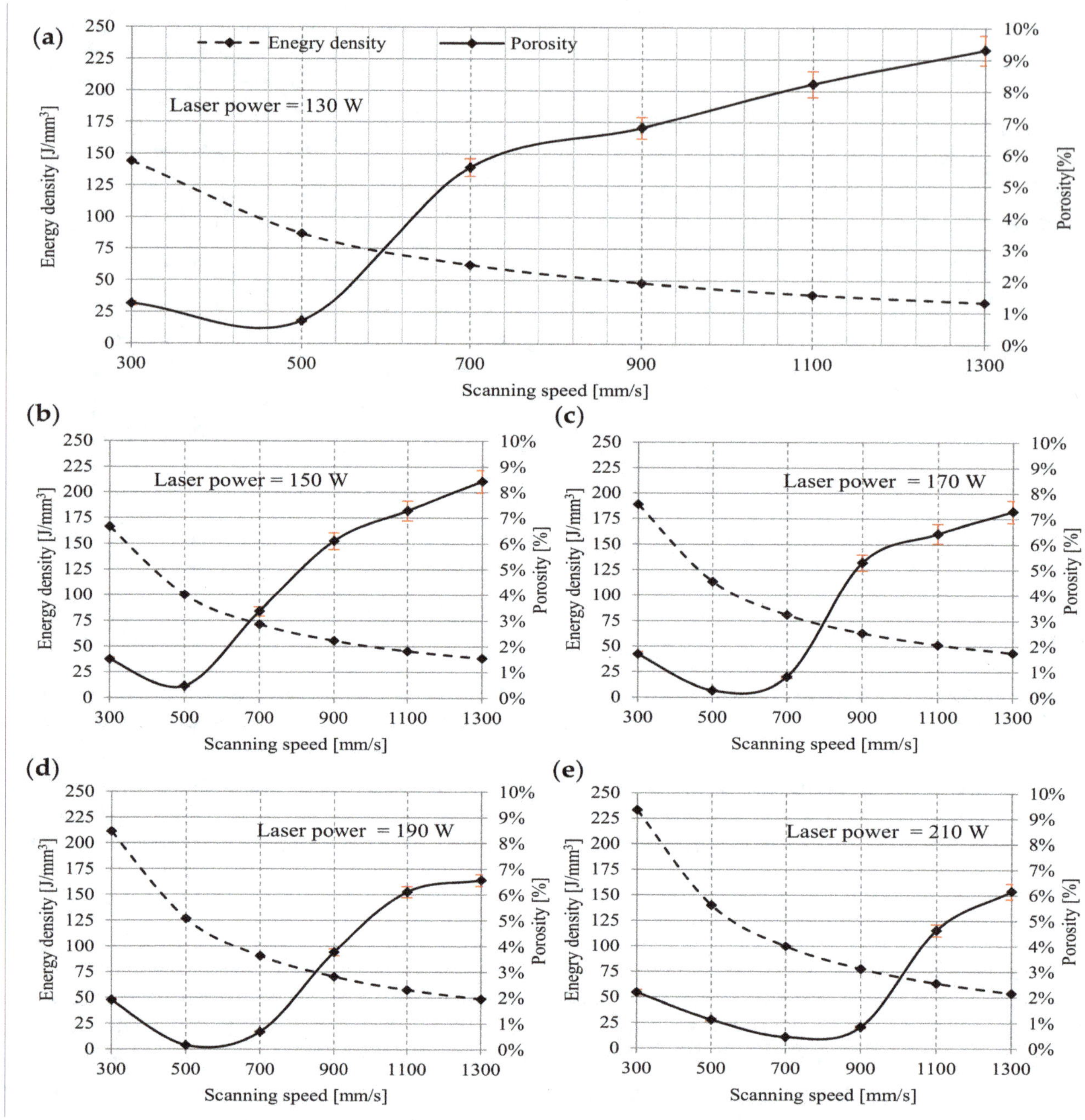

Figure 3. The influence of scanning speed and energy density on the porosity: (**a**) 130 W, (**b**) 150 W, (**c**) 170 W, (**d**) 190 W, (**e**) 210 W.

At low energy density (33–71 J/mm^3), the porosity ranges from 9.31% to 3.37%. The pores are unevenly distributed, irregular in shape, and interconnected. Porosity is characterized by large recesses filled with loose particles of unmelted grains. A possible explanation for this is a low energy density and relatively small depth of laser penetration, which make the size of the melt pool too small as the powder particles are not sufficiently liquefied to completely melt, but provides a sufficient bond between the layers. The increase in energy density from 78 J/mm^3 to 127 J/mm^3 generates a relatively high temperature, which facilitates the flow of liquid and fills the space between already melted grains, causing the porosity in the range of 0.84–0.16%.

At higher energy densities, the pores are small and mostly spherical, and their formation is most often associated with gas bubbles trapped under the molten powder layer. An increase in the laser energy density above 127 J/mm^3 causes changes in the pore morphology and an increase in porosity from 1.12% for 140 J/mm^3 to 2.18% for 233 J/mm^3 (Figure 4).

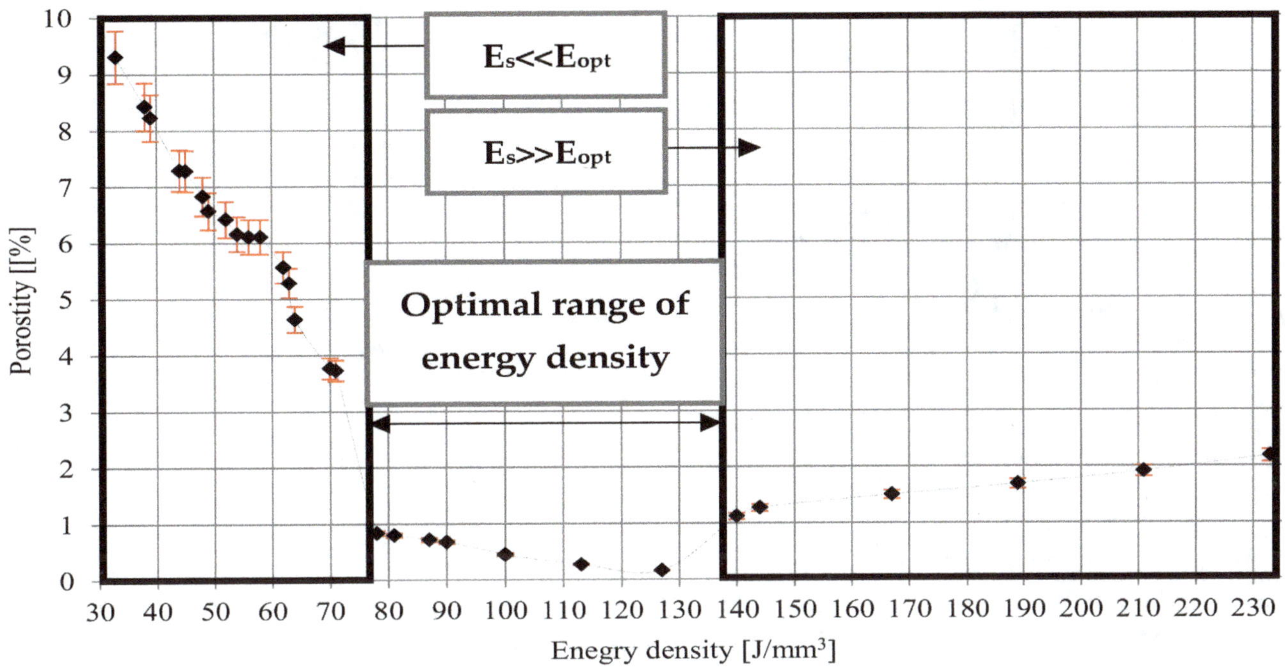

Figure 4. Relation of porosity and energy density for Ti6Al4V DMLS alloy.

The influence of energy density on porosity was also investigated by Han et al. [44], Laquai et al. [45], and Dilip et al. [46]. While the range of the optimal power density indicated by Han and Lagui is similar to that obtained in the present study (120–180 J/mm^3 and 120–195 J/mm^3, respectively), significant differences were observed. Both authors state that the porosity in the tested samples did not exceed 0.05%. What is more, Han also revealed that, in the range of much lower (60 J/mm^3) and much higher (240 J/mm^3) energy density, the density of melted material is not less than 99.75%. Lagui, on the other hand, observed an increase in porosity just above 1% for only energy densities below 50 J/mm^3 and above 300 J/mm^3. Completely different characteristics were presented by Dilip et al. [47]. They showed that the optimal range of energy density was between 50 and 66 J/mm^3 (porosity below 0.5%), for energy densities around 40 J/mm^3, the porosity increased to about 5%, while at higher energy densities between 90 and 130 J/mm^3, the porosity was about 10%.

3.2. Mechanical Properties

The layered structure obtained in DMLS technology makes the samples characterized by anisotropic mechanical properties. For this purpose, two types of samples were printed—vertically oriented samples (V, ZX) and horizontally orientated samples (H, XZ; Figure 5). The layering in both samples was perpendicular to the building direction (Z), while the tensile forces acting on the samples were oriented perpendicular to the layers in the ZX samples and parallel to the layers in the XZ samples. The tensile strength results presented in Figures 6–10 were calculated on the basis of five consecutive tests.

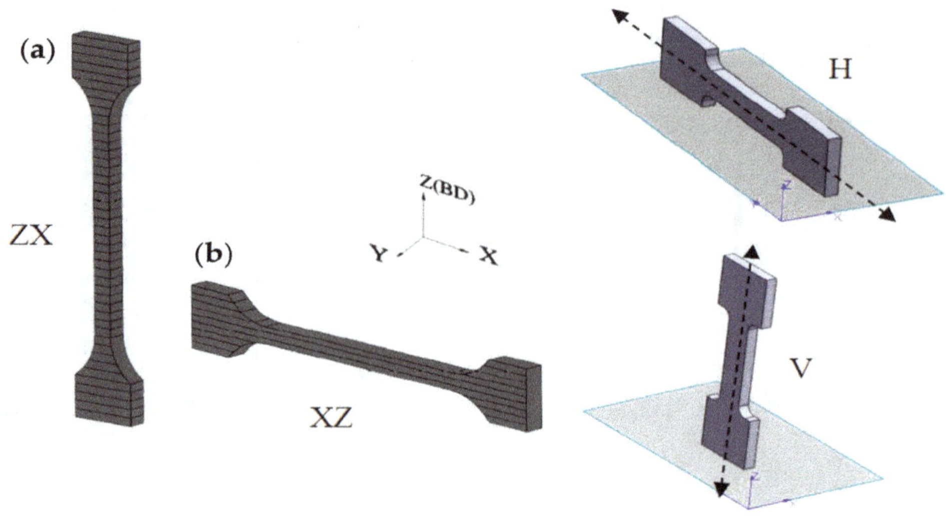

Figure 5. Tensile samples oriented in: (**a**) XZ plane and (**b**) ZX plane.

3.2.1. As-build Samples

Based on ASTM F 1472 specifications for the forged Ti6Al4V alloy used as medical materials, YS and UTS should not be lower than 868 and 930 MPa, respectively, and elongation at break should be no less than 10%. For all as-built samples (Figure 6a–c), the yield strength and tensile strength significantly exceeded the minimum requirements for the forged material described in the standard and were equal to 1065.46 ± 127.91 MPa and 1100.13 ± 126.17 MPa, respectively. The highest strength was characterized by samples melted with 190 W power and 500 mm/s speed (Re max = 1261 ± 5.65 MPa and Rm max = 1288 ± 28.28 MPa), while the lowest was the samples melted at 130 W and a speed of 1300 mm/s (Re min = 885 ± 7.07 MPa; Rm min = 918.5 ± 28.99 MPa). In the group of samples melted with 130 W and 1100–1300 mm/s, strength parameters did not meet the criteria of ASTM F 472.The fragility of the martensitic microstructure and the presence of residual stresses are responsible for the lower ductility.

It can be determined that the samples elongation was definitely lower than required in this standard, and its average value was 4.23 ± 1.24%, with the maximum elongation in this group of samples being A max = 5.8 ± 0.84%, and the minimum A min = 2.2 ± 0.56%. The tensile strength of Ti6Al4V samples produced by the DMLS method is only slightly higher than their yield strength, which indicates the brittleness of the material and its low ductility. An increase scanning speed above 700 mm/s in almost every sample group influences the reduction of the strength parameters and elongation. This is due to the fact that higher speeds cause the generation of a lower energy density, which results in structural defects and the weakening of bonds between layers. Additionally, the increase in power affected the changes of mechanical parameters—tensile strength increased from 1050 ± 136.97 MPa (130 W) to 1148.83 ± 106.74 MPa (210 W). YS and A also increased—from 1013.58 ± 134.95 MPa to 1112.41 ± 109.85 MPa and from 3.72 ± 1.43% to 4.72 ± 0.99%.

The surfaces fracture of non-heat treated samples showed mixed characteristic of brittle and ductile fracture, accompanied by very small plastic deformation. Fracture surfaces were characterized by the presence of shallow dimples on quasi cleavage surface, delamination, or stepped cracks, suggesting intergranular destruction along hard, prone to cracking, brittle needles α', which then propagated due to decohesion caused by further deformation of the sample. A large number of gas defects and pores caused the concentration of stress and violent crack propagation, and the mixed nature of cracking to a limited elongation (Figure 6d).

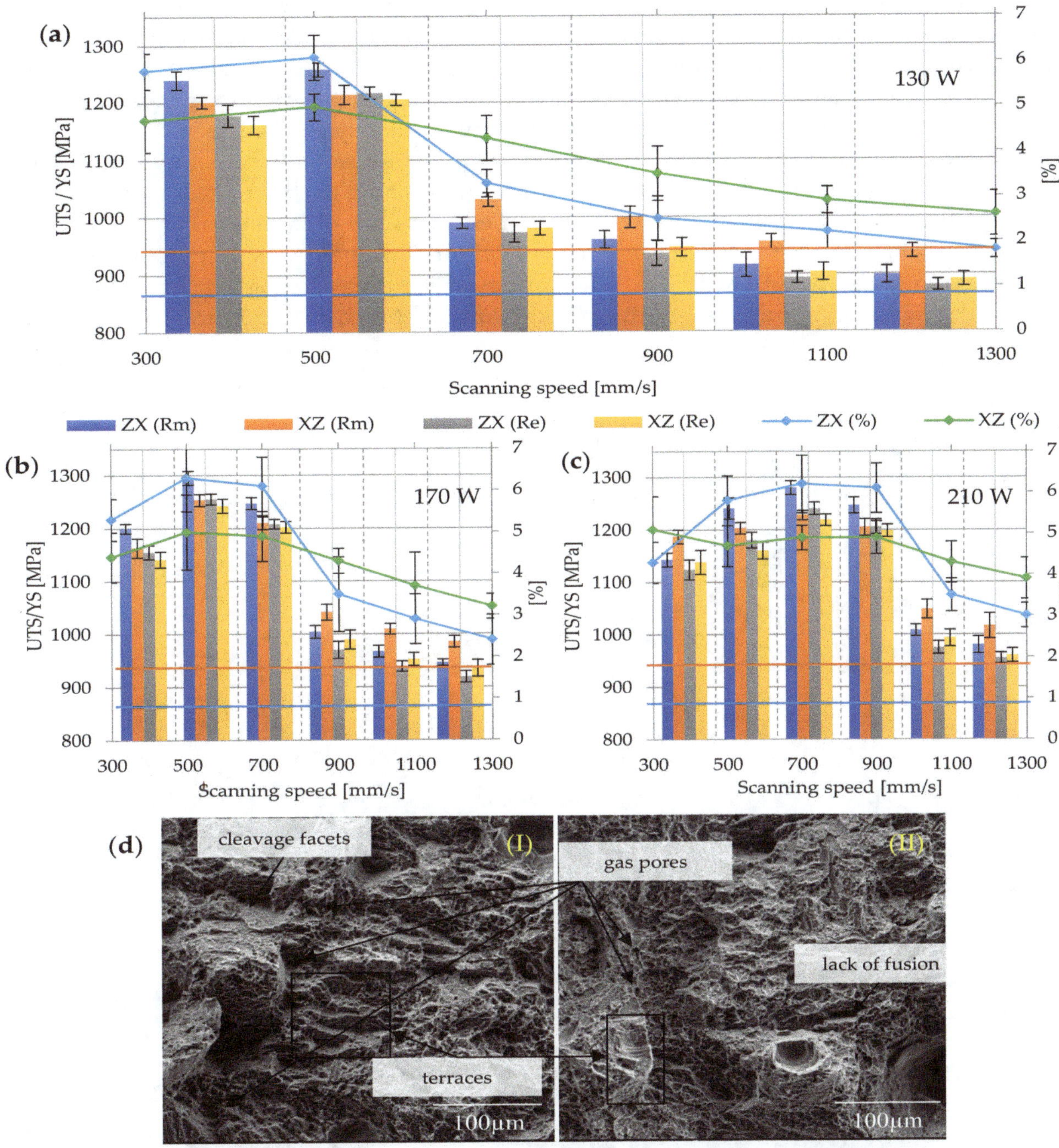

Figure 6. Strength parameters of as–built samples with different laser speeds and powers: (**a**) 130 W, (**b**) 170 W, (**c**) 210 W, and (**d**) fracture surface: (I) 130 W, 300 mm/s, ZX; (II) 130 W, 300 mm/s, XZ; 900×; Rm min — and Re min — for Ti6Al4V in accordance with ASTM F 1472.

3.2.2. Heat Treatment at 650 °C

Despite heat treatment, the results of tensile and yield strength were still higher than the minimum determined by the ASTM F 1472 standard (Rm = 1071.7 ± 128.08 MPa; Re = 994.85 ± 124.91 MPa), and the elongation was also unsatisfactory and almost a half lower than required (A = 4.24 ± 1.25%). The highest strength was characterized by samples melted with the power of 190 W and the speed of 500 mm/s (Rm max = 1237 ± 26.87 MPa; Re max = 1192.5 ± 6.36 MPa), the lowest was the samples melted with the power of 130 W at a speed of 1300 mm/s (Rm min = 864.5 ± 24.74 MPa; Re min = 810 MPa). The tensile strength of ZX samples decreased to an average of 1050.73 ± 145.97 MPa, and XZ samples to 1023.86 ± 206.64 MPa. With the decrease in strength properties, the elongation increased for ZX samples to 4.27 ± 1.57%, and for XZ samples to 4.21 ± 0.83%. The differences in tensile strength between the samples printed in the XZ plane and ZX plane was approx. 3.3% (Figure 7a–c). Obtained results clearly indicate that annealed samples had higher elongation at break—regardless of their orientation, and thus better ductility, in comparison to as-build samples. A large range of values from average elongation at break indicates that the improvement is not as significant as in other works presented in the literature [24,25,45]. The minimum elongation value, according to the standard, cannot be lower than 10%, which in the case of the applied heat treatment, was not obtained for any of the samples, therefore reducing the stresses turned out to be beneficial for DMLS Ti6Al4V, but is still insufficient to meet the criteria imposed by ASTM F 1472. The surface of the breakthrough remained mixed, with features of brittle and ductile fractures, with shallow dimples staircase cracks and pores (Figure 7d).

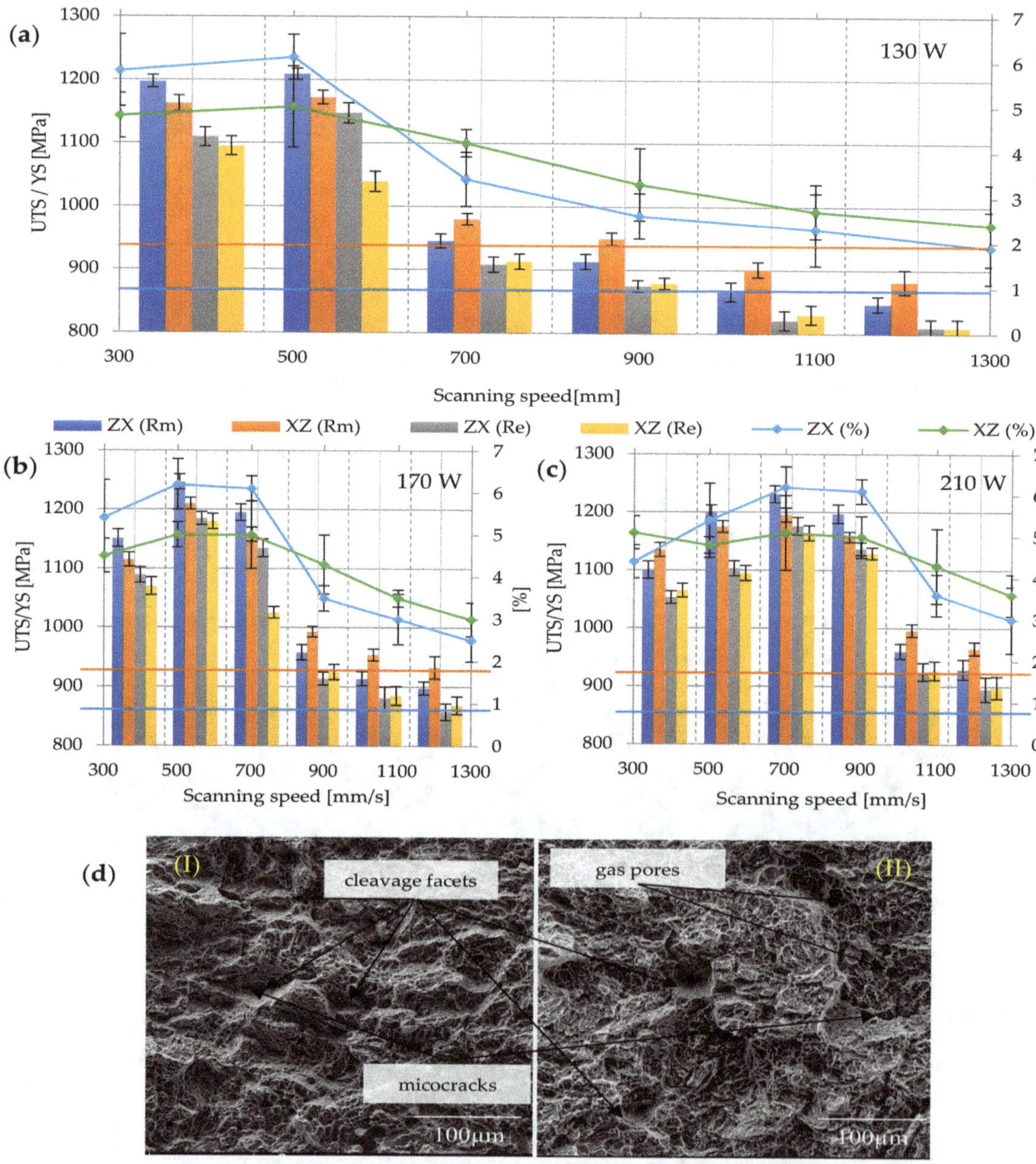

Figure 7. Strength parameters of samples heat treated at 650 °C with different laser speeds and powers: (**a**) 130 W, (**b**) 170 W, (**c**) 210 W, and (**d**) fracture surface: (I) 130 W, 300 mm/s, ZX; (II) 130 W, 300 mm/s, XZ; 900×; Rm min — and Re min — for Ti6Al4V in accordance with ASTM F 1472.

3.2.3. Heat Treatment at 750 °C

Annealing at 750 °C for 2 h significantly reduced the strength parameters and increased the plasticity of the material, as a result of partial phase transformation $\alpha' \rightarrow \alpha + \beta$ and at the same time caused the growth of grain α, thus changing the phase composition and grain morphology (in relation to as-build samples).

For heat treatment at 750 °C, the Rm of the samples was equal to 1002.88 ± 119.42 MPa, while Re = 900.07 ± 77.43 MPa. The highest strength was again achieved in samples melted with a power of 190 W and a speed of 500 mm/s (Rm max = 1169.5 ± 6.36 MPa; Re max = 1085.5 ± 13.43 MPa). The lowest tensile strength and yield strength were obtained in samples melted with a power of 130 W and a speed of 1300 mm/s again—the average value of Rm min = 812 ± 11.31 MPa; Re min = 723 ± 12.72 MPa. Heat treatment also had a slight influence on the elongation—increased from A = 5.24 ± 1.25% to A = 5.71 ± 1.69%. The difference in the strength of the ZX and XZ samples also decreased: ZX Rm = 1002.27 ± 126.06 MPa, XZ Rm = 998.72 ± 113.82 MPa, similar to the yield strength—Re = 899.53 ± 133.26 MPa (for ZX), Re = 900.6 ± 115.76 MPa (for XZ). The elongation for ZX samples increased to 5.75 ± 2.07%, while for XZ samples, to 5.67 ± 1.23% (Figure 8a–c). The nature of the fractures area has changed slightly, showing more features of a ductile fracture than in the case of previous samples. On the fracture surfaces, defects of the microstructure, i.e., pores, cracks, and discontinuities of the material, were visible (Figure 8d).

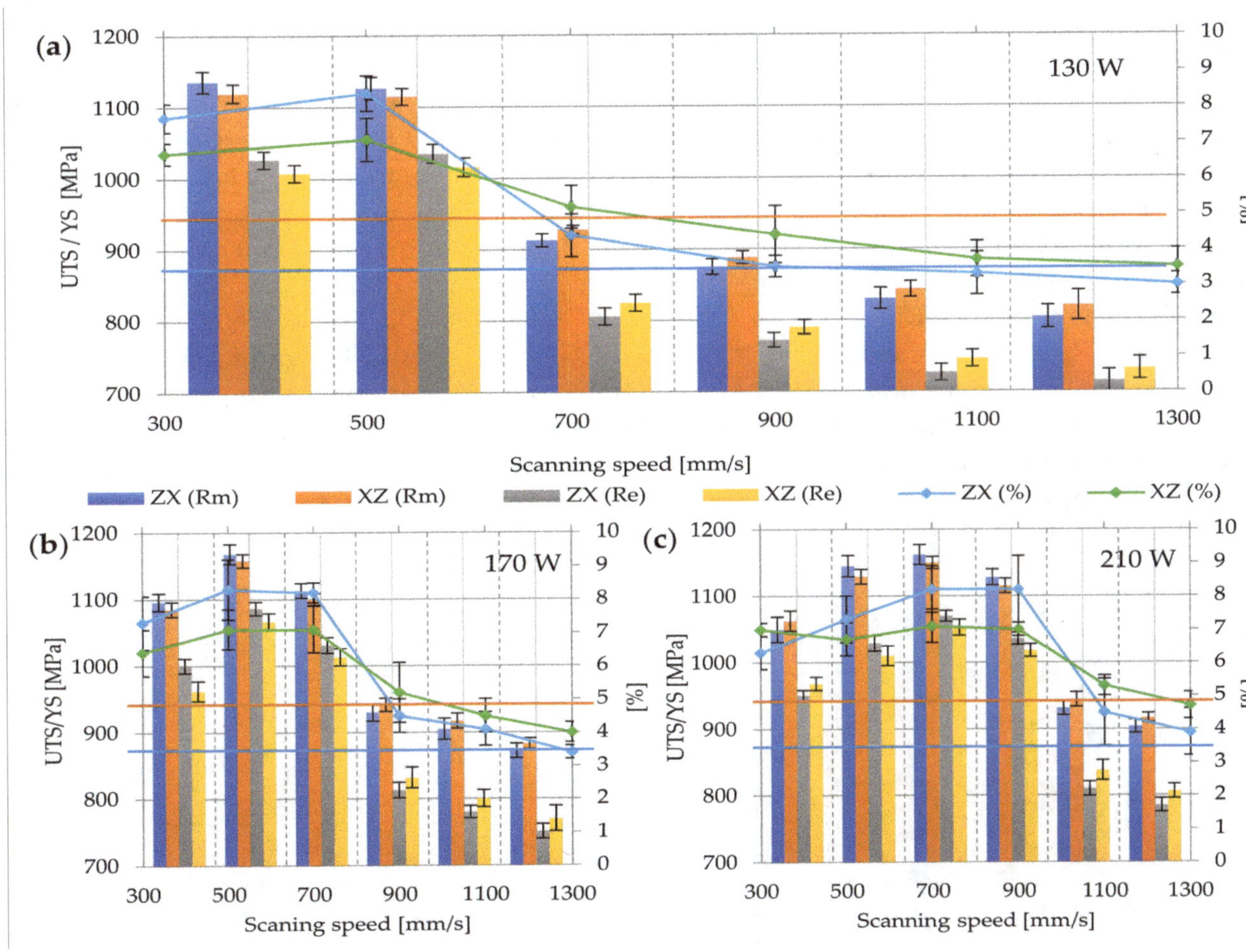

Figure 8. *Cont.*

(d)

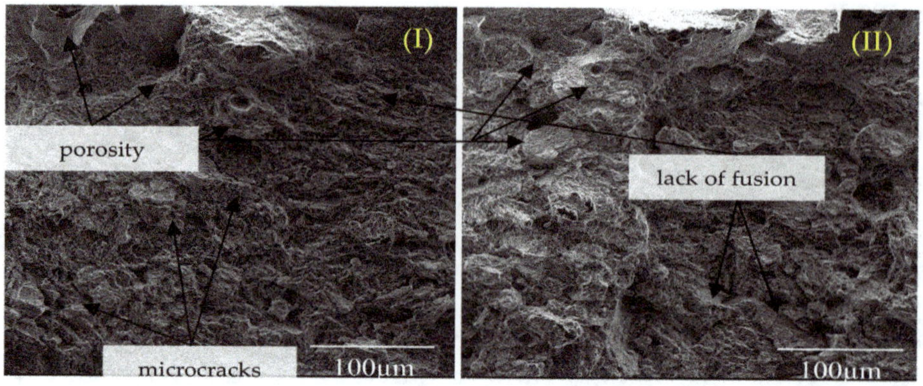

Figure 8. Strength parameters of samples heat treated at 750 °C with different laser speeds and powers: (**a**) 130 W, (**b**) 170 W, (**c**) 210 W, and (**d**) fracture surface: (I) 130 W, 300 mm/s, ZX; (II) 130 W, 300 mm/s, XZ; 900×; Rm min — and Re min — for Ti6Al4V in accordance with ASTM F 1472.

3.2.4. Heat Treatment at 850 °C

Heat treatment at 850 °C led to a change in the microstructure and decomposition of the α′phase to the α + β. Therefore, it can be assumed that the samples annealed at this temperature presented the best relationship between strength and elongation. The average tensile strength value for all analyzed samples was equal to 908.63 ± 119.49 MPa, yield strength 795.9 ± 159.32 MPa, and elongation at break 8.72 ± 2.51%. The highest tensile and yield strength were again characterized by samples of 190 W/500 mm/s (Rm max = 1058 ± 4.94 MPa; Re max = 958 ± 4.95 MPa), the lowest was again the samples of 130 W/1300 mm/s. The average value of Rm min was 724.5 ± 4.95 MPa, and Re min = 625.5 ± 6.36 MPa. A significant part of the samples treated at this temperature does not meet the criteria of ASTM F 1472 in terms of tensile strength and yield strength, but they still meet the criteria of ASTM F 1108-14.

What is more, processing at 850 °C resulted in homogenization of the microstructure, and as a result, anisotropic properties of differently orientated samples have disappeared. The tensile strength of ZX samples was therefore Rm = 908.36 ± 122.79 MPa, samples XZ Rm = 908.97 ± 118.198 MPa, the yield strength Re for both orientations was equal to: 807.83 ± 124.05 MPa and 810.56 ± 124.05 MPa, and elongation A: 8.75 ± 2.65% and 8.68 ± 2.41% (Figure 9a–c). The surface fracture is typically ductile, with dimples and voids, in the middle of which there are particles of inclusions. In the central part of the crack, the dimples are equi-axial, while on the sides they have a strong shearing character and a parabolic shape (Figure 9d).

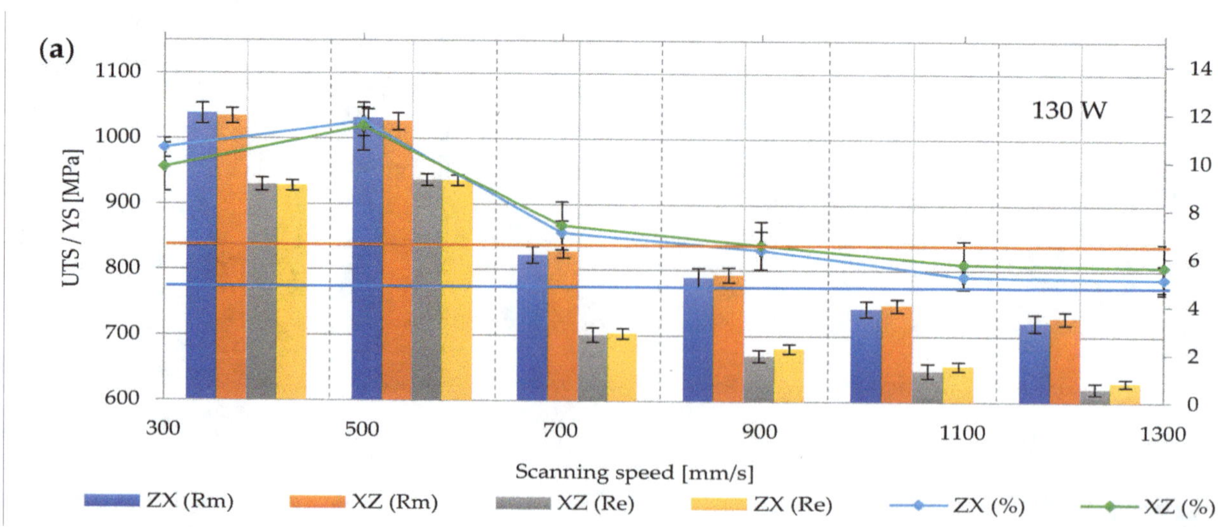

Figure 9. *Cont.*

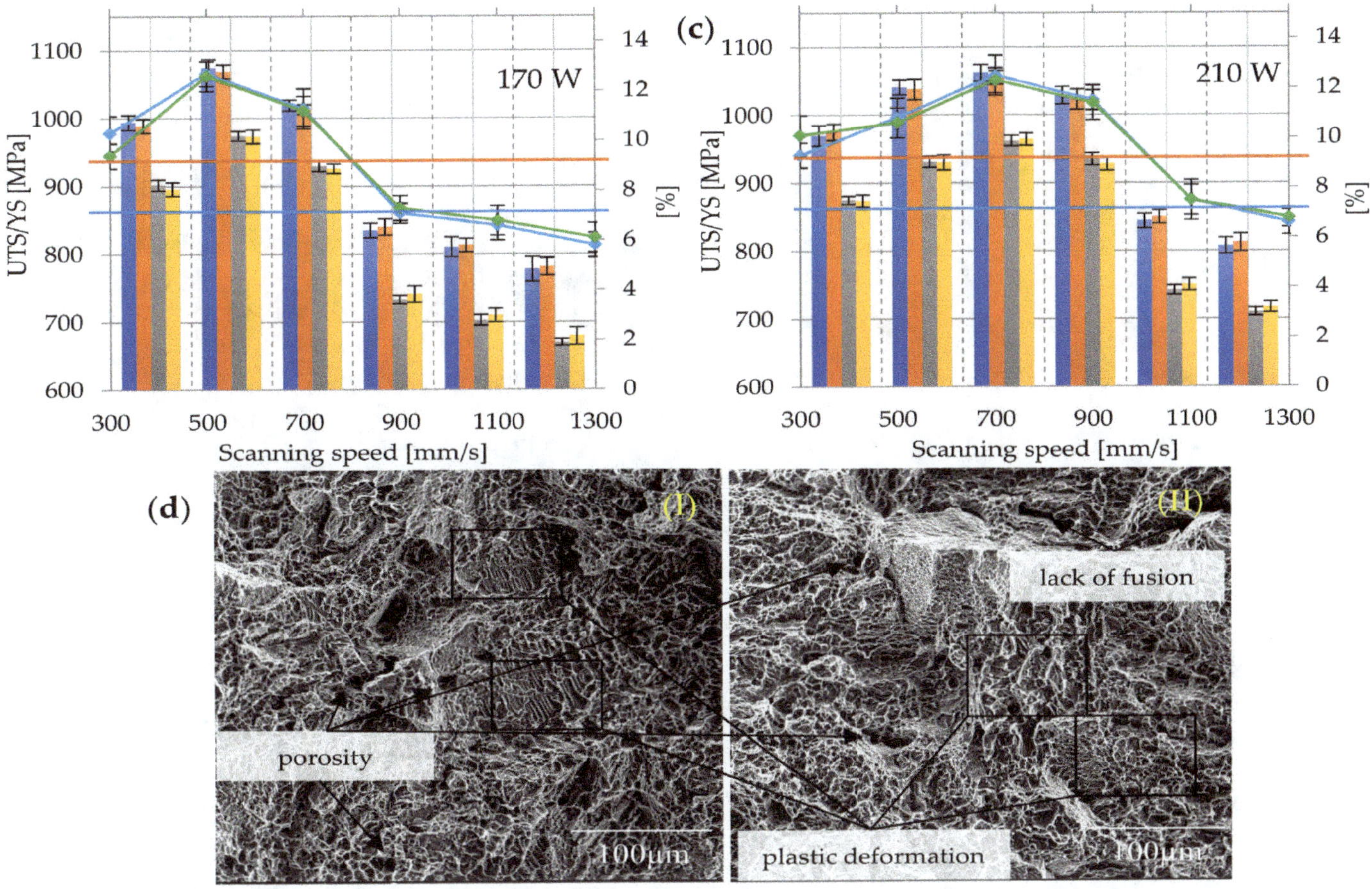

Figure 9. Strength parameters of samples heat treated at 850 °C with different laser speeds and powers: (**a**) 130 W, (**b**) 170 W, (**c**) 210 W, and (**d**) fracture surface: (I) 130 W, 300 mm/s, ZX; (II) 130 W, 300 mm/s, XZ; 900×; Rm min — and Re min — for Ti6Al4V in accordance with ASTM F 1472.

3.2.5. Heat Treatment at 950 °C

Heat treatment at 950 °C significantly affected the change in the microstructure—similarly to that in the lower temperature treatment, the α′martensitic phase decomposed into the α + β phase mixture, but temperature close to β-trasus caused increased grain size and deterioration of plastic properties. Therefore, along with the decrease in the value of strength properties, the elongation at break decreases. As a result, the analyzed properties have the following values: Tensile strength Rm for all analyzed samples is 848.48 ± 86.56 MPa, yield strength 781.35 ± 96.3 MPa, and elongation at break 7.75 ± 2.69%. The highest measured values of tensile strength and yield stress are, respectively, Rm max = 931 ± 1.41 MPa; Re max = 927.5 ± 3.54 MPa, while the lowest—Rm min = 702.5 ± 12.5 MPa and Re min = 615.5 ± 6.36 MPa (Figure 10a–c). The character of the fracture surface remains ductile (Figure 10d).

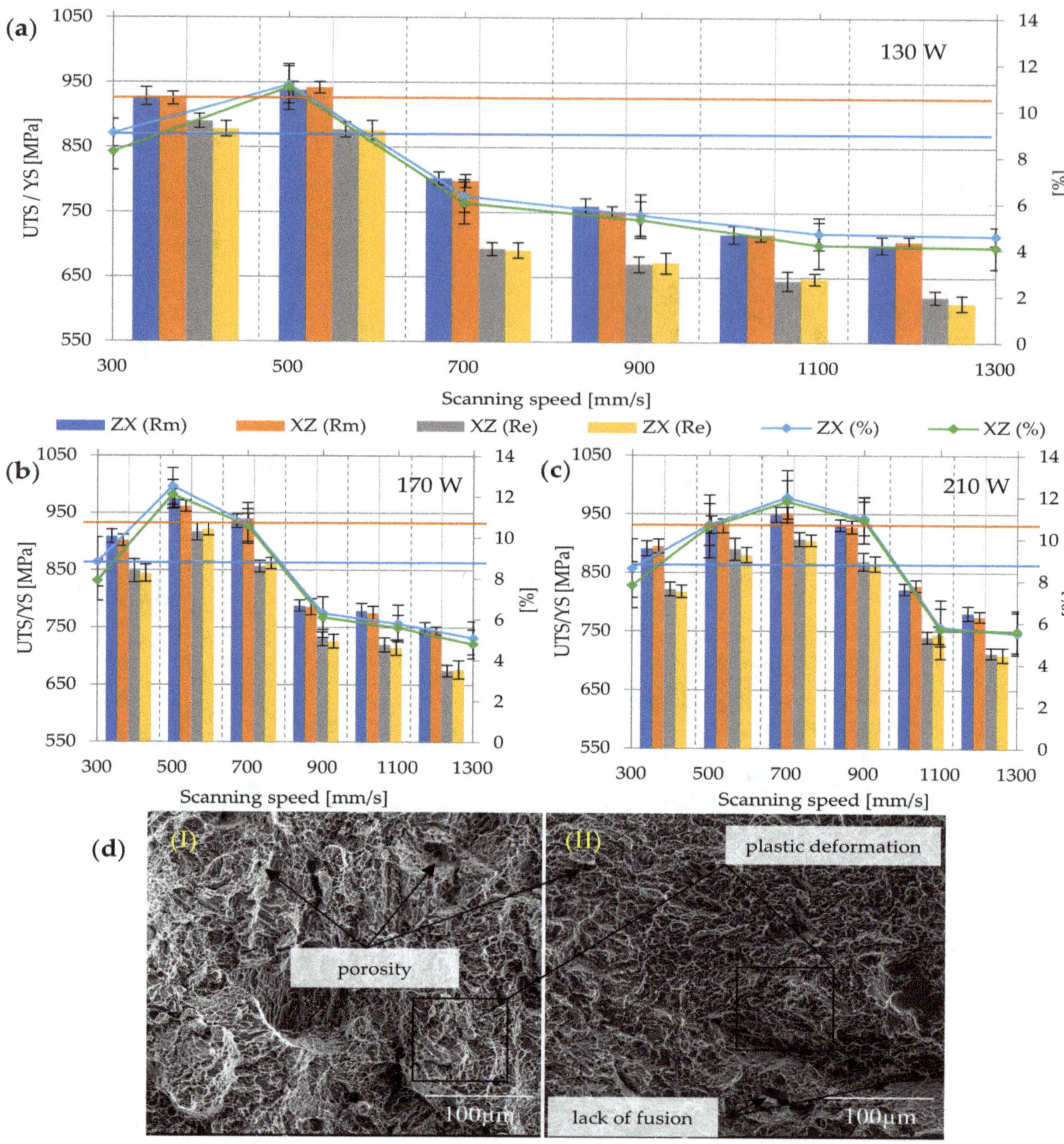

Figure 10. Strength parameters of samples heat treated at 650 °C with different laser speeds and powers: (**a**) 130W, (**b**) 170W, (**c**) 210W, and (**d**) fracture surface: (I) 130 W, 300 mm/s, ZX; (II) 130 W, 300 mm/s, XZ; 900×; Rm min — and Re min — for Ti6Al4V in accordance with ASTM F 1472.

The obtained data is supplemented by the assessment of the influence of porosity on the strength and elongation of samples, the yield point and Young's modulus (Figures 11 and 12). With the increase of porosity, all these parameters revealed a downward trend, which clearly indicates that defects of the microstructure strongly affect the mechanical properties of the material.

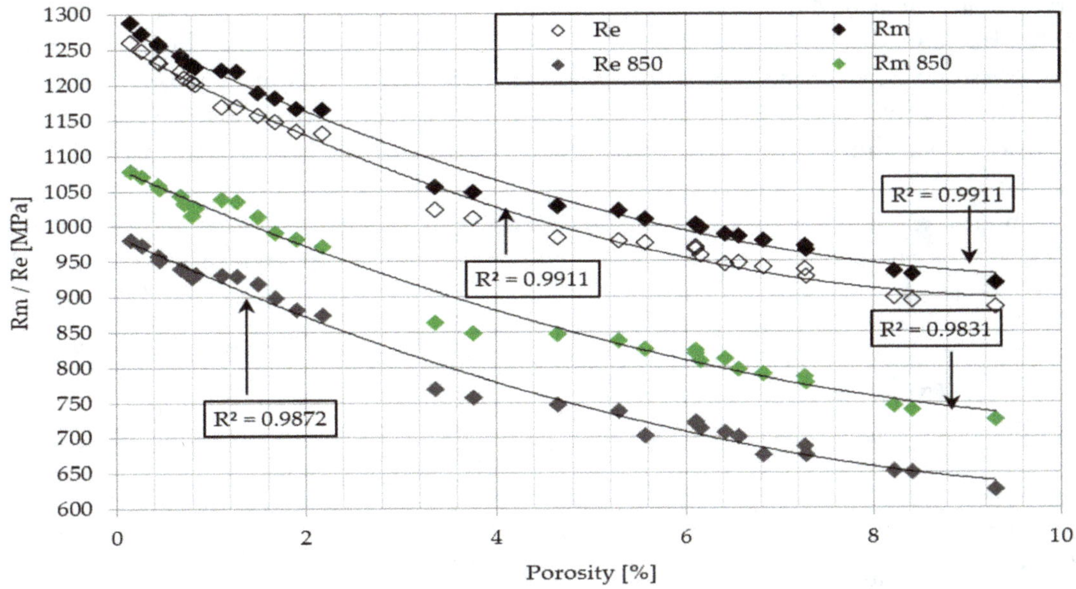

Figure 11. Influence of porosity on Ultimate Tensile Strength and Yield Strength of as-build and heat treated at 850 °C samples.

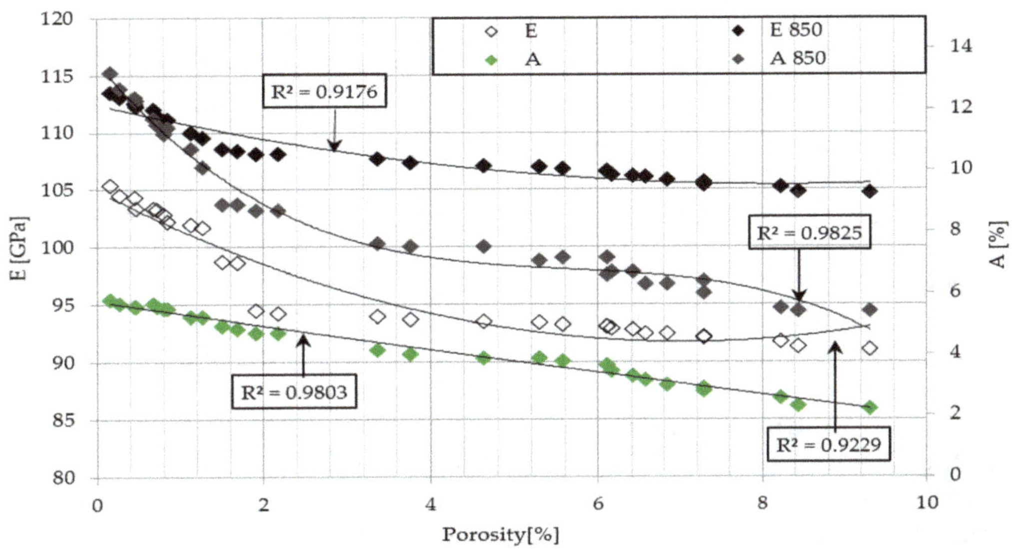

Figure 12. Influence of porosity on Young modulus and elongation of as-build and heat treated at 850 °C samples.

The analysis of the obtained results revealed that samples build in the ZX orientation compared with XZ had a higher yield strength, tensile strength, and elongation, if the volume of the microstructure defects does not exceed 2%. Vertical samples (ZX)—due to the layered structure—are seemingly more prone to initiation and cracks propagation than horizontal samples (XZ), however, they showed higher tensile strength and yield strength. The explanation of this phenomenon is related to the microstructure, especially to the columnar β grains. These grains grown perpendicular to successive layers of molten powder and in accordance with the direction of building the element. As a result, in the XZ samples, tensile force direction was perpendicular to the β grains, whereas in the ZX samples, the direction of the force was parallel. In vertical samples, the grains were axially extended, which had a positive effect on the strength properties of the whole sample. The same orientation between the columnar grains and the direction of the tensile forces led to a reduction of the grain boundary resistance, which no longer constituted an effective obstacle to the dislocation movement and which could be subject to greater distortion [48,49]. Reducing the energy density by reducing the laser beam power and increasing the scanning speed resulted in defects between successive layers of material [50,51]. For highly porous samples, force was applied parallel to the layers and caused pores deformation consistent with the direction of force, whereby the stress concentration around the pores was several times lower, and consequently, the material was less susceptible to the initiation and propagation of cracks.

Based on the microstructure and changes in mechanical properties analysis, presented in the paper, DMLS parameters, application of which guarantees the achievement of a biomaterial with properties consistent with ASTM F 1142, were indicated in Table 4.

Table 4. List of DMLS parameters and properties of Ti6Al4V alloy heat treated at 850 °C meeting the criteria of ASTM F 1142 standard for implantable biomaterials.

P [W]	V [mm/s]	Rm [MPa]		Re [MPa]		A [%]		E [GPa]		Es [J/mm³]	P [%]
		ZX	XZ	ZX	XZ	ZX	XZ	ZX	XZ		
150	500	1056 ± 13	1052 ± 12	954 ± 10	950 ± 8	13.4 ± 0.5	13.2 ± 0.6	106.5 ± 1.3	106.2 ± 0.6	100	0.46
170	500	1074 ± 13	1069 ±10	974 ± 9	973 ± 7	13.7 ± 0.6	13.6 ± 0.5	107.5 ± 0.7	107.5 ± 0.8	113	0.27
190	500	1080 ± 10	1077 ± 11	982 ± 9	980 ± 9	14.3 ± 06	14.1 ± 0.7	108.0 ± 1.2	108.7 ± 0.5	127	0.16
210	700	1062 ± 12	1055 ± 10	962 ± 9	954 ± 8	13.5 ± 0.5	13.3 ± 0.8	107.2 ± 1.0	107.4 ± 0.9	100	0.45

3.3. Microstructure Characterisation

Unique thermal features, such as heat input, large temperature gradients, and high cooling ratesdramatically affected as-built martensitic α′microstructures and led to high residual stresses. Annealing at 650 °C for 2 h was intended to remove residual stress from the material. The use of this heat treatment resulted in the decomposition of a small amount of the martensitic phase in the α + β equilibrium phase, as well as the nucleation and slow increase of the α phase at the boundaries of martensitic needles. Nevertheless, the microstructure has not changed significantly compared to untreated, and the columnar grain structure has been retained. This is due to the fact that rapid cooling during the DMLS process leads to the formation of dislocation within the alloy. These defects have an inhibitory effect on the α-phase distribution. Furthermore, during annealing at 650 °C, which is significantly below than β–transus, the driving force of the phase distribution is insufficient. The microstructure after heat treatment at 650 °C still remained needle-shaped (Figure 13a). The only noticeable change was the increase in grain thickness to 0.6 μm (Table 5).

The microstructure of samples annealed at 750 °C for 2 h and cooled together with the furnace clearly indicate the decomposition of fine martensite into α and β mixture, in which the α phase occurs in the form of fine needles (Figure 13b). The analyzed microstructure consisted of a smaller amount of α′ martensite embedded in the more stable α and β phase. According to the findings of Shunmugavel et al., the upper limit of martensite decay in the Ti6Al4V alloy is 800 °C, which means that only above this temperature martensite is completely decomposed into the phases α and β [14]. The average thickness of α′ plates was 1.2 μm.

Heating of samples at 850 °C for 2 h significantly influenced the changes of the microstructure—the α′ phase completely decomposed into the mixture of α and β phases. The α grain thickness increased to the average value 1.5 μm. Heat treatment carried out at 850 °C did not change the morphology of the primary β grains. The reason for this is the coexistence of the α + β phases, which mutually inhibit their further growth. Different orientation of the growth of adjoining grains prevents the migration of boundaries in the axial direction, which leads to slight changes in their shape (Figure 13c).

The increase of the annealing temperature to 950 °C resulted in the reduction of the inhibitory effect of the grain boundaries—the structure was transformed into coarse grains. The average width of the plate grains of the α-phase after annealing was approximately 2.3 μm. This was the result of the increase in the driving force of the α → β phase decay and the joining of the adjacent β grains under the influence of high temperature. In the fully lamellar microstructure, the size of the α colony and the alternately packed α and β plates with a clear orientation define the grain and have a strong influence on the size and length of the slip, determining the ductility of the Ti6Al4V alloy (Figure 13d). Thus, after a heat treatment at 950 °C, a lower strain was expected during the static tensile test.

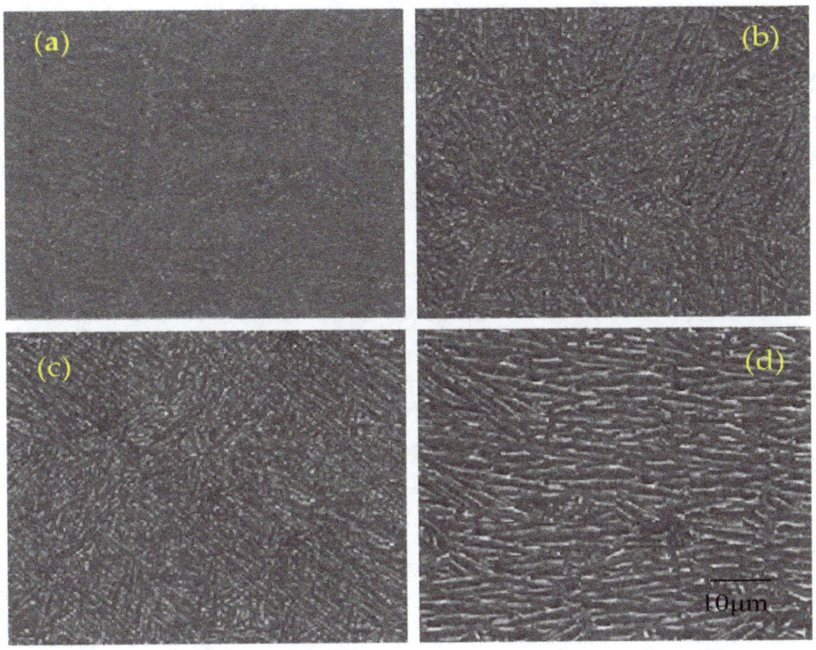

Figure 13. SEM images of microstructure of heat treated samples: (**a**) 650 °C, (**b**) 750 °C, (**c**) 850 °C, and (**d**) 950 °C.

Table 5. Change the grain size in respect of energy density and temperature.

Heat Treatment	Energy Density [J/mm^3]			
	33	100	233	Average
AB	0.17 ± 0.05	0.25 ± 0.08	0.38 ± 0.06	0.27 ± 0.11
650 °C	0.42 ± 0.11	0.57 ± 0.12	0.81 ± 0.11	0.60 ± 0.22
750 °C	0.81 ± 0.10	1.16 ± 0.15	1.63 ± 0.09	1.20 ± 0.41
850 °C	1.17 ± 0.12	1.49 ± 0.13	2.11 ± 0.11	1.59 ± 0.48
950 °C	1.83 ± 0.15	2.31 ± 0.18	2.80 ± 0.21	2.31 ± 0.49

The analysis of the microstructure made of Ti6Al4V alloys produced under heat treatment was conducted by phase analysis (Figure 14). XRD spectra clearly presented that the α′ phase was the dominant fraction in as-build samples. All peaks untreated material were indexed as the α′ phase, while the β phase was not detected. Both martensitic phases α and α′ have similar crystallographic cell parameters. However, since fast cooling may promote martensitic transformation, it was expected that the hexagonal hcp phase in the material was acicular martensite. Therefore, metastable martensite remained as the only phase present at room temperature in the alloy Ti6Al4V produced by DMLS technology. In the material heat treated at 650 °C, the main peaks remained the same as in the as-build, however peaks (110) β-Ti2θ = 38.57° and (211) β-Ti (2θ = 71.02°) corresponded to the β phase. A similar pattern was obtained for heat treatment at 750 °C, only the intensity of α–peaks increased due to the increase in grain thickness. Figure 9 presented phase analysis for V oriented samples melted with an energy density of 100 J/mm^3.

Heat treatment at 850 °C resulted in complete decomposition of α′ martensite into α + β phase and this influenced the XRD pattern obtained in the study, because peaks 2θ = 35.40°, 39.37°, 40.47°, 53.31°, and 63.54° corresponded to the plate α-phase, not the α′ phase. The peaks of this phase showed strong intensity, which was related to the increase in grain size. The intensity of peaks (110) β-Ti

(2θ = 38.57°) and (211) β-Ti (2θ = 71.02°) also increased, which clearly indicates that a significant amount of β phase increased due to the redistribution of alloying elements. The XRD of the annealed material at 950 °C showed that the microstructure of the DMLS alloy formed a mixture of α + β phases. This unambiguously confirms that the transformation temperature of β–transus is higher than 950 °C.

The change of microstructure as a result of heat treatment affects not only mechanical properties, but also corrosion resistance. According to the literature, as-build samples show a poorer corrosion resistance compared to heat treated samples. Based on published studies, it can be concluded that the corrosion resistance depends on the volume of β phase—the more that is in the structure, the higher the corrosion resistance [52,53].

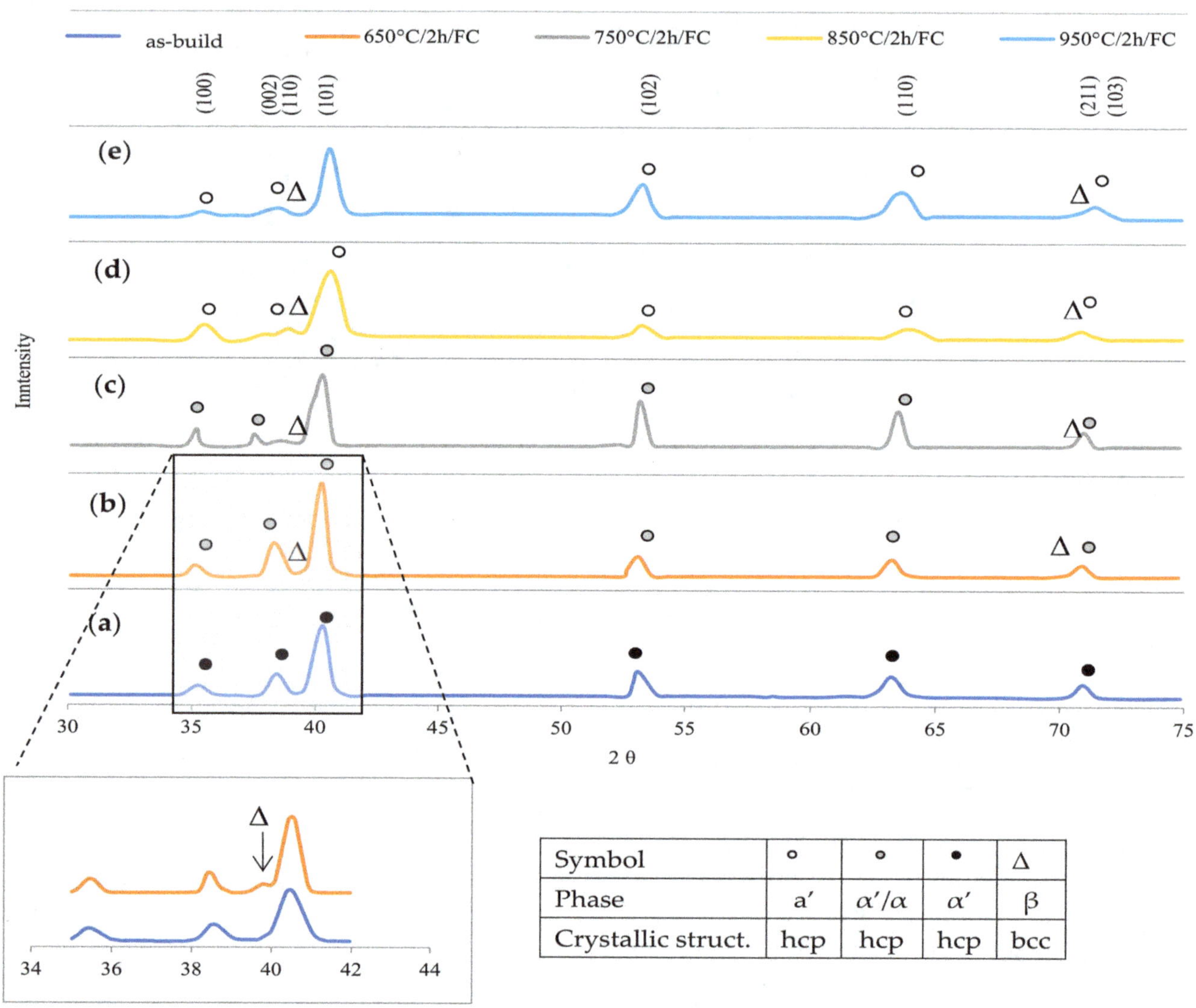

Figure 14. XRD spectrum of Ti6Al4V alloy DMLS: (**a**) as-build, (**b**) annealing at 650 °C, (**c**) annealed at 750 °C, (**d**) 850 °C, and (**e**) 950 °C for 2 h, cooled with a furnace.

4. Conclusions

This work aimed to determine the influence of DMLS parameters on the resulting properties of the obtained material and to assess the effect of different heat treatment temperatures on the structure and mechanical properties ofsamples oriented vertically and horizontally. The results of completed research are the following conclusions:

- The results of porosity in samples made with DMLS technology differs from those presented in the literature; however, it should be noted that the micro-CT porosity analysis, which was carried out in this work, allowed the assessment of total porosity, whereas in studies presented in the data of the reference, these measurements were made on the basis of fragmentary image analysis or the Archimedes method, which allows the estimation of apparent density.
- At low energy density (33–71 J/mm^3), the porosity varies from 9.31% to 3.37%; the increase in energy density from 78 J/mm^3 to 127 J/mm^3 causing the porosity in the range of 0.84–0.16%; above 127 J/mm^3, the porosity increase again as the effect of the material overheating.
- The microstructure created in the DMLS process is fine-grained α' martensite, which determines high strength properties and low ductility; this microstructure—due to the ferromagnetic properties of martensite—should not be considered as a biomaterial and requires operations whose aim is to change the microstructure to a biphasic phase and to obtain parameters compliant with the normative ones.
- The tests showed that the most favorable combination of mechanical properties and structure without the α' phase may be obtained by annealing the material in the temperature range 850–950 °C for 2 h, cooled together with the furnace.
- After heat treatment, the samples showed YS and UTS similar to those for wrought and annealed Ti6Al4V—this was the effect of the coexistence of the α and β phases.
- Tensile strength tests showed the sensitivity of the as-build material for porosity and orientation of samples, which results from the creation of columnar grains growing along the boundaries of the prior β grains.
- Heat treatment influenced the reduction of tensile (Rm) and yield strength (Re) parameters with a simultaneous increase of elongation (A) and Young's modulus (E), additionally, heat treatment at 850 °C resulted in homogenization of the microstructure and elimination of anisotropy resulting from different directions of stretching samples and layering.
- The highest density of samples (porosity not exceeding 0.5%) was obtained for samples melted with energy density in the range of 100–127 J/mm^3.
- The analysis of the obtained results revealed that samples build in the ZX orientation compared with XZ had a higher yield strength, tensile strength, and elongation, if the volume of microstructure defects does not exceed 2%.
- Regardless of the energy density, the microstructure obtained in the DMLS process consists of martensite needles, however, the higher the energy density, the larger the grain size; the size of grains also grows with the increasing temperature of heat treatment, which affects the reduction of strength properties and increase of elongation.

Acknowledgments: Studies have been financed from the funds for science of Ministry of Science and Higher Education of Republic of Poland, project no. No S/WM/1/2017.

References

1. Wu, S.Q.; Lu, Y.J.; Gan, Y.L.; Huang, T.T.; Zhao, C.Q.; Lin, J.J.; Lin, J.X. Microstructural evolution and microhardness of a selective-laser-melted Ti-6Al-4V alloy after post heat treatments. *J. Alloy. Compd.* **2016**, *672*, 643–652. [CrossRef]
2. Popovich, A.; Sufiiarov, V.; Borisov, E.; Polozov, I. Microstructure and mechanical properties of Ti-6Al-4V manufactured by SLM. *Key Eng. Mater.* **2015**, *651*, 677–682. [CrossRef]
3. Galarraga, H.; Lados, D.A.; Dehoff, R.R.; Kirka, M.M.; Nandwana, P. Effects of the microstructure and porosity on properties of Ti-6Al-4V ELI alloy fabricated by electron beam melting (EBM). *Add. Manuf.* **2016**, *10*, 47–57. [CrossRef]

4. Hrabe, N.; Quinn, T. Effects of processing on microstructure and mechanical properties of a titanium alloy (Ti-6Al-4V) fabricated using electron beam melting (EBM), Part 2: Energy input, orientation, and location. *Mater. Sci. Eng. A* **2013**, *573*, 271–277. [CrossRef]
5. Sallica-Leva, E.; Caram, R.; Jardini, A.L.; Fogagnolo, J.B. Ductility improvement due to martensite α' decomposition in porous Ti-6Al-4V parts produced by selective laser melting for orthopedic implants. *J. Mech. Behav. Biomed.* **2016**, *54*, 149–158. [CrossRef] [PubMed]
6. Leuders, S.; Vollmer, M.; Brenne, F.; Tröster, T.; Niendorf, T. Fatigue strength prediction for titanium alloy TiAl6V4 manufactured by selective laser melting. *Metall. Mater. Trans. A* **2015**, *46*, 3816–3823. [CrossRef]
7. Qiu, C.; Adkins, N.J.; Attallah, M.M. Microstructure and tensile properties of selectively laser-melted and of HIPed laser-melted Ti-6Al-4V. *Mater. Sci. Eng. A* **2013**, *578*, 230–239. [CrossRef]
8. Vandenbroucke, B.; Kruth, J.P. Selective laser melting of biocompatible metals for rapid manufacturing of medical parts. *Rapid Prototyping J.* **2007**, *13*, 196–203. [CrossRef]
9. Calignano, F. Design optimization of supports for overhanging structures in aluminum and titanium alloys by selective laser melting. *Mater. Des.* **2014**, *64*, 203–213. [CrossRef]
10. Simonelli, M.; Tse, Y.Y.; Tuck, C. Effect of the build orientation on the mechanical properties and fracture modes of DMLS Ti-6Al-4V. *Mater. Sci. Eng. A* **2014**, *616*, 1–11. [CrossRef]
11. Xu, W.; Sun, S.; Elambasseril, J.; Liu, Q.; Brandt, M.; Qian, M. Ti-6Al-4V additively manufactured by selective laser melting with superior mechanical properties. *JOM* **2015**, *67*, 668–673. [CrossRef]
12. Kok, Y.; Tan, X.P.; Wang, P.; Nai, M.L.S.; Loh, N.H.; Liu, E.; Tor, S.B. Anisotropy and heterogeneity of microstructure and mechanical properties in metal additive manufacturing: A critical review. *Mater. Des.* **2018**, *139*, 565–586. [CrossRef]
13. Sallica-Leva, E.; Jardini, A.L.; Fogagnolo, J.B. Microstructure and mechanical behavior of porous Ti-6Al-4V parts obtained by selective laser melting. *J. Mech. Behav. Biomed.* **2013**, *26*, 98–108. [CrossRef] [PubMed]
14. Shunmugavel, M.; Polishetty, A.; Littlefair, G. Microstructure and Mechanical Properties of Wrought and Additive Manufactured Ti-6Al-4V Cylindrical Bars. *Proc. Tech.* **2015**, *20*, 231–236. [CrossRef]
15. Murr, L.E.; Quinones, S.A.; Gaytan, S.M.; Lopez, M.I.; Rodela, A.; Martinez, E.Y.; Wicker, R.B. Microstructure and mechanical behavior of Ti-6Al-4V produced by rapid-layer manufacturing, for biomedical applications. *J. Mech. Behav. Biomed. Mater.* **2009**, *2*, 20–32. [CrossRef] [PubMed]
16. Tao, P.; Zhong, J.; Li, H.; Hu, Q.; Gong, S.; Xu, Q. Microstructure, Mechanical Properties, and Constitutive Models for Ti-6Al-4V Alloy Fabricated by Selective Laser Melting (SLM). *Metals* **2019**, *9*, 447. [CrossRef]
17. Greitemeier, D.; Dalle Donne, C.; Syassen, F.; Eufinger, J.; Melz, T. Effect of surface roughness on fatigue performance of additive manufactured Ti-6Al-4V. *Mater. Sci. Tech. Ser.* **2016**, *32*, 629–634. [CrossRef]
18. Zhang, Y.; Bernard, A.; Harik, R.; Karunakaran, K.P. Build orientation optimization for multi-part production in additive manufacturing. *J. Intell. Manuf.* **2017**, *28*, 1393–1407. [CrossRef]
19. Wauthle, R.; Vrancken, B.; Beynaerts, B.; Jorissen, K.; Schrooten, J.; Kruth, J.P.; Van Humbeeck, J. Effects of build orientation and heat treatment on the microstructure and mechanical properties of selective laser melted Ti-6Al-4V lattice structures. *Add. Manuf.* **2015**, *5*, 77–84.
20. Carroll, B.E.; Palmer, T.A.; Beese, A.M. Anisotropic tensile behavior of Ti-6Al-4V components fabricated with directed energy deposition additive manufacturing. *Acta Mater.* **2015**, *87*, 309–320. [CrossRef]
21. Mezzetta, J.; Choi, J.P.; Milligan, J.; Danovitch, J.; Chekir, N.; Bois-Brochu, A.; Brochu, M. Microstructure-Properties Relationships of Ti-6Al-4V Parts Fabricated by Selective Laser Melting. *Int. J. Precis. Eng. Manuf. Green Technol.* **2018**, *5*, 605–612. [CrossRef]
22. Li, P.; Warner, D.H.; Fatemi, A.; Phan, N. Critical assessment of the fatigue performance of additively manufactured Ti-6Al-4V and perspective for future research. *Int. J. Fatigue* **2016**, *85*, 130–143. [CrossRef]
23. Patterson, A.E.; Messimer, S.L.; Farrington, P.A. Overhanging features and the SLM/DMLS residual stresses problem: Review and future research need. *Technologies* **2017**, *5*, 15. [CrossRef]
24. Vrancken, B.; Thijs, L.; Kruth, J.P.; Van Humbeeck, J. Heat treatment of Ti-6Al-4V produced by Selective Laser Melting: Microstructure and mechanical properties. *J. Alloys Compd.* **2012**, *541*, 177–185. [CrossRef]
25. Vilaro, T.; Colin, C.; Bartout, J.D. As-fabricated and heat-treated microstructures of the Ti-6Al-4V alloy processed by selective laser melting. *Metall. Mater. Trans. A* **2014**, *42*, 3190–3199. [CrossRef]
26. Liu, Q.C.; Elambasseril, J.; Sun, S.J.; Leary, M.; Brandt, M.; Sharp, P.K. The effect of manufacturing defects on the fatigue behavior of Ti-6Al-4V specimens fabricated using selective laser melting. *Adv. Mat. Resh.* **2014**, *891*, 1519–1524.

27. Prabhu, A.W.; Vincent, T.; Chaudhary, A.; Zhang, W.; Babu, S.S. Effect of microstructure and defects on fatigue behavior of directed energy deposited Ti-6Al-4V. *Sci. Technol. Weld. Joi.* **2015**, *20*, 659–669. [CrossRef]
28. Razavi, S.M.J.; Bordonaro, G.G.; Ferro, P.; Torgersen, J.; Berto, F. Porosity effect on tensile behavior of Ti-6Al-4V specimens produced by laser engineered net shaping technology. *Proc. Inst. Mech. Eng. Part C: J. Mech. Eng. Sci.* **2018**. [CrossRef]
29. Gong, H.; Rafi, K.; Gu, H.; Ram, G.J.; Starr, T.; Stucker, B. Influence of defects on mechanical properties of Ti-6Al-4V components produced by selective laser melting and electron beam melting. *Mater. Des.* **2015**, *86*, 545–554. [CrossRef]
30. Zhang, G.; Wang, J.; Zhang, H. Research Progress of Balling Phenomena in Selective Laser Melting. *Found. Technol.* **2017**, *2*, 2.
31. Kasperovich, G.; Hausmann, J. Improvement of fatigue resistance and ductility of TiAl6V4 processed by selective laser melting. *J. Mater. Process. Tech.* **2015**, *220*, 202–214. [CrossRef]
32. Aboulkhair, N.T.; Everitt, N.M.; Ashcroft, I.; Tuck, C. Reducing porosity in AlSi10Mg parts processed by selective laser melting. *Add. Manuf.* **2014**, *1*, 77–86. [CrossRef]
33. Thijs, L.; Verhaeghe, F.; Craeghs, T.; Van Humbeeck, J.; Kruth, J.P. A study of the microstructural evolution during selective laser melting of Ti-6Al-4V. *Acta Mater.* **2010**, *58*, 3303–3312. [CrossRef]
34. Weingarten, C.; Buchbinder, D.; Pirch, N.; Meiners, W.; Wissenbach, K.; Poprawe, R. Formation and reduction of hydrogen porosity during selective laser melting of AlSi10Mg. *J. Mater. Process. Tech.* **2015**, *221*, 112–120. [CrossRef]
35. Brånemark, P.I. Osseointegration and its experimental background. *J. Prosth. Dent.* **1983**, *50*, 399–410. [CrossRef]
36. Rack, H.J.; Qazi, J.I. Titanium alloys for biomedical applications. *Mater. Sci. Eng. C* **2006**, *26*, 1269–1277. [CrossRef]
37. Wang, J.L.; Liu, R.L.; Majumdar, T.; Mantri, S.A.; Ravi, V.A.; Banerjee, R.; Birbilis, N. A closer look at the in vitro electrochemical characterization of titanium alloys for biomedical applications using in-situ methods. *Acta Biomater.* **2017**, *54*, 469–478. [CrossRef] [PubMed]
38. Harun, W.S.W.; Kamariah, M.S.I.N.; Muhamad, N.; Ghani, S.A.C.; Ahmad, F.; Mohamed, Z. A review of powder additive manufacturing processes for metallic biomaterials. *Powder Technol.* **2018**, *327*, 128–151. [CrossRef]
39. Karlsson, J.; Norell, M.; Ackelid, U.; Engqvist, H.; Lausmaa, J. Surface oxidation behavior of Ti-6Al-4V manufactured by Electron Beam Melting (EBM®). *J. Manuf. Process.* **2015**, *17*, 120–126. [CrossRef]
40. Du Plessis, A.; Kouprianoff, D.P.; Yadroitsava, I.; Yadroitsev, I. Mechanical Properties and In Situ Deformation Imaging of Microlattices Manufactured by Laser Based Powder Bed Fusion. *Materials* **2018**, *11*, 1663. [CrossRef]
41. Maamoun, A.; Xue, Y.; Elbestawi, M.; Veldhuis, S. Effect of selective laser melting process parameters on the quality of al alloy parts: Powder characterization, density, surface roughness, and dimensional accuracy. *Materials* **2018**, *11*, 2343. [CrossRef] [PubMed]
42. Maamoun, A.; Xue, Y.; Elbestawi, M.; Veldhuis, S. The Effect of Selective Laser Melting Process Parameters on the Microstructure and Mechanical Properties of Al6061 and AlSi10Mg Alloys. *Materials* **2019**, *12*, 12. [CrossRef] [PubMed]
43. Yu, M.; Yi, J.; Liu, J.; Li, S.; Wu, G.; Wu, L. Effect of electropolishing on electrochemical behaviours of titanium alloy Ti-10V-2Fe-3Al. *J. Wuhan Univ. Technol. Mater. Sci. Ed.* **2011**, *26*, 469–477. [CrossRef]
44. Han, J.; Yang, J.; Yu, H.; Yin, J.; Gao, M.; Wang, Z.; Zeng, X. Microstructure and mechanical property of selective laser melted Ti6Al4V dependence on laser energy density. *Rapid Prototyp. J.* **2017**, *23*, 217–226. [CrossRef]
45. Laquai, R.; Müller, B.R.; Kasperovich, G.; Haubrich, J.; Requena, G.; Bruno, G. X-ray refraction distinguishes unprocessed powder from empty pores in selective laser melting Ti-6Al-4V. *Mater. Res. Lett.* **2018**, *6*, 130–135. [CrossRef]
46. Dilip, J.J.S.; Zhang, S.; Teng, C.; Zeng, K.; Robinson, C.; Pal, D.; Stucker, B. Influence of processing parameters on the evolution of melt pool, porosity, and microstructures in Ti-6Al-4V alloy parts fabricated by selective laser melting. *Progress Add. Manuf.* **2017**, *2*, 157–167. [CrossRef]

47. Singh, A.P.; Yang, F.; Torrens, R.; Gabbitas, B. Solution treatment of Ti-6Al-4V alloy produced by consolidating blended powder mixture using a powder compact extrusion route. *Mater. Sci. Eng. A* **2018**, *712*, 157–165. [CrossRef]
48. Brezinová, J.; Hudák, R.; Guzanová, A.; Draganovská, D.; Ižaríková, G.; Koncz, J. Direct Metal Laser Sintering of Ti6Al4V for Biomedical Applications: Microstructure, Corrosion Properties and Mechanical Treatment of Implants. *Metals* **2016**, *6*, 171. [CrossRef]
49. Zhao, X.; Li, S.; Zhang, M.; Liu, Y.; Sercombe, T.B.; Wang, S.; Murr, L.E. Comparison of the microstructures and mechanical properties of Ti-6Al-4V fabricated by selective laser melting and electron beam melting. *Mater. Des.* **2016**, *95*, 21–31. [CrossRef]
50. Fan, Z.; Feng, H. Study on selective laser melting and heat treatment of Ti-6Al-4V alloy. *Results Phys.* **2018**, *10*, 660–664. [CrossRef]
51. Wang, D.; Dou, W.; Yang, Y. Research on selective laser melting of Ti6Al4V: Surface morphologies, optimized processing zone, and ductility improvement mechanism. *Metals* **2018**, *8*, 471. [CrossRef]
52. Dai, N.; Zhang, L.C.; Zhang, J.; Chen, Q.; Wu, M. Corrosion behavior of selective laser melted Ti-6Al-4V alloy in NaCl solution. *Corros. Sci.* **2016**, *102*, 484–489. [CrossRef]
53. Dai, N.; Zhang, J.; Chen, Y.; Zhang, L.C. Heat treatment degrading the corrosion resistance of selective laser melted Ti-6Al-4V alloy. *J. Electrochem. Soc.* **2017**, *164*, 428–434. [CrossRef]

7

Does the Hirsch Index Improve Research Quality in the Field of Biomaterials? A New Perspective in the Biomedical Research Field

Saverio Affatato * and Massimiliano Merola

Laboratorio di Tecnologia Medica, IRCCS-Istituto Ortopedico Rizzoli, Via di Barbiano, 1/10 40136 Bologna, Italy; massimiliano.merola@tecno.ior.it

* Correspondence: affatato@tecno.ior.it

Abstract: Orthopaedic implants offer valuable solutions to many pathologies of bones and joints. The research in this field is driven by the aim of realizing durable and biocompatible devices; therefore, great effort is spent on material analysis and characterization. As a demonstration of the importance assumed by tribology in material devices, wear and friction are two of the main topics of investigation for joint prostheses. Research is led and supported by public institutions, whether universities or research centers, based on the laboratories' outputs. Performance criteria assessing an author's impact on research contribute somewhat to author inflation per publication. The need to measure the research activity of an institution is an essential goal and this leads to the development of indicators capable of giving a rating to the publication that disseminates them. The main purpose of this work was to observe the variation of the Hirsch Index (h-index) when the position of the authors is considered. To this end, we conducted an analysis evaluating the h-index by excluding the intermediate positions. We found that the higher the h value, the larger the divergence between this value and the corrected one. The correction relies on excluding publications for which the author does not have a relevant position. We propose considering the authorship order in a publication in order to obtain more information on the impact that authors have on their research field. We suggest giving the users of researcher registers (e.g., Scopus, Google Scholar) the possibility to exclude from the h-index evaluation the objects of research where the scientist has a marginal position.

Keywords: h-index; bibliometric indicators; biomaterials; quality of research; citations

---

1. Introduction

Joint replacement surgery is a successful and consolidated branch of orthopaedics. Its progressive achievement in alleviating pain and disability, helping patients to return to an active life, is reliant on efficient relationships between clinicians and researchers working across transverse areas of medicine and science [1]. The purpose of tribology research applied to orthopaedics is the minimization and elimination of losses resulting from friction and wear [2]. The research of new biomaterials plays an important role, and as a consequence, in vitro tests for such materials are of great importance [3]. The knowledge of the laboratory wear rate is an important aspect in the preclinical validation of prostheses. Research and development of wear-resistant materials continues to be a high priority [4–6]. Clinical research designed to carefully evaluate the performance of new materials intended to reduce wear is essential to ascertaining their efficacy and preventing the possibility of unexpected failure [7,8]. Unfortunately, failures and revision surgeries still constitute the main clinical problems related to total joint replacement [9]. The research is therefore constantly pushed to find new solutions to wear-related issues and to identify new high-standard materials. The public institutions of research receive national funding on the bases of their results and are therefore constrained to obtain high levels of quality assessment [10]. Evaluation of scientific publications is the criterion used by the universities and research institutes to measure the merit and value of researchers and academics [11], and it has a crucial impact on research funds distribution [12–14]. The need to measure the research quality of institutions is an essential goal, which has led to the development of indicators capable of giving a rating to publications. These indicators are used in bibliometric disciplines to quantitatively evaluate the quality and diffusion of scientific production within the scientific community. In order to obtain funds within the orthopaedic community, there is a strong pressure on researchers to publish even if the merit of the study is unreliable; this is because objectives are set to achieve a certain number of publications instead of focusing on the quality of the research [15].

There are two main ways to evaluate scientific research:

- Bibliometric indicators are quantitative methods based on the number of times a publication is cited. The higher the number of citations, the larger the group of researchers who have used this work as a reference and, thus, the stronger its impact on the scientific community;
- Peer review is a qualitative method based on the judgement of experts. A small number of researchers, specialized in the field of the work, analyze and evaluate the scientific value of a publication.

Eugene Garfield proposed the Impact Factor (IF) in 1955 [16,17] with the intent to help scientists look for bibliographic references; the IF indicator was quickly adopted to assess the influence of journals and, not long after, of individual scientists. A journal's impact factor is the ratio of two elements: the numerator is the number of citations in the current year to items published in the previous two years, and the denominator is the total number of articles published in the same two years [16,17]. It is published by the ISI-Thomson publisher on the basis of the Web of Science database and measures the frequency with which an article published in a journal is cited by other periodicals over a specific period of time (two years after its release). This measure is used as an appraisal of the importance of a magazine compared with others in the same sector: the higher the impact factor, the more authoritative the magazine [18]. The impact factors of each magazine can be consulted on the website of the Journal of Citation Reports (JCR) [19].

The impact factor is widely used as an index of academic research quality. It is also applied as a winning criterion for the granting of funds and incentives, or as a basis for the evaluation of a scholar or a professional in public competitions [11]. Yet the impact factor is an indicator for measuring the impact of a magazine in its specific disciplinary area, certainly not for evaluating the authors, and this latter use has been criticized for many reasons. In order to overcome the problems of the impact factor, in 2005, Jorge E. Hirsch [20] proposed a new index, known as the h-index or Hirsch index, as a single-number criterion to evaluate the scientific output of a researcher. It combines a measure of quantity (publications) and impact (citations). In other words, a scientist has index h if h-many of his articles have at least h-many citations each, and the other articles have fewer than h-many citations each [21]. It performs better than other single-number criteria previously used to evaluate the scientific output of a researcher (impact factor, total number of documents, total number of citations, citation per paper rate, and number of highly cited papers) [22]. The h-index is easy to understand and can be easily gained by anyone with access to the Thomson ISI Web of Science [22]. Actually, the h-index has been reviewed as one of the most reliable criteria for evaluating the scientific outputs of researchers [23]. This index has many flaws: the articles with citations less than the h-index value are excluded from the calculation. The number of citations is influenced by self-citations and colleague citations, meaning that its value can be increased by recommendation to friends and colleagues [23–25]. There are many circumstances where the h-index provides misleading information on the impact of an author. However, this popular bibliometric indicator does not consider multiple co-authorship nor author position [11,26]. To our knowledge, no policy guides author order in biomedical publications. The position of an author, controversies about author order, and disagreements on the involvement of the last author are constantly debated; thus, it is worth analyzing the relationship between author position and bibliometric indicators [27]. The contribution of an author to a research project is not always clear, especially when a manuscript is attributed to a large group [28].

Rating and weighting of research value is not an easy task, as history shows; often, what is believed to be modern and mainstream research will yield highly rated papers but is not always a guarantee of innovation and scientific progress [15]. With this in mind, and to go more into depth in this matter, we produced a statistical evaluation of the h-index on a cohort of 60 authors belonging to the biomedical field, accounting for only given positions. In detail, three modified h-values were evaluated: considering only the First (F) and Second (S) authorships (referred to as FS); only the F and the Last (L) authorships (referred to as FL); and the F, S, and L positions (referred to as FSL). The main goal of this work was to implement an algorithm that can calculate a modified h-index considering the author's position in an article.

Different approaches are available to decide the author order, like sorting them alphabetically or listing them in descending order according to their contribution [29]. Several approaches may be used to assess the contribution of an author to a paper [30]. In the "sequence-determines-credit" (SDC) system, the author order reflects the declining importance of their contribution. The "equal contribution" approach uses alphabetical order and implies identical involvement. The "first-last-emphasis" norm underlines the importance of the last author. Using the "percent-contribution-indicated" implies detailing each author's impact.

The convention used in the biomedical field of research, as reported in the literature [27], is as follows: the first author conducts the majority of the work; the last author could be the senior member of the group and usually leads the research; co-authors, those between the first and last, are ranked in order of their input to the work; the corresponding authors—typically senior scholars—communicate with editors and readers. With this premise, we considered the first, the second, and the last authors as the main contributors to biomedical research.

2. Methods

A total of 60 authors from the biomedical field were selected as a cohort; 30 of them were obtained from an Italian scientist ranking system [31] and the other 30 were chosen from all around the world.

To obtain the modified h-index, an algorithm was implemented in MATLAB (MathWorks, Natick, MA, USA). The complete list of articles attributed to an author was extracted from the scopus.com webpage using the implemented feature called "Export all". The information extracted was limited to Authors, Title, and Citation Count. Each list was obtained in the csv extension; these lists were then imported into the workspace of MATLAB using the Import Tool App. Each author entry was analyzed to find out their position; thus, according to the excluding criterion, the publication was considered or not for the evaluation of h. Given that authors are frequently cited in different ways (e.g., Surname, Name; Surname, N.; Surname M.N., etc.), the investigation considered all different options. If a publication respected the inclusion criterion, its citation count was taken into account. The list of included citation counts was sorted in ascending order; thus, the h value was by evaluated considering the last position at which the citation count was higher than or equal to the position itself. In Figure 1, a flow chart of the exclusion process is shown.

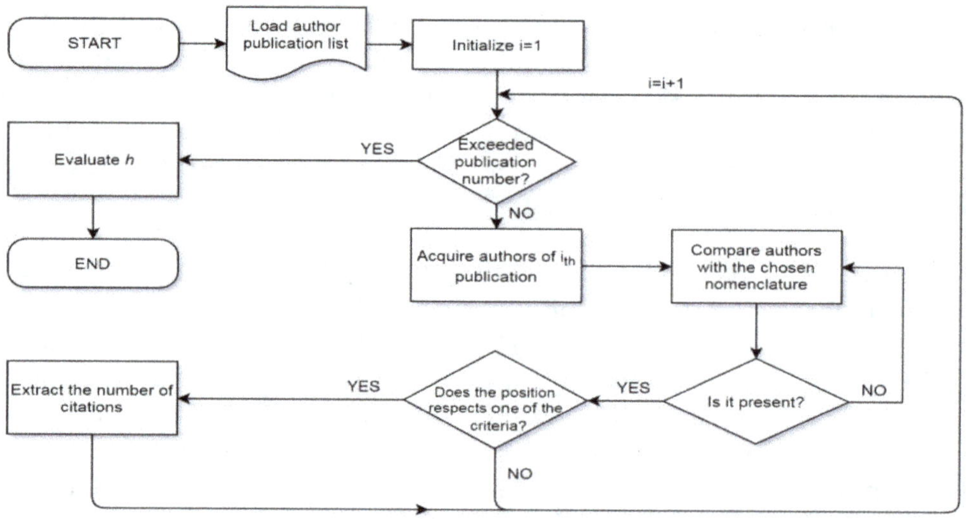

Figure 1. Flowchart of the process to obtain the corrected h-value.

3. Results

In Figure 2 are summarized the results obtained through the different exclusion criteria here studied. It is worth underlining the large divergences obtained comparing the higher h-values with their respective corrected ones.

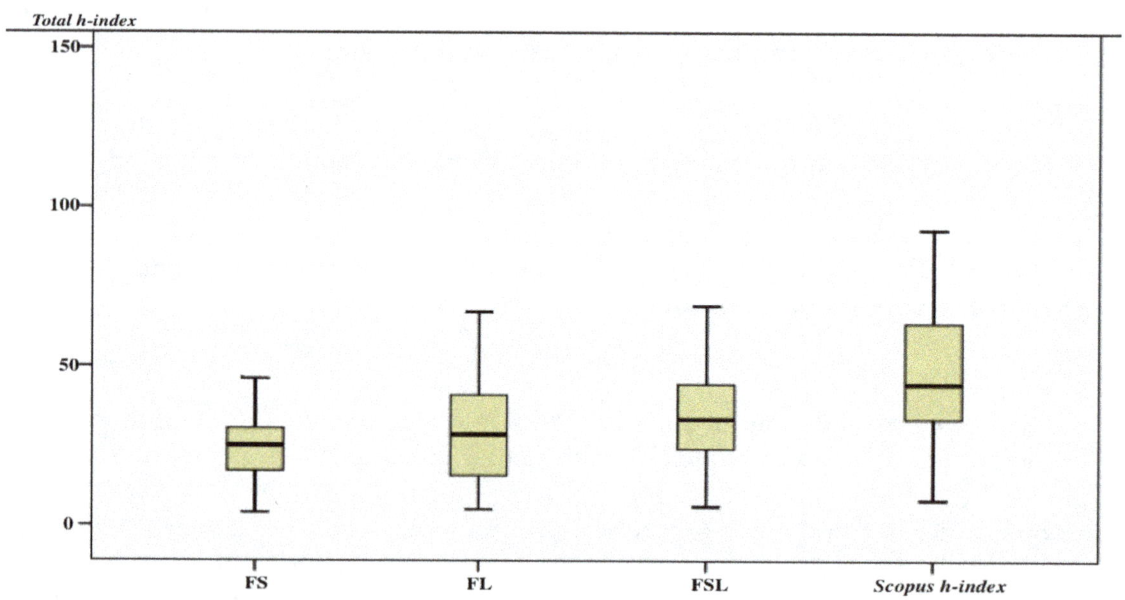

Figure 2. A box plot shows the modified h-index values (± standard deviation) for all authors considered in this study. The total h-index retrieved from Scopus is the highest of the four classifications.

From the results in Figure 2, we emphasize that on the basis of our exclusion criteria, the modified h-value decreases significantly.

To highlight these differences, the entire cohort was divided into three sub-cohorts. A first group of authors with h-value ranging from 0 to 35 (called Low), a second group from 36 to 50 (Middle), and a third group from 51 up to the maximum of 181 (High) were extracted, as shown in Figure 3.

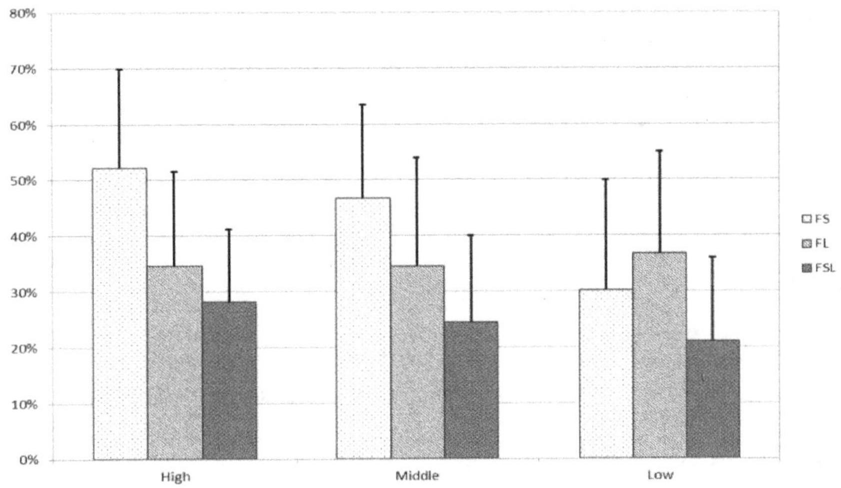

Figure 3. Histogram of the influence of the exclusion criteria on the h-values in sub-cohorts based on the starting h from Scopus.

In Figure 3 it is underlined that the High sub-cohort, starting from the highest value of h, is the most affected by all the exclusion criteria. This is especially true in the FS case, where it reaches a mean reduction of more than 50%. On the contrary, for the Low group, this exclusion criterion only decreases the h-value by roughly 30%. The Low group is more influenced by the exclusion of the publications where the authors are present as second authors (35% of decrease). The Middle group is more affected by the FS criterion, followed by the FL and the FSL.

In Figure 4, another histogram of the influence of the exclusion criteria is presented. In this case, the sub-cohorts were obtained based on the number of articles each author has. Considering the large range (from a minimum of 15 to a maximum of 1241), we chose to obtain a further group, yielding a total of four. The Low group collected the authors with up to 150 publications, the Middle group ranged from 151 to 300, High from 301 to 500, and Super High (S. High) from 501 to the maximum.

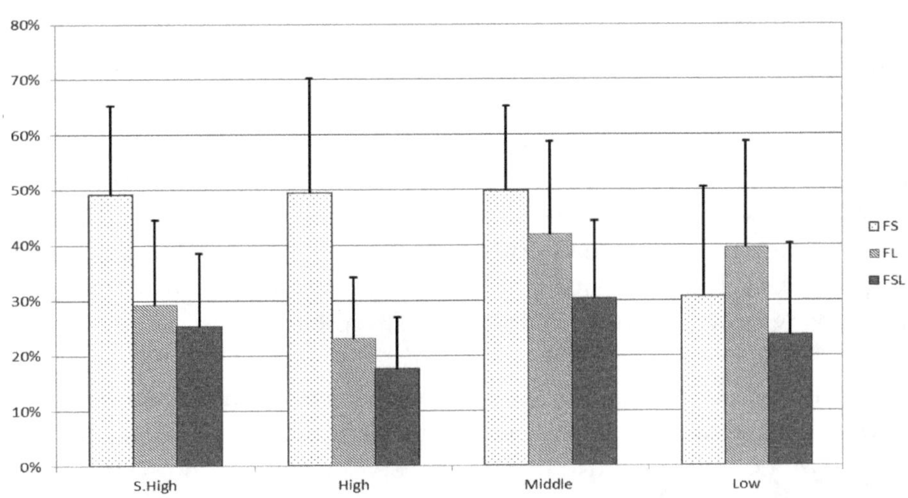

Figure 4. Histogram of the influence of the exclusion criteria on the h-values with sub-cohorts based on the number of publications.

This representation also outlined how the authors with a great number of publications are more affected by the exclusion criteria that do not take into consideration the articles where they are listed last among the authors. The first three sub-cohorts have a mean reduction of around 50% from their starting h-value when the FS criterion is applied. On the counter side, the FL criterion more greatly affects the Middle and the Low cohorts, reaching roughly 40% against the 30% and 20% of the Super High and High, respectively. The FSL criterion has a similar outcome on the group, but is stronger on the Middle and the Super High sub-cohorts, where it is about 30%.

4. Discussion and Conclusions

The term "impact factor" has gradually evolved to describe both journals' and authors' impacts. Journal impact factors generally involve relatively large populations of articles and citations. There are some ambiguities in the use of the h-index that could provoke changes in the publishing behaviour of scientists, such as increasing the number of self-citations distributed among the documents on the edge of the h-index [32]. Another disadvantage of the h-index is that not all citations of a researcher are involved in the calculation and its value may not increase with a rise in citations. Highly cited papers are significant for the evaluation of the h-index, but once they belong to the top h-many papers, the effect of number of citations they get is negligible [22]. Considering that the evaluators reduce scientific success to a single value, researchers can change their behaviour to increase these values, even by using unethical strategies [33]. Moreover, the scientific independent criterion of peer-review evaluation is going to be replaced by a system of private companies whose only feedback is the indicator number [11]. The authors believe that it is essential to continue analyzing the bibliometric indicators in order to establish their drawbacks and limitations and to propose improvements where necessary. It is especially relevant to determine in which cases this index could be biased, since it could have serious consequences for the assessment of scientists and academics. Our work proposes to be an insight into the bibliometric indicators and to help the scientific community and research institutions consider how authorship position impacts on the h-value.

The main purpose of this work was to observe the variation of the h-value when the position of authorship is considered. Therefore, an empirical analysis was conducted to assess the influence of an author's intermediate positions on their h-index. The results of this study showed that when the h-value is high, there is a large divergence between this value and the "corrected" one. We propose an improved method to consider the importance of the authorship in a publication in order to obtain a more profound understanding of the effective impact that an author has on their research field. This could be realized by giving users of researcher registers (e.g., Scopus, Google Scholar, etc.) the possibility to select which version of the h-index they want to analyze. The users should have the possibility, along with the already-implemented exclusion of self-citations, to exclude the publications where the authors have an intermediate position. It is worth noting that this correction should be considered for senior researchers, whereas young ones often have difficulties obtaining a relevant position in authorship. Thus, this exclusion can negatively affect the process of researcher renewal, discouraging young ones who would not see their efforts rewarded.

We believe that bibliometric indices should evolve with the aim of fairer evaluation of scientific productions. This would also be beneficial for funding distribution in the biomedical and orthopaedic research spheres, above all considering the threat of research cuts being to the detriment of patients' health. Alternatively, there is the risk that research toward new and more efficient biomaterials could stagnate due to a lack of capital granted to deserving scientists.

Author Contributions: S.A. conceived and designed the experiments; M.M. performed the software analyses; S.A. wrote the first draft of the manuscript; S.A. and M.M. analyzed the data; S.A. and M.M. wrote the final paper.

Acknowledgments: The authors thank Barbara Bordini for her help with statistical analyses.

References

1. Affatato, S. *Perspectives in Total Hip Arthroplasty: Advances in Biomaterials and their Tribological Interactions;* Affatato, S., Ed.; Elsevier Science: New York, NY, USA, 2014.
2. Viceconti, M.; Affatato, S.; Baleani, M.; Bordini, B.; Cristofolini, L.; Taddei, F. Pre-clinical validation of joint prostheses: A systematic approach. *J. Mech. Behav. Biomed. Mater.* **2009**, *2*, 120–127. [CrossRef] [PubMed]
3. Matsoukas, G.; Willing, R.; Kim, I.Y. Total Hip Wear Assessment: A Comparison Between Computational and In Vitro Wear Assessment Techniques Using ISO 14242 Loading and Kinematics. *J. Biomech. Eng.* **2009**, *131*, 41011. [CrossRef] [PubMed]
4. Oral, E.; Neils, A.; Muratoglu, O.K. High vitamin E content, impact resistant UHMWPE blend without loss of wear resistance. *J. Biomed. Mater. Res. B Appl. Biomater.* **2015**, *103*, 790–797. [CrossRef] [PubMed]
5. Ansari, F.; Ries, M.D.; Pruitt, L. Effect of processing, sterilization and crosslinking on UHMWPE fatigue fracture and fatigue wear mechanisms in joint arthroplasty. *J. Mech. Behav. Biomed. Mater.* **2016**, *53*, 329–340. [CrossRef] [PubMed]
6. Kyomoto, M.; Moro, T.; Yamane, S.; Saiga, K.; Watanabe, K.; Tanaka, S.; Ishihara, K. High fatigue and wear resistance of phospholipid polymer grafted cross-linked polyethylene with anti-oxidant reagent. In Proceedings of the 10th World Biomaterials Congress, Montréal, QC, Canada, 17–22 May 2016.
7. Essner, A.; Schmidig, G.; Wang, A. The clinical relevance of hip joint simulator testing: In vitro and in vivo comparisons. *Wear* **2005**, *259*, 882–886. [CrossRef]
8. Affatato, S.; Spinelli, M.; Zavalloni, M.; Mazzega-Fabbro, C.; Viceconti, M. Tribology and total hip joint replacement: Current concepts in mechanical simulation. *Med. Eng. Phys.* **2008**, *30*, 1305–1317. [CrossRef] [PubMed]
9. Ulrich, S.D.; Seyler, T.M.; Bennett, D.; Delanois, R.E.; Saleh, K.J.; Thongtrangan, I.; Stiehl, J.B. Total hip arthroplasties: What are the reasons for revision? *Int. Orthop.* **2008**, *32*, 597–604. [CrossRef] [PubMed]
10. Geuna, A.; Martin, B.R. University Research Evaluation and Funding: An International Comparison. *Minerva* **2003**, *41*, 277–304. [CrossRef]
11. Carpenter, C.R.; Cone, D.C.; Sarli, C.C. Using publication metrics to highlight academic productivity and research impact. *Acad. Emerg. Med.* **2014**, *21*, 1160–1172. [CrossRef] [PubMed]
12. Rezek, I.; McDonald, R.J.; Kallmes, D.F. Is the h-index Predictive of Greater NIH Funding Success Among Academic Radiologists? *Acad. Radiol.* **2011**, *18*, 1337–1340. [CrossRef]
13. Ciriminna, R.; Pagliaro, M. On the use of the h-index in evaluating chemical research. *Chem. Central J.* **2013**, *7*, 132. [CrossRef] [PubMed]
14. Narin, F.; Olivastro, D.; Stevens, K.A. Bibliometrics: Theory, practice and problems. *Eval. Rev.* **1994**, *18*, 65–76. [CrossRef]
15. Fayaz, H.C.; Haas, N.; Kellam, J.; Bavonratanavech, S.; Parvizi, J.; Dyer, G.; Smith, M. Improvement of research quality in the fields of orthopaedics and trauma—A global perspective. *Int. Orthop.* **2013**, *37*, 12051212. [CrossRef] [PubMed]
16. Garfield, E. The history and meaning of the journal impact factor. *JAMA* **2006**, *295*, 90–93. [CrossRef] [PubMed]
17. Garfield, E. The meaning of the Impact Factor. *Int. J. Clin. Health Psychol.* **2003**, *3*, 363–369.
18. Bordons, M.; Fernández, M.T.; Gómez, I. Advantages and limitations in the use of impact factor measures for the assessment of research performance. *Scientometrics* **2002**, *53*, 195–206. [CrossRef]
19. How Do I Find the Impact Factor and Rank for a Journal ?. Available online: https://guides.hsl.virginia.edu/faq-jcr (accessed on 12 October 2018).
20. Hirsch, J.E. An index to quantify an individual's scientific research output. *Proc. Natl. Acad. Sci. USA* **2005**, *102*, 16569–16572. [CrossRef] [PubMed]
21. Bornmann, L.; Daniel, H.D. Does the h-index for ranking of scientists really work? *Scientometrics* **2005**, *65*, 391–392. [CrossRef]
22. Costas, R.; Bordons, M. The h-index: Advantages, limitations and its relation with other bibliometric indicators at the micro level. *J. Informetr.* **2007**, *1*, 193–203. [CrossRef]
23. Ahangar, H.G.; Siamian, H.; Yaminfirooz, M. Evaluation of the scientific outputs of researchers with similar h index: A critical approach. *Acta Inform. Med.* **2014**, *22*, 255–258. [CrossRef] [PubMed]

24. Martin, B.R. Whither research integrity? Plagiarism, self-plagiarism and coercive citation in an age of research assessment. *Res. Policy* **2013**, *42*, 1005–1014. [CrossRef]
25. Foo, J.Y.A. Impact of excessive journal self-citations: A case study on the folia phoniatrica et logopaedica journal. *Sci. Eng. Ethics* **2011**, *17*, 65–73. [CrossRef] [PubMed]
26. Kreiman, G.; Maunsell, J.H.R. Nine Criteria for a Measure of Scientific Output. *Front. Comput. Neurosci.* **2011**, *5*, 1–6. [CrossRef] [PubMed]
27. Du, J.; Tang, X.L. Perceptions of author order versus contribution among researchers with different professional ranks and the potential of harmonic counts for encouraging ethical co-authorship practices. *Scientometrics* **2013**, *96*, 277–295.
28. Tarkang, E.E.; Kweku, M.; Zotor, F.B. Publication practices and responsible authorship: A review article. *J. Public Health Afr.* **2017**, *8*, 36–42. [CrossRef] [PubMed]
29. Kissan, J.; Laband, D.N.; Patil, V. Author order and research quality. *South. Econ. J.* **2005**, *7*, 545–555.
30. Tscharntke, T.; Hochberg, M.E.; Rand, T.A.; Resh, V.H.; Krauss, J. Author sequence and credit for contributions in multiauthored publications. *PLoS Biol.* **2007**, *5*, 18. [CrossRef] [PubMed]
31. Degli Esposti, M.; Boscolo, L. Top Italian Scientists Biomedical Sciences. 2018. Available online: http://www.topitalianscientists.org/TIS_HTML/Top_Italian_Scientists_Biomedical_Sciences.htm (accessed on 17 April 2018).
32. Van Raan, A.F. Comparison of the Hirsch-index with standard bibliometric indicators and with peer judgment for 147 chemistry research groups. *Scientometrics* **2006**, *67*, 491–502. [CrossRef]
33. Masic, I. H-index and how to improve it? *Donald Sch. J. Ultrasound. Obstet. Gynecol.* **2016**, *10*, 83–89. [CrossRef]

8

Wear Behaviours and Oxidation Effects on Different UHMWPE Acetabular Cups Using a Hip Joint Simulator

Saverio Affatato [1,*], Alessandro Ruggiero [2], Sami Abdel Jaber [1], Massimiliano Merola [2] and Pierangiola Bracco [3]

1 Medical Technology Laboratory, IRCCS—Rizzoli Orthopaedic Institute, Via di Barbiano, 1/10, 40136 Bologna, Italy; jaber@tecno.ior.it

2 Department of Industrial Engineering, University of Salerno, 84084 Fisciano, Italy; ruggiero@unisa.it (A.R.); mmerola@unisa.it (M.M.)

3 Chemistry Department and Nanostructured Interfaces and Surfaces (NIS) Centre, University of Turin, Via Giuria 7, 10125 Turin, Italy; pierangiola.bracco@unito.it

* Correspondence: affatato@tecno.ior.it

Abstract: Given the long-term problem of polyethylene wear, medical interest in the new improved cross-linked polyethylene (XLPE), with or without the adding of vitamin E, has risen. The main aim of this study is to gain further insights into the mutual effects of radiation cross-linking and addition of vitamin E on the wear performance of ultra-high-molecular-weight polyethylene (UHMWPE). We tested four different batches of polyethylene (namely, a standard one, a vitamin E-stabilized, and two cross-linked) in a hip joint simulator for five million cycles where bovine calf serum was used as lubricant. The acetabular cups were then analyzed using a confocal profilometer to characterize the surface topography. Moreover; the cups were analyzed by using Fourier Transformed Infrared Spectroscopy and Differential Scanning Calorimetry in order to assess the chemical characteristics of the pristine materials. Comparing the different cups' configuration, mass loss was found to be higher for standard polyethylene than for the other combinations. Mass loss negatively correlated to the cross-link density of the polyethylenes. None of the tested formulations showed evidence of oxidative degradation. We found no correlation between roughness parameters and wear. Furthermore, we found significantly differences in the wear behavior of all the acetabular cups. XLPEs exhibited lower weight loss, which has potential for reduced wear and decreased osteolysis. However, surface topography revealed smoother surfaces of the standard and vitamin E stabilized polyethylene than on the cross-linked samples. This observation suggests incipient crack generations on the rough and scratched surfaces of the cross-linked polyethylene liners.

Keywords: vitamin-E stabilized PE; cross-linked PE; standard PE; hip simulator; FTIR analysis

---

1. Introduction

Ultra-high-molecular-weight polyethylene (UHMWPE) is a particular type of polyethylene (PE) with an exceptionally high molecular mass. It is a unique polymer with outstanding properties, in terms of chemical inertness, lubricity, impact, and abrasion resistance. Despite coming from a family of polymers with an extremely simple chemical composition, consisting of only hydrogen and carbon, UHMWPE shows a complex hierarchy of organizational structures at the molecular and supermolecular length scales [1]. Besides the molecular mass, the microstructure of the polymer also plays an important role in determining its physical, chemical, and mechanical properties. UHMWPE, as most polyethylenes, is a semi-crystalline polymer, composed of at least two interpenetrating phases: a crystalline, ordered phase, and an amorphous disordered one, possibly intercalated by a partially ordered interphase. Such a precise combination of chemical structure, molecular mass, and microstructure is at the basis of the peculiar balance of high mechanical properties and wear resistance that has made UHMWPE the material of choice in arthroplasty [2].

Thanks to its unique properties, UHMWPE is the most used material in hip joint replacement, being the soft insert coupled with harder materials (typically ceramics and metals). Such coupling shows very good tribological performances in terms of friction and wear [3,4]. Unfortunately, oxidative degradation can decrease its mechanical properties, leading to debris production and eventual osteolysis and implant loosening [5–7]. It is believed that wear of UHMWPE is to take place via plastic deformation of the polymer, with molecular alignment in the direction of motion that results in the formation of fine, drawn-out fibrils oriented parallel to each other. As a result of this arrangement, the UHMWPE wear surface may strengthen along the direction of sliding, while it weakens in the transverse direction [2]. Many efforts were done to improve the mechanical and molecular characteristic of the UHMWPE, as by cross-linking its molecular chains or by doping it with vitamin E [8]. Radiation cross-linking was demonstrated to improve the wear resistance of UHMWPE. On the other hand, irradiated polyethylene has also shown an unacceptably low oxidation stability [2]. As a consequence, stabilization strategies were developed in order to minimize post-irradiation oxidative ageing. Basically, two different strategies were adopted: one involved a thermal treatment of the polyethylene (re-melting or annealing), while the other included the addition of an anti-oxidant stabilizer. Oral and co-workers [9], suggested that the re-melting of the polyethylene reduces crystallinity and fatigue properties. Therefore, vitamin E was introduced to solve the oxidation problem [10]. Some authors [11–13], suggest to incorporate vitamin E in UHMWPE through blending the vitamin in the UHMWPE powder and then cross-link the blend through irradiation. With this process, the presence of vitamin E should protect the radiation-cross-linked polymer from oxidation, thus avoiding re-melting.

Preclinical evaluation of new biomaterials is necessary, and it could be considered as an extension of the risk analysis [14,15]. The wear performance of these improved biomaterials is often evaluated using hip joint simulators. Hip wear simulation tests are used since 40 years ago, and they represent a powerful system to assess the improvement in wear resistance before clinical use [16,17]. Some authors [18–20] observed a reduction in wear rate by the addition of vitamin E to highly cross-linked UHMWPE compared to conventional UHMWPE. However, there is a trade-off in determining the oxidation stability and the reduction in wear rate between the radiation dose applied for cross-linking and the amount of vitamin E incorporated into the polymer. Affatato and co-workers [21], using a hip joint simulator, found that the cross-linked polyethylene (XLPE) blended with vitamin E wore more than XLPE and conventional UHMWPE.

Each potential innovation has been accompanied by a great deal of pre-clinical trials, performed by researchers all over the world, often with very different methods and sometimes with contradictory results. In this regard, to go more in depth in the wear and oxidation behavior of new formulations of UHMWPE, we asked whether the addition of vitamin E on conventional UHMWPE could improve its wear performance in comparison with highly cross-linked polyethylene.

2. Materials and Methods

2.1. Specimens Tested

Four different batches of UHMWPE acetabular cups (32 mm inner × 50 mm outer dimensions; 6 specimens for each batch) coupled with 32 mm cobalt–chromium–molybdenum (CoCrMo) femoral heads have been investigated using a hip joint simulator. Three components of each batch run onto the simulator following a standardized procedure [22], another three acetabular cups for each type of material used were stored (non-loaded) in bovine calf serum to compensate for weight changes due to fluid absorption. All polyethylenes tested in this study were machined from polymer bars Chirulen GUR 1020 (Polymax, Adler, Milan, Italy). Cross-linked acetabular cups were firstly γ-ray irradiated with 50 and 75 kGy ($\pm$10%), then thermally treated at 150 °C (re-melted), in order to remove free radicals formed during irradiation (hereinafter called XL-50 and XL-75). After these treatments, the cups were machined to their final shape. Similarly, vitamin E-containing (0.1% mass), UHMWPE acetabular cups (hereinafter called VE) were machined from a vitamin E-blended UHMWPE bars (Polymax, Adler, Milan, Italy). The UHMWPE that not received any treatment were called standard PE (STD). All the cups were then subjected to ethylene oxide sterilization (ETO). All polyethylene acetabular cups were pre-soaked for four weeks in a bath of deionized water prior the wear tests.

2.2. Experimental Wear Details

Wear test was performed using a 12-station hip joint simulator (IORSynthe, Bologna, Italy) [9]. The test was carried out applying the kinematic inputs and outputs as recommended by ISO 14242-1:2012. The simulator utilizes hydraulic actuators to apply the cyclic vertical compressive loads (oscillating between 300 and 3000 N). The lubricant used was 25 vol % newborn calf serum balanced with distilled water, with 0.2% (mass) sodium azide in order to retard bacterial growth, and 20 mM EDTA (ethylenediaminetetraacetic acid) to minimize precipitation of calcium phosphate. The mass loss of the cups was determined every 0.5 million cycles (Mc) using a microbalance (Sartorius Cubis Mse 225 S-000-DU, Goettingën, Germany) with a resolution of 0.01 mg and an uncertainty of 0.01 mg. Before the weighting operation, the specimens were cleaned from dust and possible debris using a dedicated detergent (Clean 70, Elma GmbH, Düsseldorf, Germany) in an ultrasonic bath maintained at 40 °C for 10 min. After rinsing, the cups were put back in the ultrasonic bath with deionized water for an additional 15 min. The cups were then dried with nitrogen gas. During any interruption of the test (every 500×10^5 cycles), the cups were stored in a closed, dust-free container at 70% of relative humidity. The test was re-started with fresh serum solution.

The test lasted five Mc, as recommended by the international guidelines [23], under environmental temperature conditions. The wear trend was determined from the mass loss of each acetabular cup, corrected by acetabular soak control. The wear rates, calculated from the steady-state slopes of the mass loss versus number of cycles, were obtained using least squares linear regression. The mass loss data were analyzed using a nonparametric Kruskall–Wallis (K–W) test; statistical significance was set at $p < 0.05$.

2.3. Surface Topography Characterization

The topographic analyses were performed using a PLu Neox profilometer (Sensofar, Terrassa, Spain), capable to gain three-dimensional images of a surface, operating either as confocal microscope or as white light interferometer with a vertical resolution, declared by the manufacturer, of less than 0.1 nm. In this study, we selected the confocal lens of 20× magnifications, while the acquisition lengths were adjusted to compensate the inner curvature of the surfaces. Such a non-contact instrument was selected to measure the roughness of the polyethylene cups as optical techniques do not risk damaging the surface under investigation. On the other hand, a traditional roughness profilometer can scratch the surface of a soft material, such as the UHMWPE. The acquisition process followed an established procedure [24], where the polyethylene liners were first cleaned from debris, as described for the wear measurement, and—right before each acquisition—cleaned with ethanol and allowed to dry under a controlled environment in ambient air. In Figure 1, a schematic representation of the acquisition apparatus is shown.

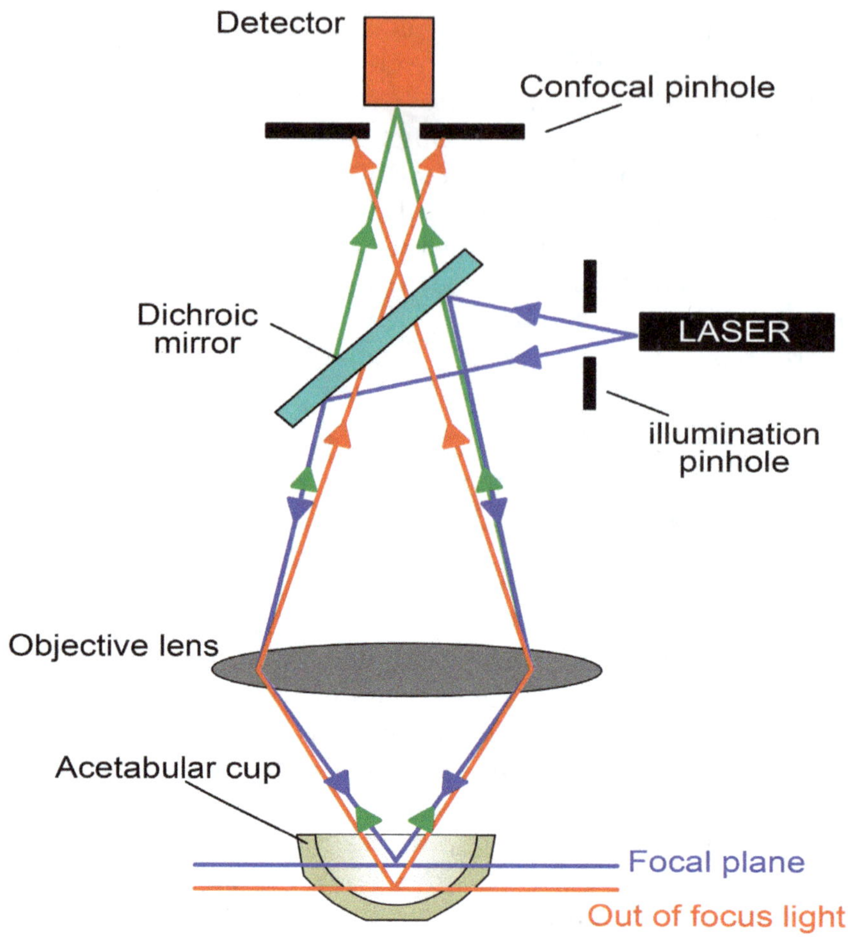

Figure 1. Schematic representation of the confocal apparatus for the topography acquisitions.

The topography characterization was realized on eight selected UHMWPE acetabular cups. In particular, we analyzed the most worn acetabular cups for each configuration, plus the corresponding check-control, to compare worn and unworn acetabular cups. The topographical acquisitions were realized to gain qualitative information on the surface condition of the samples after five Mc of test running. Furthermore, it was obtained a quantitative analysis in term of surface roughness. To do so, a Gaussian filter was applied according to the international guidelines in ISO 4287:1997 [25]. A cut-off wavelength of 80 μm was selected along with an evaluation length of 400 μm—equivalent to 5 times the cut-off. The roughness parameters selected were Ra, Rq, Rz, and Rt. Ra defines the absolute of the mean deviation of the irregularities from the mean line, over a sampling length. Rq is the standard deviation of the distribution of surface heights. Rz is the difference in height between the average of the five highest peaks and the five deepest valleys. Rt is the maximum height of the profile, defined as the vertical distance between the highest peak and the lowest valley along the measurement length.

2.4. FTIR Spectroscopy

All four different biomaterials were characterized by means of a Fourier Transformed Infrared Spectroscopy (FTIR) Microscope (Spectrum Spotlight 300, Perkin-Elmer, Shelton, CT, USA). A series of 180 μm thick slices was obtained from the cups cross section, using a PolyCuts Microtome (Leica Microsystem, Wetzlar, Germany) at 10 mm/s in air at room temperature. Line-scan spectra were collected on a 100×100 μm^2 area (resolution 4 cm^{-1}, 16 scans per spectrum), every 100 μm along the mapping direction, starting from the articulating surface towards the bulk. All spectra were normalized at 2020 cm^{-1} at an absorption of 0.05, corresponding to a film thickness of ca. 100 μm.

The combination band at 2020 cm^{-1}, associated with the twisting of CH_2, was used as an internal standard, since it can be regarded as unaffected by minor changes in the polymer structure. The molar concentration of trans-vinylene double bonds was calculated from the 965 cm^{-1} absorption bands, using the well-established molar absorptivity proposed by De Kock and Hol [26].

2.5. Determination of Cross-Link Density and Crystallinity

The cross-link density of each sample was quantified by gravimetric swelling. Small cylinders with diameter of 5 mm and approximate weight of 15 mg were cut from the control cups and immersed in 25 mL of xylene at 135 °C for 3 h to reach the equilibrium swelling. The initial weight and xylene uptake were used to calculate the swell ratio and the cross-link density, using a validated protocol [21].

The crystallinity of the test samples was determined using a differential scanning calorimetry (DSC 6-Perkin-Elmer, Waltham, MA, USA) at a heating rate of 10 °C/min. The sample weights varied around 5 mg. The heat of fusion was calculated by integrating the DSC endotherm from 60 to 160 °C. The crystallinity was calculated by normalizing the heat of fusion to the heat of fusion of 100% crystalline polyethylene (293 J/g) [27].

3. Results

All the polyethylene acetabular cups completed the planned five Mc. As showed in Figure 2, where the different polyethylene liners are compared, a higher mass loss rate for the standard polyethylene (STD) than for the other combinations was found. Close to this trend, the VE cups have a slightly smaller wear rate.

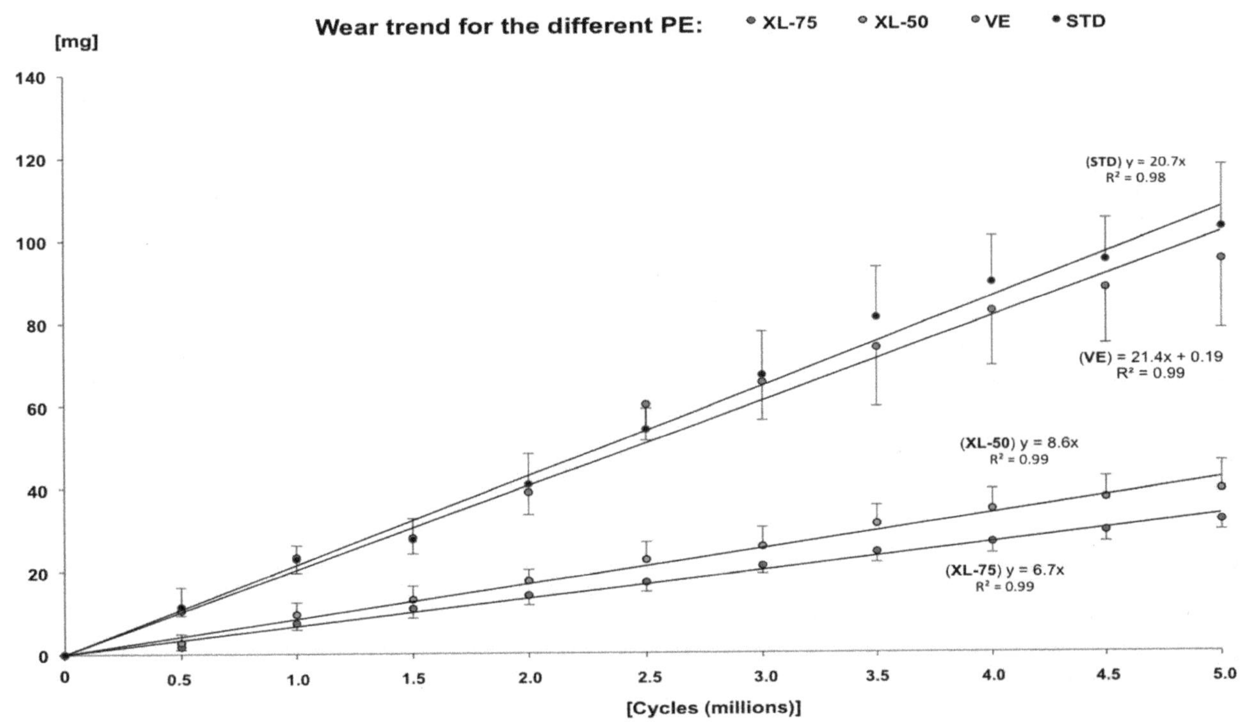

Figure 2. Wear behavior for the different configurations of polyethylene tested.

The polyethylene named XL-75 maintained the lowest mass loss than the other configurations during the whole test, as confirmed by the results of the post hoc test (Table 1). Statistical significant differences were observed between XL-75 vs UHMWPE and VE ($p = 0.015$ and $p = 0.02$, respectively). No statistically significant differences ($p > 0.05$) were observed between the other configurations of polyethylene cups using the K-S statistical test (Table 1).

Table 1. Cumulative mass loss (mean ± standard deviation) for the four sets of polyethylene (PE) acetabular cups tested. Values and statistical analysis performed using a Kruskall–Wallis nonparametric test.

Cycles (Mc)	Mean ± Standard Deviation (mg)				K–W Test	Post Hoc Test (p-Value)					
	STD	VE	XL-50	XL-75	(p-Value)	STD vs. VE	STD vs. XL-50	STD vs. XL-75	VE vs. XL-50	VE vs. XL-75	XL-50 vs. XL-75
0.5	11.4 ± 4.8	10.5 ± 1.2	2.7 ± 2.1	1.7 ± 0.7	0.037	0.821	0.079	0.036	0.047	0.020	0.734
1.0	22.9 ± 3.4	23.3 ± 3.8	9.6 ± 2.8	7.5 ± 1.6	0.035	0.910	0.089	0.024	0.070	0.017	0.571
1.5	27.6 ± 5.2	28.1 ± 3.9	13.0 ± 3.4	10.9 ± 2.3	0.038	0.910	0.070	0.031	0.054	0.024	0.734
2.0	40.9 ± 7.3	39.0 ± 5.5	17.4 ± 2.7	13.9 ± 2.4	0.030	0.910	0.089	0.013	0.113	0.017	0.428
2.5	54.1 ± 5.0	60.13 ± 8.8	22.5 ± 4.3	17.2 ± 2.4	0.026	0.571	0.174	0.031	0.054	0.007	0.428
3.0	67.0 ± 10.5	65.2 ± 9.1	25.7 ± 4.6	21.0 ± 1.9	0.035	0.910	0.070	0.017	0.089	0.024	0.571
3.5	80.8 ± 12.2	73.7 ± 14.2	31.2 ± 4.5	24.3 ± 2.6	0.030	0.910	0.089	0.013	0.113	0.017	0.428
4.0	89.4 ± 11.3	82.4 ± 13.3	34.6 ± 4.9	26.6 ± 2.8	0.030	0.910	0.089	0.013	0.113	0.017	0.428
4.5	94.8 ± 10.0	88.1 ± 13.6	37.3 ± 5.1	29.3 ± 2.7	0.030	0.910	0.089	0.013	0.113	0.017	0.428
5.0	102.6 ± 15.1	94.9 ± 16.7	39.3 ± 6.7	31.8 ± 2.6	0.032	0.910	0.079	0.015	0.100	0.020	0.496

Statistical significance: $p < 0.05$.

3.1. Surface Topography Analysis

Surface topography of the samples is shown in Figures 3 and 4, where contour images for each analyzed cup are presented. The different range of the height scales is influenced by the inner curvature of the cups. In Figure 3, the image shows the inner surfaces of the soak cups, which did not undergo wear simulation. The contours images of the topography present a similar pattern, typical of a clear UHMWPE surface for hip implants. In fact, the polymer has a lamellar shape, characterized by fine scratches, deriving from the polishing phase. Nevertheless, few long and transversal scratches are visible all over the images.

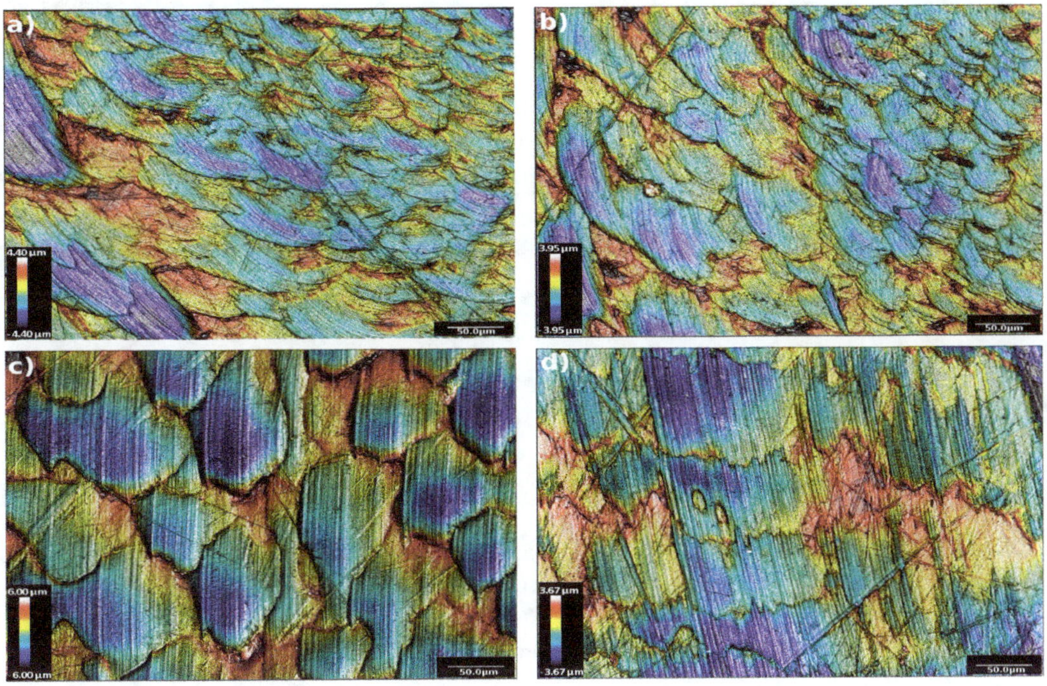

Figure 3. Contour images of the topographies acquired on the inner surfaces of four non-loaded specimens: (**a**) VE; (**b**) STD; (**c**) XL-75; (**d**) XL-50.

In Figure 4 are presented the contour topographies of the worn cups, after five million cycles of wear test. The images highlight that the inner surface of the cups is mainly characterized by the presence of grooves and scratches. In Figure 4a, a VE cup presents an almost smooth surface crossed by long and fine scratches; no signs of depth wear nor delamination are visible. In Figure 4b the inner surface of an STD cup is characterized by more frequent and larger grooves than on the VE. These paths are crossed in different directions. Also, signs of delamination are found along the border of these scratches. Figure 4c presents a worn area relative to a XL-75 cup. In this case, rough scratches are visible along with a deep groove (on the right side) and a worn crater (left side). In Figure 4d is shown a worn surface of a XL-50 cup, the surface presents many scratches in multiple directions and recurrent signs of wear along the side of these lines. Further worn images on the different configurations of the polyethylene tested, are shown in the supplementary section (Figure S1).

These qualitative analyses were combined with roughness measurements that are summarized in Figure 5. Ra values are equal to 0.09, 0.10, 0.25, and 0.45 µm respectively for the VE, STD, XL-75 and XL-50 cups. Rq is 0.19, 0.13, 1.5, and 2.1 µm, respectively, for VE, STD, XL-75, and XL-50; these values highlight how the deviation from the mean line is higher on the rougher surfaces of the cross-linked polyethylene. Rz and Rt provide evidence of the presence of elevate peaks and deep valleys along the measured profiles, and our analysis shows considerably higher values for the cross-linked polyethylene than the standard and the vitaminized ones. The values of Rz are 0.48, 0.57,

0.78, and 1.07 μm, respectively, for VE, STD, XL-75 and XL-50, whereas for the Rt parameters these are 1.69, 0.85, 22.7, and 30.7 μm, in the same order of correspondence.

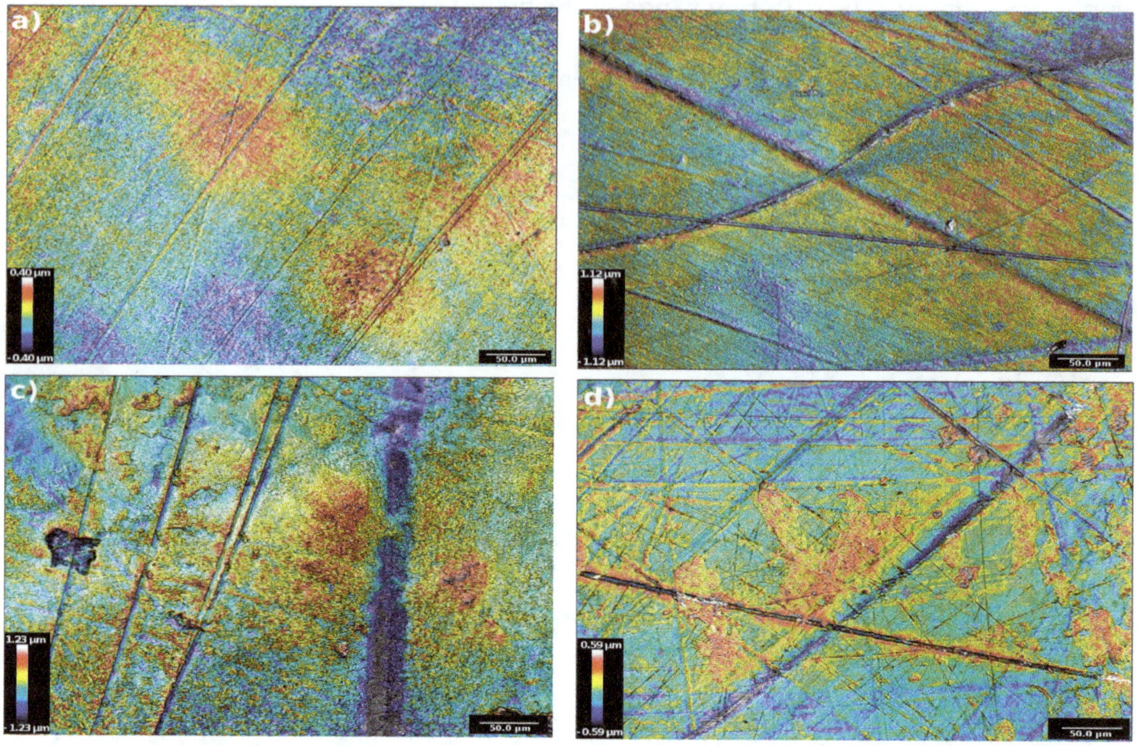

Figure 4. First set of contour images of the topographies acquired on the worn inner surfaces of four loaded specimens: (**a**) VE; (**b**) STD; (**c**) XL-75; (**d**) XL-50.

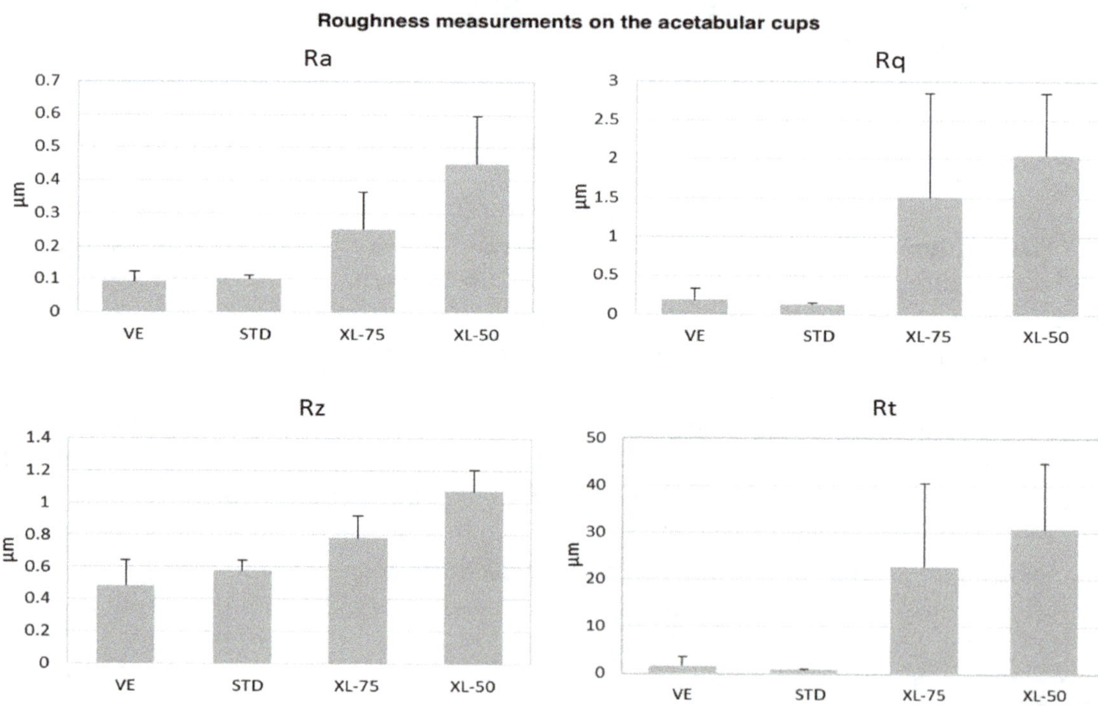

Figure 5. Roughness histograms of the worn surfaces on the mentioned cups. The parameters are Ra, Rq, Rz, and Rt.

3.2. *FTIR Spectroscopy and Cross-Link Density Results*

The physical–chemical characteristics of the control samples, resulting from FTIR, DSC, and cross-link density measurements, are summarized in Table 2.

Table 2. Physical–chemical characteristics of the control samples, resulting from FTIR, DSC, and cross-link density measurements.

Polyethylene	Crystallinity (%)	Trans-Vinylene (mmol/L)	Cross-Link Density (mol/dm^3)
STD	50.3 ± 0.9	-	-
VE	51.2 ± 1.2	-	-
XL-50	40.8 ± 1.0	5.2	0.132 ± 0.009
XL-75	35.5 ± 0.9	5.8	0.139 ± 0.010

Figure 6 shows the FTIR spectra of all materials. The VE sample spectrum does not show any significant difference from that of virgin UHMWPE (STD). On the contrary, the spectra of the irradiated samples show a decrease in the vinyl double bonds absorption at 909 cm^{-1} and the appearance of an additional absorption at 965 cm^{-1}, attributed to the formation of trans-vinylene double bonds, whose concentration is constant along the cup section, and increases with the radiation dose (see Table 2). No traces of oxidation products in the 1700 cm^{-1} area were observed in any of the samples (not shown). No significant differences in crystallinity were found between the STD and VE samples, while a significant decrease was observed in the crystallinity of the cross-linked polyethylenes. The cross-link density (ν_d) was measurable on the irradiated samples only (XL-50 and XL-75) and was found to increase as the radiation dose increases.

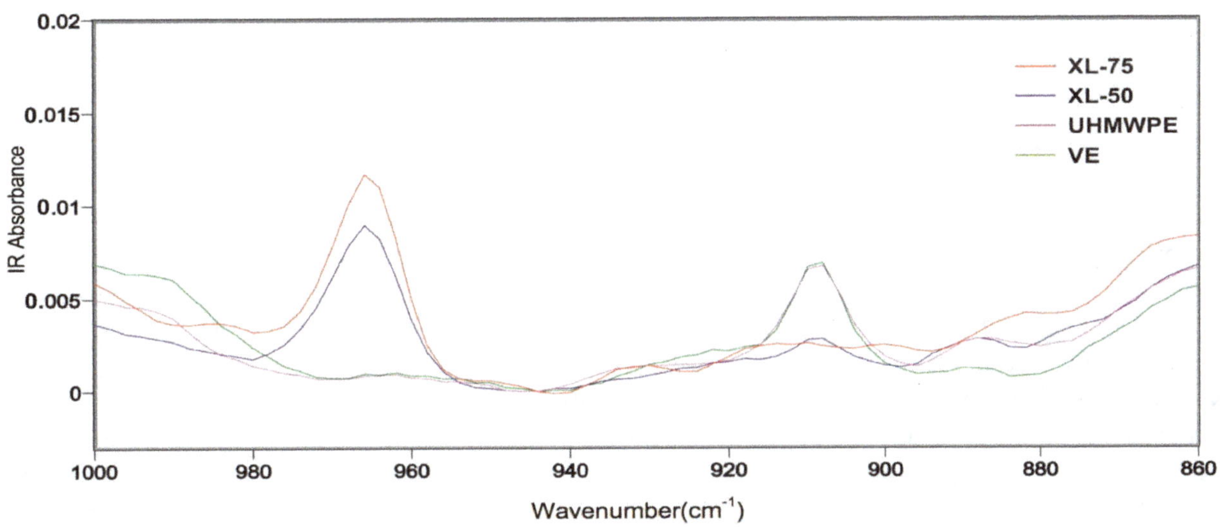

Figure 6. FTIR spectra of the investigated materials.

4. Discussion

The main purpose of this work was to characterize the wear performance of four different polyethylenes coupled with CoCrMo femoral heads using a 12-stations hip joint simulator for five million cycles. In particular, we asked whether the sole addition of vitamin E on conventional UHMWPE could improve its wear performance in comparison with high cross-linked polyethylene. We observed the highest wear rate on the STD polyethylene cups, followed closely by the VE, whereas the wear rate of XL-50 and XL-75 were sensibly lower than the former, but close to each other. In his research, McKellop et al. [6] found that the process of cross-linking highly improved the wear resistance, and the wear rate decreased markedly with increasing radiation dose, reaching a reduction of the 87% for the cup irradiated at 9.5 Mrad compared to the one irradiated at 3.3 Mrad. Affatato et al. [22] found that the wear of conventional UHMWPE was 40 times higher than for cross-linked polyethylene (XLPE), testing these materials against femoral heads of CoCrMo deliberately scratched.

The adding of vitamin E into the microstructure of conventional polyethylene used for hip components should prevent oxidative degradation and reduce the incidence of fatigue crack, confirming the results obtained by other authors [13]. The clinical consequence of the oxidation is an increased wear rate, starting approximately between 2 and 10 years postoperative [28].

Trans-Vinylene groups are known to be formed in UHMWPE upon irradiation, and can be used to assess the absorbed radiation dose [29]. The concentration of vinylene double bonds measured in our irradiated samples increases with the irradiation dose, as expected. At the same time, vinyl groups, normally present in virgin UHMWPE, are consumed as a consequence of irradiation, being involved in the formation of Y-shaped cross-links, as shown in Figure 7 [30].

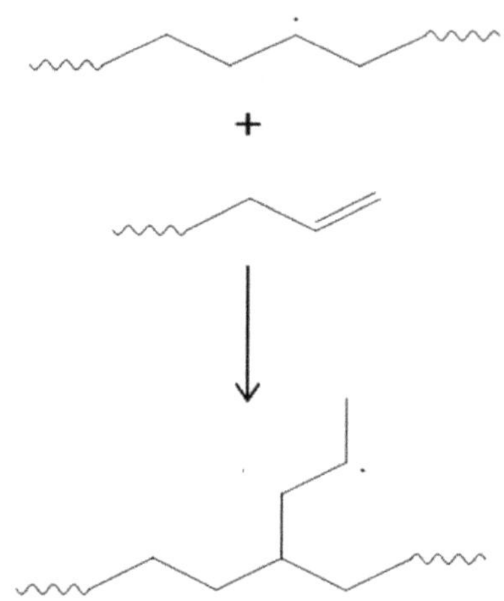

Figure 7. Mechanism of cross-linking of ultra-high-molecular-weight polyethylene (UHMWPE) through consumption of vinyl double bonds.

Accordingly, the FTIR analysis of both irradiated samples demonstrates consumption of the vinyl double bonds, while the cross-linking density measurements indicates that those samples have been cross-linked as a consequence of irradiation. Since cross-linking is known to increase the abrasion resistance, this explains the reduced wear, compared to the STD configuration, observed in the wear test. Nevertheless, both XLPE samples showed a significant decrease in crystallinity, and this is known to be correlated with a decrease in fatigue resistance, which creates concerns on their in vivo durability.

On the contrary, VE sample does not show any significant difference in the chemical and physical characteristics, compared to STD UHMWPE, indicating that the addition of vitamin E, which is intended as a stabilizer against oxidation, does not induce any modification to other properties. This also explains the similar behavior observed between VE and STD in the wear test.

From the topographical analysis, a very similar surface pattern of the unworn surfaces of the different polyethylene was found, verifying an almost equal initial condition for all of the cups that underwent the in vitro wear simulation. On the contrary, the inner surface of the worn samples showed large differences, both in terms of qualitative observation and in terms of rigorous measurement of the roughness. The contour images of the cross-linked polyethylene presented a more rough surface, with many signs of delamination and incipient cracks, which are symptoms of the fatigue wear phenomena [31]. On the other side, the non-cross-linked polyethylene presented a smoother surface than the XL ones, which suggests an abrasive wear occurrence that lead to a setting-in phase of the non-cross-linked polyethylene surfaces to the CoCrMo counterbody.

The roughness analysis emphasized these differences in the wear behavior of the polyethylene cups. In fact, higher roughness values on the cross-linked cups than on the standard and vitaminized ones were found. As grooves and scratches are assessed as origin points for surface-initiated micro-cracks, a high roughness value can be an indicator of the fatigue wear mechanism. As expressed in literature, cross-linking affects the compression and tension fatigue of the UHMWPE. Baker et al. [32] found growth of fatigue cracks under fully compressive cyclic loading in notched samples of UHMWPE. Cole et al. [33], in their experimental investigation on the fracture toughness and fatigue-crack resistance of two kinds of molded UHMWPE, found that "gamma irradiation decreased each material's resistance to fatigue-crack growth, and that the decreases were greater with increased irradiation dose".

5. Conclusions

All the acetabular cups studied in this work showed significant differences with respect to their wear behavior. Lower weight loss was exhibit by the XLPEs, which has potential for reduced wear and decreased osteolysis. The amount of weight loss after five million cycles in a hip joint wear simulator did not correlate with the roughness parameters, while cross-link density is strongly correlated with the wear resistance of UHMWPE. Nevertheless, the sensible higher presence of grooves and scratches on the cross-linked surfaces than on the standard ones is believed to be a plausible cause of fatigue wear. This, with the continuous cyclical compression of the element, could lead to an increased wear rate after elevate amount of working cycles.

Little is known or understood about the relationship between particle debris from PE wear and the biological response leading to osteolysis, and less is known about the role of cross-linking [12,28]. The promise of improved clinical performance in respect to osteolysis is a matter to be determined by long-term (>10 years) clinical follow-up studies. An increased understanding of the related biological processes and osteolysis is needed to provide the ability to better evaluate the STD, XLPEs, and VE performance in vivo.

Acknowledgments: The authors would like to thank Barbara Bordini (Rizzoli Orthopaedic Institute) for her help with statistical analyses and Pasquale Cutino for his help during the topography acquisition. This work was supported by the Italian Program of Donation for Research "5 per mille", year 2014.

Author Contributions: S.A. and PB conceived and designed the experiments; S.A. and S.A.J. performed the wear tests; A.R. and M.M. performed the optical measurements and data analysis; S.A. and S.A.J. contributed materials and analysis tools; S.A., A.R., M.M. and P.B. wrote the paper.

References

1. Kurtz, S.M. A Primer on UHMWPE. *UHMWPE Biomater. Handb.* **2016**, 1–6. [CrossRef]
2. Bracco, P.; Bellare, A.; Bistolfi, A.; Affatato, S. Ultra-High Molecular Weight Polyethylene: Influence of the Chemical, Physical and Mechanical Properties on the Wear Behavior. A Review. *Materials* **2017**, *10*, 791. [CrossRef] [PubMed]
3. Ruggiero, A.; D'Amato, R.; Gómez, E.; Merola, M. Experimental comparison on tribological pairs UHMWPE/TIAL6V4 alloy, UHMWPE/AISI316L austenitic stainless and UHMWPE/AL2O3 ceramic, under dry and lubricated conditions. *Tribol. Int.* **2016**, *96*, 349–360. [CrossRef]
4. Ruggiero, A.; D'Amato, R.; Gómez, E. Experimental analysis of tribological behavior of UHMWPE against AISI420C and against TiAl6V4 alloy under dry and lubricated conditions. *Tribol. Int.* **2015**, *92*, 154–161. [CrossRef]
5. Brach del Prever, E.M.; Bistolfi, A.; Bracco, P.; Costa, L. UHMWPE for arthroplasty: Past or future? *J. Orthop. Traumatol.* **2009**, *10*, 1–8. [CrossRef] [PubMed]

6. McKellop, H.; Shen, F.W.; Lu, B.; Campbell, P.; Salovey, R. Development of an extremely wear-resistant ultra high molecular weight polyethylene for total hip replacements. *J. Orthop. Res.* **1999**, *17*, 157–167. [CrossRef] [PubMed]
7. Harris, W.H.; Muratoglu, O.K. A Review of Current Cross-linked Polyethylenes Used in Total Joint Arthroplasty. *Clin. Orthop. Relat. Res.* **2005**, 46–52. [CrossRef]
8. Affatato, S.; Freccero, N.; Taddei, P. The biomaterials challenge: A comparison of polyethylene wear using a hip joint simulator. *J. Mech. Behav. Biomed. Mater.* **2016**, *53*, 40–48. [CrossRef] [PubMed]
9. Oral, E.; Malhi, A.S.; Muratoglu, O.K. Mechanisms of decrease in fatigue crack propagation resistance in irradiated and melted UHMWPE. *Biomaterials* **2006**, *27*, 917–925. [CrossRef] [PubMed]
10. Oral, E.; Godleski Beckos, C.; Malhi, A.S.; Muratoglu, O.K. The effects of high dose irradiation on the cross-linking of vitamin E-blended ultrahigh molecular weight polyethylene. *Biomaterials* **2008**, *29*, 3557–3560. [CrossRef] [PubMed]
11. Azzi, A.; Stocker, A. Vitamin E: Non-antioxidant roles. *Prog. Lipid Res.* **2000**, *39*, 231–255. [CrossRef]
12. Oral, E.; Muratoglu, O.K. Vitamin E diffused, highly crosslinked UHMWPE: A review. *Int. Orthop.* **2011**, *35*, 215–223. [CrossRef] [PubMed]
13. Tomita, N.; Kitakura, T.; Onmori, N.; Ikada, Y.; Aoyama, E. Prevention of Fatigue Cracks in Ultrahigh Molecular Weight Polyethylene Joint Components by the Addition of Vitamin E. *J. Biomed. Mater. Res.* **1999**, *48*, 474–478. [CrossRef]
14. Trommer, R.M.; Maru, M.M. Review article Importance of preclinical evaluation of wear in hip implant designs using simulator machines. *Rev. Bras. Ortop.* **2016**, *52*, 251–259. [CrossRef] [PubMed]
15. Viceconti, M.; Affatato, S.; Baleani, M.; Bordini, B.; Cristofolini, L.; Taddei, F. Pre-clinical validation of joint prostheses: A systematic approach. *J. Mech. Behav. Biomed. Mater.* **2009**, *2*, 120–127. [CrossRef] [PubMed]
16. Affatato, S.; Spinelli, M.; Zavalloni, M.; Mazzega-Fabbro, C.; Viceconti, M. Tribology and total hip joint replacement: Current concepts in mechanical simulation. *Med. Eng. Phys.* **2008**, *30*, 1305–1317. [CrossRef] [PubMed]
17. Taddei, P.; Ruggiero, A.; Pavoni, E.; Affatato, S. Transfer of metallic debris after in vitro ceramic-on-metal simulation: Wear and degradation in Biolox® Delta composite femoral heads. *Compos. Part B Eng.* **2016**. [CrossRef]
18. Oral, E.; Christensen, S.D.; Malhi, A.S.; Wannomae, K.K.; Muratoglu, O.K. Wear resistance and mechanical properties of highly cross-linked, ultrahigh-molecular weight polyethylene doped with vitamin E. *J. Arthroplast.* **2006**, *21*, 580–591. [CrossRef] [PubMed]
19. Wannomae, K.K.; Christensen, S.D.; Micheli, B.R.; Rowell, S.L.; Schroeder, D.W.; Muratoglu, O.K. Delamination and adhesive wear behavior of alpha-tocopherol-stabilized irradiated ultrahigh-molecular-weight polyethylene. *J. Arthroplast.* **2010**, *25*, 635–643. [CrossRef] [PubMed]
20. Micheli, B.R.; Wannomae, K.K.; Lozynsky, A.J.; Christensen, S.D.; Muratoglu, O.K. Knee Simulator Wear of Vitamin E Stabilized Irradiated Ultrahigh Molecular Weight Polyethylene. *J. Arthroplast.* **2012**, *27*, 95–104. [CrossRef] [PubMed]
21. Affatato, S.; Bracco, P.; Costa, L.; Villa, T.; Quaglini, V.; Toni, A. In vitro wear performance of standard, crosslinked, and vitamin-E-blended UHMWPE. *J. Biomed. Mater. Res. A* **2012**, *100*, 554–560. [CrossRef] [PubMed]
22. Affatato, S.; Bersaglia, G.; Rocchi, M.; Taddei, P.; Fagnano, C.; Toni, A. Wear behaviour of cross-linked polyethylene assessed in vitro under severe conditions. *Biomaterials* **2005**, *26*, 3259–3267. [CrossRef] [PubMed]
23. *Implants for Surgery—Wear of Total Hip-Joint Prostheses—Part 1: Loading and Displacement Parameters for Wear-Testing Machines and Corresponding Environmental Conditions for Test*, 2nd ed.; ISO 14242-1:2012; International Organization for Standardization: Geneva, Switzerland, 2012.
24. Ruggiero, A.; Merola, M.; Affatato, S. On the biotribology of total knee replacement: A new roughness measurements protocol on in vivo condyles considering the dynamic loading from musculoskeletal multibody model. *Meas. J. Int. Meas. Confed.* **2017**, *112*. [CrossRef]
25. ISO 4287:1997. In *Geometrical Product Specifications (GPS)—Surface Texture: Profile Method—Terms, Definitions and Surface Texture Parameters*; International Organization for Standardization: Geneva, Switzerland, 1997.
26. De Kock, R.J.; Hol, P.A.H.M.; Bos, H. Infrared determination of unsaturated bonds in polyethylene. *Fresenius' Zeitschrift Für Analytische Chemie* **1964**, *205*, 371–381. [CrossRef]

27. Wunderlich, B.; Dole, M. Specific heat of synthetic high polymers. VIII. Low pressure polyethylene. *J. Polym. Sci.* **1957**, *24*, 201–213. [CrossRef]
28. Kurtz, S.M.; Dumbleton, J.H.; Siskey, R.S.; Wang, A.; Manley, M. Trace concentrations of vitamin E protect radiation crosslinked UHMWPE from oxidative degradation. *J. Biomed. Mater. Res. A* **2009**, *90*, 549–563. [CrossRef] [PubMed]
29. *Standard Test Method for Evaluating Trans-Vinylene Yield in Irradiated Ultra-High-Molecular-Weight Polyethylene Fabricated Forms Intended for Surgical Implants by Infrared Spectroscopy*; ASTM F2381-04; ASTM International: West Conshohocken, PA, USA, 2004.
30. Bracco, P.; Brunella, V.; Luda, M.P.P.; Zanetti, M.; Costa, L. Radiation-induced crosslinking of UHMWPE in the presence of co-agents: Chemical and mechanical characterisation. *Polymer* **2005**, *46*, 10648–10657. [CrossRef]
31. Nélias, D.; Dumont, M.L.; Champiot, F.; Vincent, A.; Girodin, D.; Fougéres, R. Role of Inclusions, Surface Roughness and Operating Conditions on Rolling Contact Fatigue. *J. Tribol.* **1999**, *121*, 240. [CrossRef]
32. Baker, D.A.; Hastings, R.S.; Pruitt, L. Study of fatigue resistance of chemical and radiation crosslinked medical grade ultrahigh molecular weight polyethylene. *J. Biomed. Mater. Res.* **1999**, *46*, 573–581. [CrossRef]
33. Cole, J.C.; Lemons, J.E.; Eberhardt, A.W. Gamma irradiation alters fatigue-crack behavior and fracture toughness in 1900H and GUR 1050 UHMWPE. *J. Biomed. Mater. Res.* **2002**, *63*, 559–566. [CrossRef] [PubMed]

9

Biomechanical Effect of UHMWPE and CFR-PEEK Insert on Tibial Component in Unicompartmental Knee Replacement in Different Varus and Valgus Alignments

Yong-Gon Koh [1], Hyoung-Taek Hong [2] and Kyoung-Tak Kang [2,*]

1 Joint Reconstruction Center, Department of Orthopaedic Surgery, Yonsei Sarang Hospital, 10 Hyoryeong-ro, Seocho-gu, Seoul 06698, Korea; osygkoh@gmail.com

2 Department of Mechanical Engineering, Yonsei University, 50 Yonsei-ro, Seodaemun-gu, Seoul 03722, Korea; hyoungtaekhong@gmail.com

* Correspondence: tagi1024@gmail.com

Abstract: The current study aims to analyze the biomechanical effects of ultra-high molecular weight polyethylene (UHMWPE) and carbon-fiber-reinforced polyetheretherketone (CFR-PEEK) inserts, in varus/valgus alignment, for a tibial component, from 9° varus to 9° valgus, in unicompartmental knee replacement (UKR). The effects on bone stress, collateral ligament force, and contact stress on other compartments were evaluated under gait cycle conditions, by using a validated finite element model. In the UHMWPE model, the von Mises' stress on the cortical bone region significantly increased as the tibial tray was in valgus >6°, which might increase the risk of residual pain, and when in valgus >3° for CFR-PEEK. The contact stress on other UHMWPE compartments decreased in valgus and increased in varus, as compared to the neutral position. In CFR-PEEK, it increased in valgus and decreased in varus. The forces on medial collateral ligaments increased in valgus, when compared to the neutral position in UHMWPE and CFR-PEEK. The results indicate that UKR with UHMWPE showed positive biomechanical outputs under neutral and 3° varus conditions. UKR with CFR-PEEK showed positive biomechanical outputs for up to 6° varus alignments. The valgus alignment should be avoided.

Keywords: computational model; biomechanics; unicompartmental knee replacement; UHMWPE; CFR-PEEK; varus and valgus alignments

---

1. Introduction

Unicompartmental knee replacement (UKR) has become a popular alternative to total knee replacement (TKR), owing to favorable patient satisfaction reports and functional outcomes [1,2]. With a more functional anatomy being maintained, UKR can provide faster recovery and better restoration of knee kinetics, in comparison to TKR [3]. The long-term survival rates of UKR have been considerably improved, owing to refined surgical techniques and strict patient selection [4].

Various studies have shown that inaccurate alignment or technical errors in prosthetic components might cause early wear of polyethylene, periprosthetic fractures, and high revision rates to correct residual pain that is caused by implant failure [5–7]. The main complications are caused by abnormal tibial bone stress, which is thought to result from coronal malalignments of the tibial component. Therefore, UKR can be considered as a more technically demanding surgical treatment. In addition, numerous authors have suggested the relative malalignment of the knee in medial UKR, to avoid progressive osteoarthritis (OA) in the opposite compartment [8–10]. The effects of knee alignment on the long-term outcome of UKR have received attention in some reports [10,11].

The wear of ultra-high molecular weight polyethylene (UHMWPE), in both fixed- and mobile-bearings, continues to be a significant factor in the long-term performance of UKR [12]. Alternative polymers to replace UHMWPE in UKR or TKR have been proposed and they include the use of carbon-fiber reinforced polyetheretherketone (CFR-PEEK). In most cases, the carbon fibers in the CFR-PEEK materials are small, chopped fibers, and generally have no specific orientation in the polyetheretherketone (PEEK) matrix. CFR-PEEK has been classified as a low wear material in a recent in-vitro experimental study, being suitable for high-conformity scenarios, such as total hip replacement and conforming UKR [13]. However, it was recently stated that the wear rates of CFR-PEEK were very high and almost two orders of magnitude higher than the wear rate of ultra-high molecular weight polyethylene (UHMWPE) under comparable conditions for total knee replacement (TKR) [14]. S. C. Scholes and A. Unsworth stated that UKR with CFR-PEEK exhibited lower volumetric wear rates than those that were previously found in conventional metal-on-UHMWPE prostheses when tested under similar conditions [15]. Further study is required to confirm CFR-PEEK as an alternative material to UHMWPE. However, to the best of our knowledge, there has been a lack of research on the tibia bone stress when using CFR-PEEK tibial insert materials, which is an important factor determining aseptic loosening and anteromedial pain.

Most frequently, UKR is performed at a perpendicular coronal tibial position. However, various studies have reported improved results upon placing the tibial component parallel to the line of natural tibial joint, or within a few varus degrees of the epiphyseal axis [16,17]. There has been no study on the biomechanical effects of CFR-PEEK when compared to UHMWPE, with respect to varus and valgus alignments in the tibial component. Moreover, as mentioned above, there has been no biomechanical justification for the UHMWPE insert in the varus and valgus alignments in the tibial component.

The purpose of this study is to evaluate the biomechanical effects of the various varus/valgus alignment positions of tibial components in UKR with different UHMWPE and CFR-PEEK insert materials. We evaluate the contact stress on other compartments, the bone stress, and collateral ligament force, under a gait cycle condition, by using models from 9° varus to 9° valgus, with an increment of 1°, which is centered on the neutral position.

2. Materials and Methods

2.1. Intact Knee Joint Model

The present study was conducted while using a fully validated finite element (FE) model of knee joint [18–21]. The intact knee was made from computed tomography (CT) and magnetic resonance imaging (MRI) of the left knee joint of a healthy 35-year-old male volunteer. The CT imaging was conducted with a slice thickness of 0.1 mm, while using a 64-channel CT scanner (Somatom Sensation 64, Siemens Healthcare, Erlangen, Germany). In addition, MRI imaging was conducted using a 3.0 T MRI scanner (Achieva 3.0T; Philips Healthcare, North Brabant, The Netherlands) and a custom-designed knee joint cardiac coil [21]. MRI scans with a slice thickness of 0.4 mm were obtained in the sagittal plane. A high-resolution environment was used for the spectral pre-saturation inversion recovery (SPIR) sequence (TE, 25.0 ms; TR, 3590.8 ms; acquisition matrix, 512 pixels × 512 pixels; NEX, 2.0; field-of view, 140 mm × 140 mm) and a 3-T MRI system (Discovery MR750w®, GE Healthcare, Milwaukee, WI, USA) [21].

The process of combining the reconstructed CT and MRI models through the positional alignment of each model was conducted while using the commercial software Rapid form (version 2006; 3D Systems Korea, Seoul, Korea). Subsequently, the image data were imported into the image-processing software Mimics 17.0 (Materialise Ltd., Leuven, Belgium) to extract the geometry used for the generation of the three-dimensional (3D) models of all structures. The initial graphics exchange specification (IGES) files that were exported from Mimics were entered into Unigraphics NX (version 7.0; Siemens

PLM Software, Torrance, CA, USA) to form solid models for each femur, tibia, fibula, patella, and soft-tissue segment (Figure 1). The solid model was imported into Hypermesh (version 8.0; Altair Engineering, Troy, MI, USA) to generate an FE mesh. Afterwards, the FE mesh was analyzed while using the ABAQUS software (version 6.11; Simulia, Providence, RI, USA).

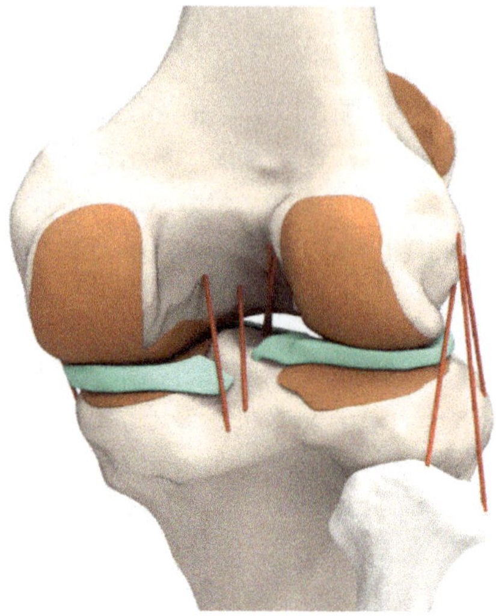

Figure 1. Developed three-dimensional finite element (3D FE) knee joint model from medical image.

In the model, the bones were assumed rigid, whereas the tibia was considered transversely isotropic as it was stiffer than soft tissue and had a minimal influence in the present study [22]. Constitutive laws were assumed for the tibia cortical and cancellous bones [23,24]. The cortical bone was considered to be transversely isotropic. The third axis was considered as parallel to the anatomical axis of each bone. The cancellous bone was considered as linear isotropic [23,24]. The articular cartilage was assumed to be an isotropic, linear elastic material, owing to the time-independent and simple compressive load applied to the knee joint [25]. The menisci were assumed to be a transversely isotropic, linearly elastic, homogeneous material [26]. The applied material properties were as shown in Table 1.

Table 1. Material properties for the 3D FE knee joint model.

Material	Material Properties
Cortical bone [23,24]	$E_1 = E_2 = 11.5$ GPa $E_3 = 17$ GPa $\nu_{12} = 0.51$, $\nu_{23} = \nu_{13} = 0.31$
Cancellous bone [23,24]	$E = 2.13$ GPa $\nu = 0.3$
Articular cartilage [25]	$E = 15$ MPa $\nu = 0.47$
Menisci [26]	$E_c = 120$ MPa (in the circumferential direction) $E_a = E_r = 20$ MPa MPa (in the axial and radial directions.) $\nu_{cr} = 0.3$ (for axial directions) $\nu_{ar} = \nu_{ac} = 0.3$ (for circumferential and radial directions)

To represent the meniscal attachments, each meniscal horn was bonded to the bone using linear spring elements (SPRINGA element type) with a total stiffness of 2000 N/mm [27]. In addition, the major ligaments were modeled while using nonlinear and tension-only spring elements [28,29].

The force-displacement relationship, based on the functional bundles in the actual ligament anatomy, is expressed in the following:

$$f(\varepsilon) = \begin{cases} \frac{k\varepsilon^2}{4\varepsilon_1}, \ 0 \le \varepsilon \le 2\varepsilon_1 \\ k(\varepsilon - \varepsilon_1), \ \varepsilon > 2\varepsilon_1 \\ 0, \ \varepsilon < 0 \end{cases}$$

$$\varepsilon = \frac{l - l_0}{l_0}$$

$$l_0 = \frac{l_r}{\varepsilon_r + 1}$$

where $f(\varepsilon)$ is the current force, k the stiffness, ε the strain, and ε_1 is assumed to be a constant equal to 0.03. The ligament bundle slack of length l_0 was calculated while using the reference bundle length l_r and the reference strain ε_r in the upright reference position.

The interfaces between the cartilage and bones were modeled as being fully bonded. The contacts between the femoral cartilage and meniscus, meniscus and tibial cartilage, and femoral cartilage and tibial cartilage were modeled for both the medial and lateral sides, and resulted in six contact pairs [18]. The contacts at all articulations adopted a finite sliding, frictionless hard contact algorithm with no penetration [18]. Convergence was defined as a relative change of more than 5% between the two adjacent meshes [20].

2.2. UKR Model

A fixed-bearing UKR (Zimmer, Inc., Warsaw, IN, USA) was virtually implanted in the medial compartment of the developed normal knee model. The bone models were imported and appropriately positioned, trimmed, and meshed with rigid elements by using surgical techniques [30].

Based on the dimensions of the femur and tibia, size 6 and 5 devices were chosen for the femoral and tibial components, respectively. The devices were aligned with the mechanical axis and positioned at the medial edge of the tibia. The neutrally aligned tibial baseplate was defined as having a square (0°) inclination in the coronal plane with a 5° posterior slope. The rotating axis was defined as a line parallel to the lateral edge of the tibial component passing through the center of the femoral component peg. A neutral femoral component distal cut, which was perpendicular to the mechanical axis of the femur and parallel to the tibial cut, was reproduced. The 19 different cut surfaces of the medial tibial plateau were created with different inclinations in the coronal plane (from 9° varus to 9° valgus, in increments of 1°) (Figure 2).

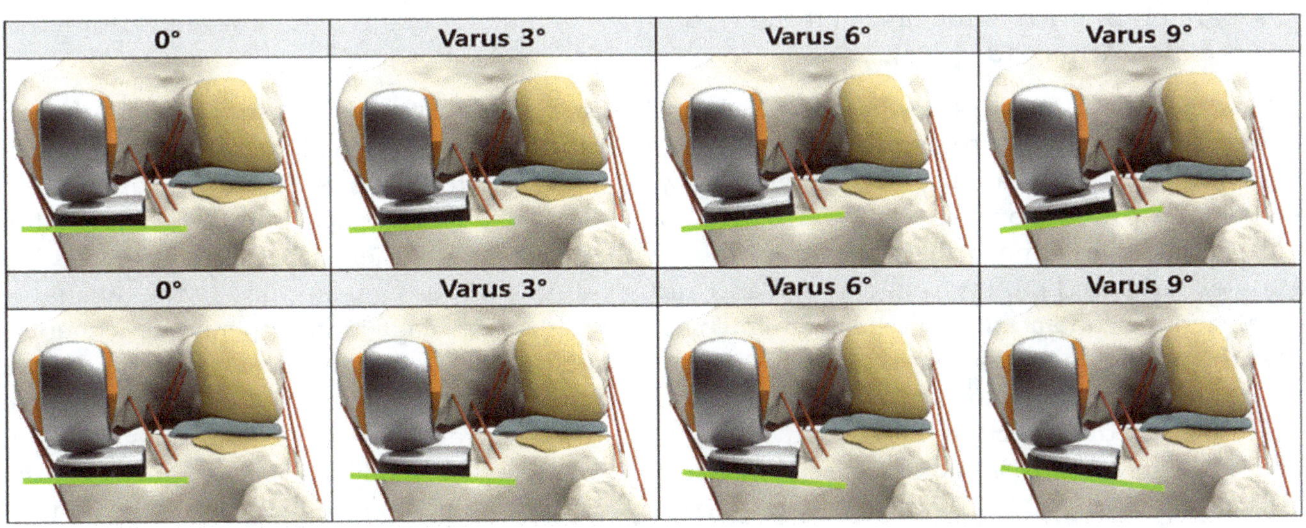

Figure 2. Schematic of varus/valgus conditions for tibial insert.

With respect to the implanted model, a cement gap of 1 mm was simulated between the bone and component. The femoral and tibial components, bone cement, and tibia insert (UHMWPE and CFR-PEEK) were modeled as linear elastic isotropic materials [31–35]. The materials of the femoral component, tibia insert, tibial component, and bone cement corresponded to a cobalt chromium alloy (CoCr), UHMWPE, CFR-PEEK, a titanium alloy (Ti6Al4V), and poly(methyl methacrylate) (PMMA), respectively. Compared to pure PEEK, CFR-PEEK contains a 30% proportion of carbon fiber reinforcement [35].

In terms of Young's modulus and Poisson's ratio, the material properties were shown in Table 2 [31–35]. The friction coefficients between the articulating surfaces were assumed to be 0.07 for UHMWPE and 0.04 for CFR-PEEK in accordance with the range that was reported in the literature [33,36,37].

Table 2. Material properties for the implanted model.

Materials	Material Properties
CoCr	E = 195 GPa v = 0.3
Ti6Al4V	E = 110 GPa v = 0.3
UHMWPE	E = 685 MPa v = 0.47
CFR-PEEK	E = 18000 MPa v = 0.4
PMMA	E = 1940 MPa and v = 0.4

2.3. Loading and Boundary Conditions

The FE investigation included two types of loading conditions, which corresponded to the loads that were used in the experimental part of the study, for the validation of the UKR model and its predictions under gait cycle loading conditions.

A validation of the intact model was conducted in a previous study, and the UKR model was validated through a comparison with models in previous experimental studies [18–21,38]. The validation of the UKR model was conducted for the flexion angles of 0°, 30°, 60°, and 90°, by using a passive flexion simulation. Additionally, anterior and posterior drawer loads of 134 N were separately applied to the tibia at the knee center, in a manner that is similar to that adopted in a previous experimental study [38].

Gait cycle loading was applied as a second loading to compare the biomechanical effects of the three different tibial insert materials [39]. A computational analysis was conducted while using the force controls of the anterior-posterior force with respect to the compressive load applied to the hip [40,41]. A proportional-integral derivative controller was incorporated into the computational model to make allowance for the control of the quadriceps, in a manner that is similar to that in an existing experiment [42]. Internal-external and varus/valgus torques were applied to the tibia [40,41]. We analyzed the contact stress on the lateral meniscus and tibial cartilage in the other compartments, as well as the tibial bone stress, which influences residual pain. Additionally, we analyzed the collateral ligament force. We defined five regions of interest (ROIs) on the proximal tibia (Figure 3). ROIs 1 and 4 were defined at the resection corner between the sagittal and transverse tibia bone cuts. The other three ROIs were located on the cancellous bone surface, beneath the tibial baseplate, with ROIs 2 and 4 being lateral and medial to the keel slot, respectively. ROI 5 was defined to investigate the source of residual pain. For all models, ROI 5 was located on the proximal anteromedial cortical bone surface.

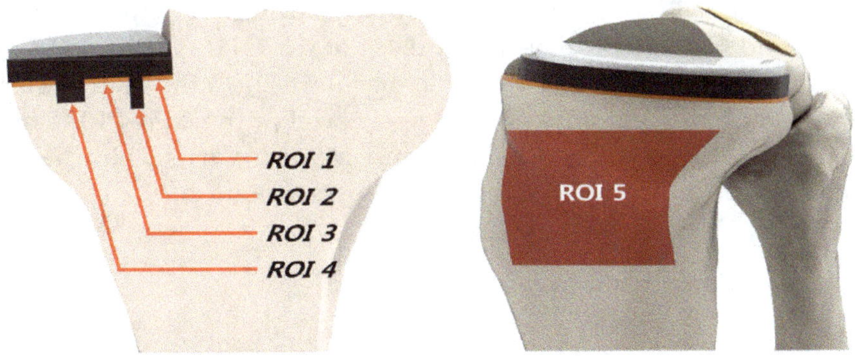

Figure 3. Five locations for the interests of this study.

Interventionary studies involving humans or animals, and other studies requiring ethical approval, must list the authority that provided approval and the corresponding ethical approval code.

3. Results

3.1. FE Model Validation

In a previous study, an intact model was validated and explained while using an in vivo laxity test for a subject identical to the FE model. We compared it with the results of the experiment on our own subject to validate the intact FE model. The anterior tibial translation was calculated at 2.83 mm in the experiment, and at 2.54 mm in the FE model under the 30° flexion loading condition; the posterior tibial translation was calculated at 2.12 mm in the experiment and 2.18 mm in the FE model for validation. Good agreement was observed between the experimental results and the FE model [19]. The UKR model validation was conducted while using the anterior and posterior tibial translations in the anterior and posterior drawer tests at 134 N for 6.1, 9.9, 8.7, and 8.5 mm, and 5.8, 4.3, 3.8, and 4.9 mm at 0°, 30°, 60°, and 90° knee flexion, respectively (Figure 4). These show good agreement with previous experimental data within the value ranges under the anterior and posterior drawer loadings [38].

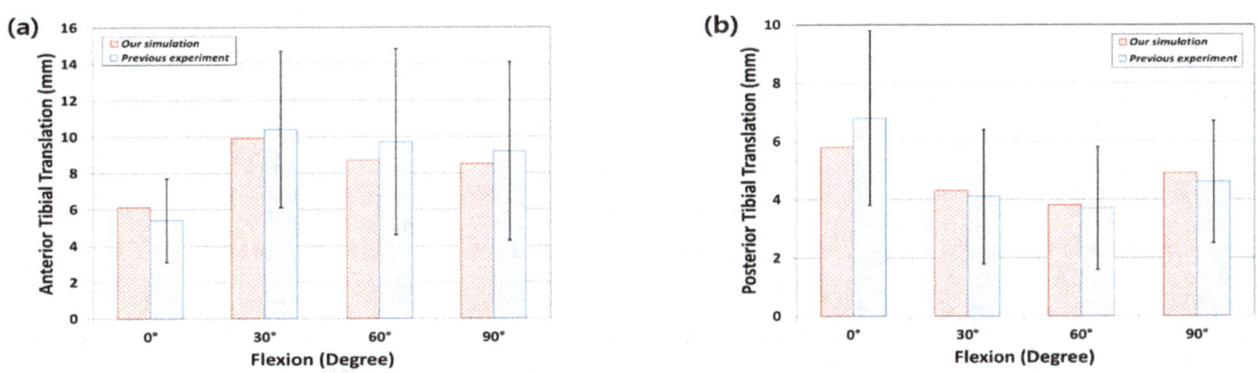

Figure 4. Comparison with previous experimental study for validation of unicompartmental knee replacement (UKR) model: (**a**) anterior tibial translation; and, (**b**) posterior tibial translation.

3.2. Comparison of Contact Stress on Other Compartments in UHMWPE and CFR-PEEK Tibial Component in Varus/Valgus Alignment

Figure 5 shows the contact stress on the other compartments (articular cartilage and lateral meniscus) in the UHMWPE and CFR-PEEK tibial insert with the varus/valgus tibial component. The contact stress on the articular cartilage and lateral meniscus increased in varus and decreased in valgus, in comparison to the neutral position in the UHMWPE insert. However, the contact stress on the articular cartilage and lateral meniscus decreased in varus and increased in valgus, in comparison to the neutral position of the CFR-PEEK insert. There was different contact stress during the stance phase in the UHMWPE and CFR-PEEK insert models. For the UHMWPE model, it increased by 11% and 8% for varus 9°, and decreased by 11% and 9% for valgus 9° in the lateral meniscus and articular cartilage, respectively, in comparison to the neutral position. For the CFR-PEEK model, it increased by 21% and 18% for valgus 9°, and decreased by 19% and 16% for varus 9° in the lateral meniscus and articular cartilage, respectively, in comparison to the neutral position.

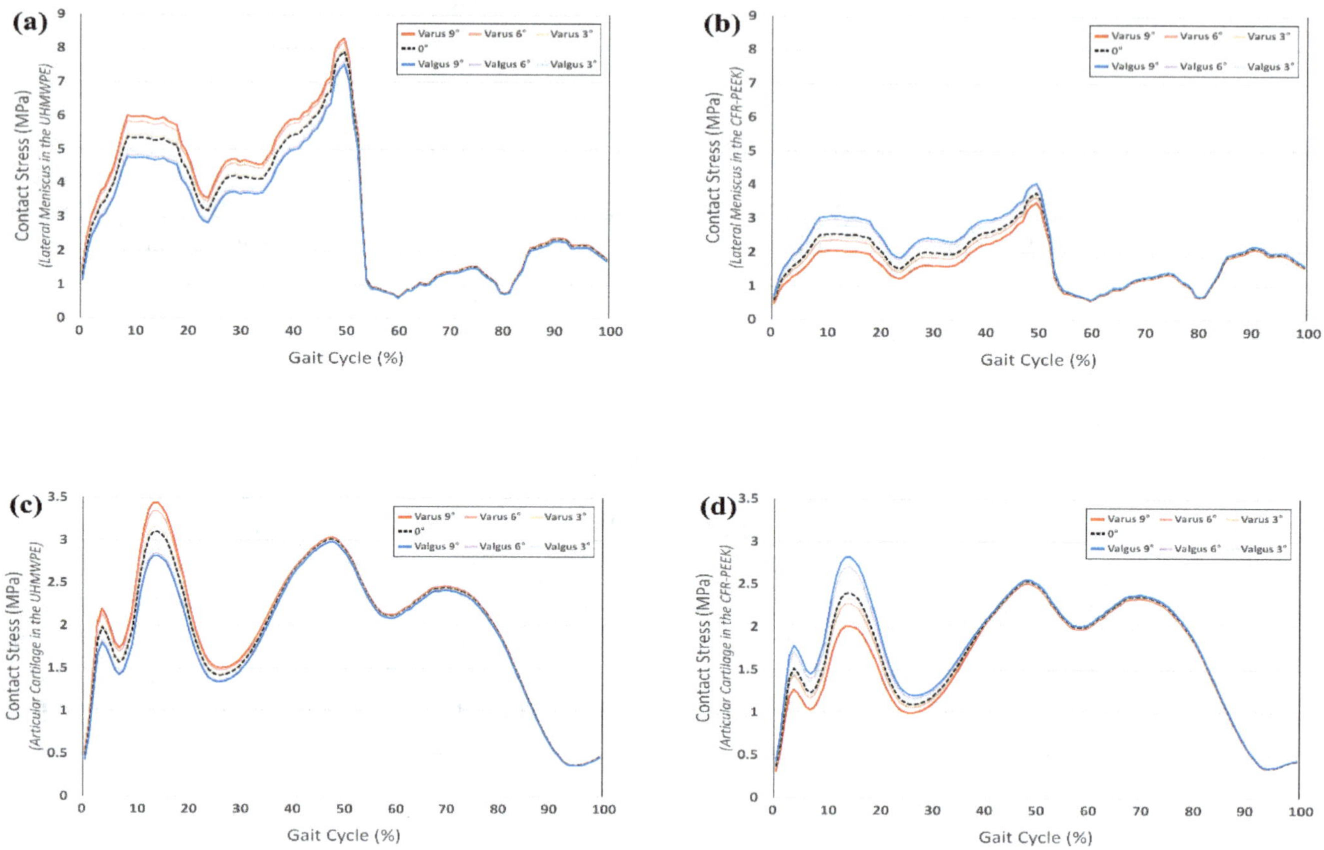

Figure 5. Comparison of contact stress on other compartments in varus/valgus condition with respect to different tibial insert materials during gait cycle: (**a**) lateral meniscus in the ultra-high molecular weight polyethylene (UHMWPE); (**b**) lateral meniscus in the carbon-fiber reinforced polyetheretherketone (CFR-PEEK); (**c**) articular cartilage in the UHMWPE; and, (**d**) articular cartilage in the CFR-PEEK.

3.3. Comparison of Von-Mises Stress in Tibial Bone and Collateral Ligament Force in UHMWPE and CFR-PEEK Tibial Component in Varus/Valgus Alignment

Figure 6 indicates the von-Mises stress on the tibia bone in the UHMWPE and CFR-PEEK tibial inserts with the varus/valgus tibial component. The greatest stress was exerted on ROI 1 and 2 (cancellous bone), in both the UHMWPE and CFR-PEEK. This trend did not change with varus and valgus in the tibial component. In addition, the bone stress in ROI 1–4, in the CFR-PEEK, was higher than in the UHMWPE. The von-Mises stress on the UHMWPE in the tibial bone showed a similar value from the neutral position to the varus 3° model. The CFR-PEEK model showed a similar value from the neutral position to varus 6°; however, it rapidly decreased afterwards, under the valgus condition. The stress in ROI 5 (cortical bone) with UHMWPE was greater than with CFR-PEEK. In addition, a similar trend was observed in ROI 1–4, for both UHMWPE and CFR-PEEK, under the varus and valgus conditions. Figure 7 indicates the force on the collateral ligament in the UHMWPE and CFR PEEK tibial insert with a varus/valgus tibial component. The force on the medial collateral ligament with the UHMWPE and CFR-PEEK increased under the valgus condition, in comparison to the neutral position. The force in the UHMWPE model with valgus 9° increased by 19% in the medial- collateral ligament, as compared to the neutral position. Moreover, the force on the medial-collateral ligament increased more in the CFR-PEEK model under the valgus condition. The force in the UHMWPE model with valgus 9° increased by 27% in the medial collateral ligament, in comparison to the neutral position. A complex pattern was observed in the lateral collateral ligament for the UHMWPE and CFR-PEEK. Under the valgus conditions, the force on the lateral collateral ligament increased during the swing and stance phases, respectively.

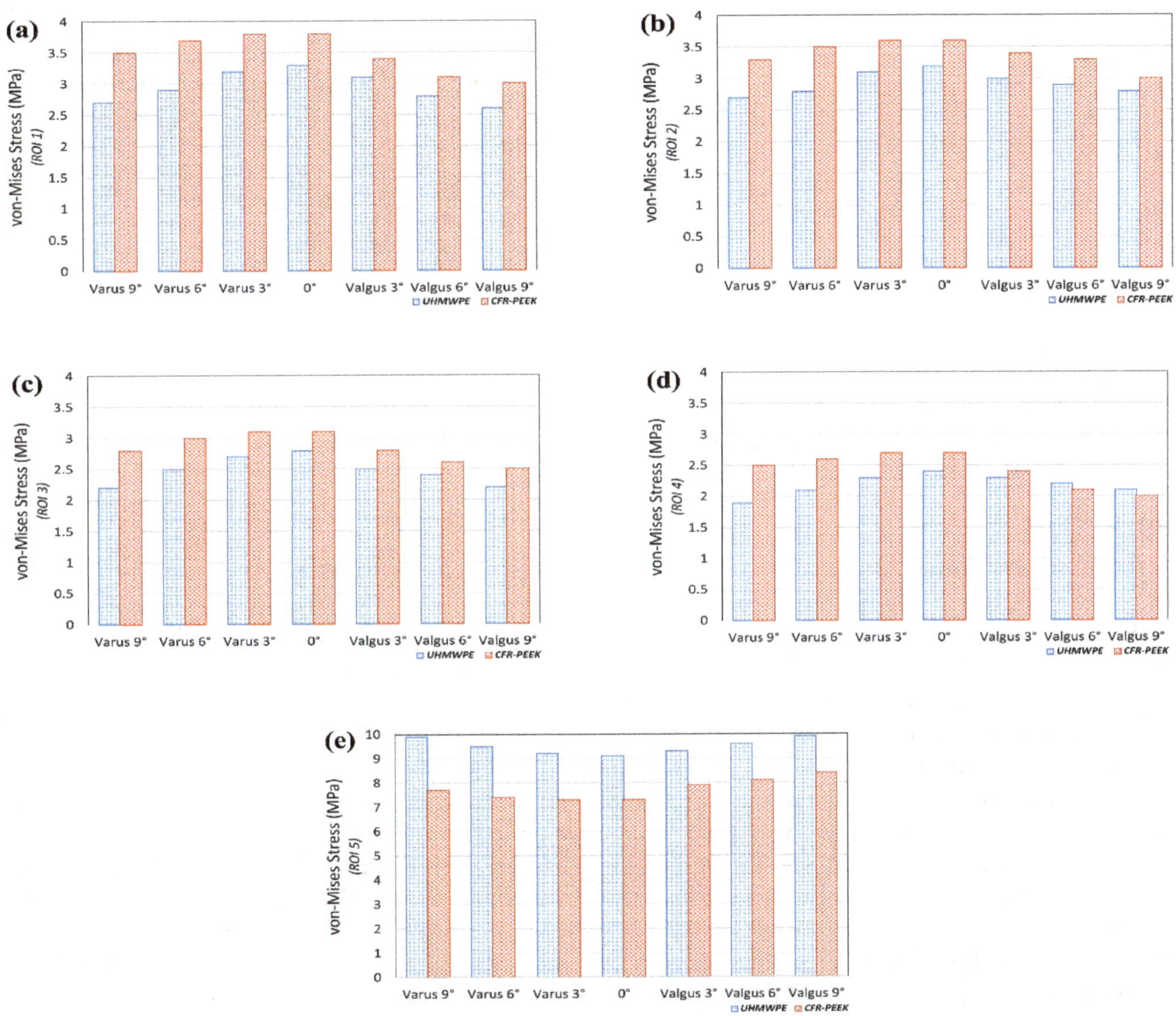

Figure 6. Comparison of von-Mises stress in ROI 1–5 in varus/valgus condition with respect to different tibial insert materials during gait cycle: (**a**) ROI 1; (**b**) ROI 2; (**c**) ROI 3; (**d**) ROI 4; and, (**e**) ROI 5.

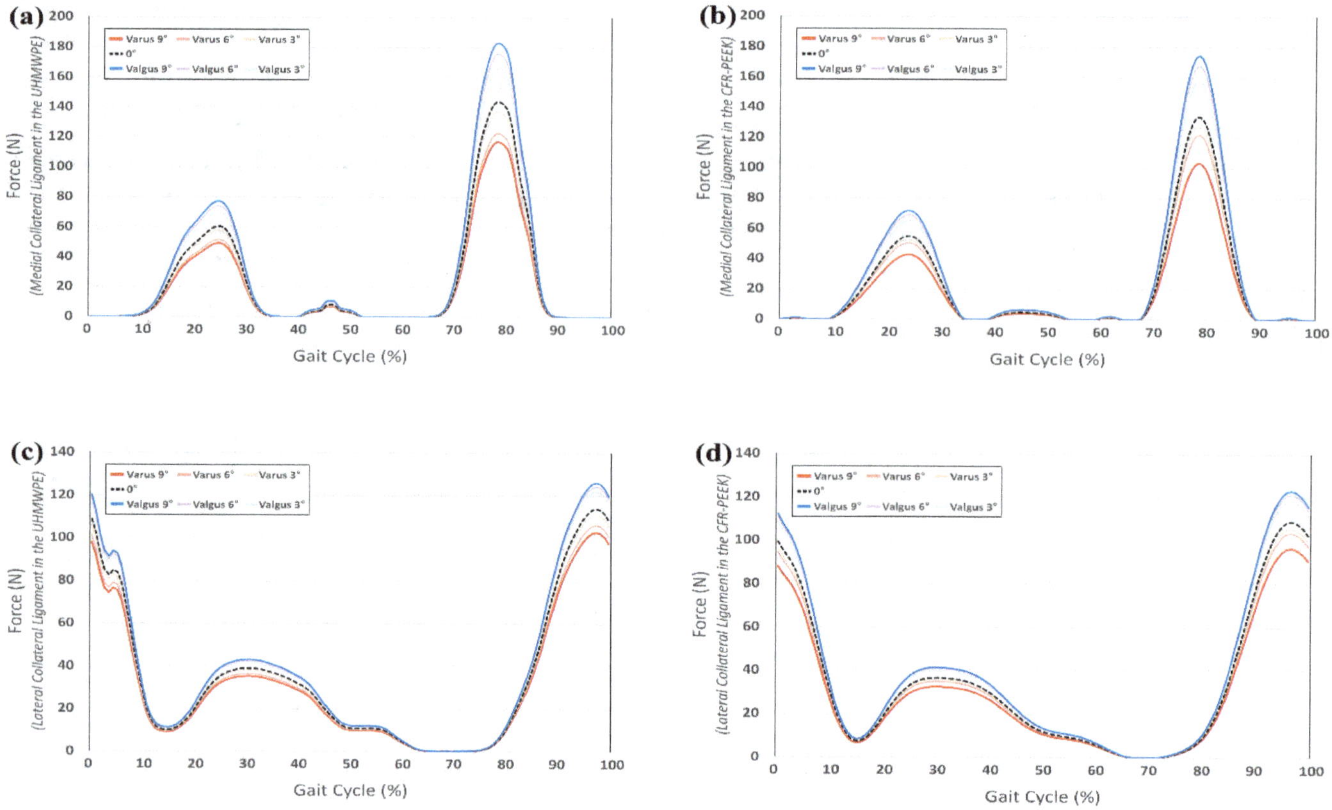

Figure 7. Comparison of ligament force in varus/valgus condition with respect to different tibial insert materials during gait cycle: (**a**) medial-collateral ligament in the UHMWPE; (**b**) medial-collateral ligament in the CFR-PEEK; (**c**) lateral-collateral ligament in the UHMWPE; and, (**d**) lateral-collateral ligament in the CFR-PEEK.

4. Discussion

The positive biomechanical effect that was observed in the UHMWPE tibial insert at the neutral position and with slight varus malalignment was the most important finding of the current study. Additionally, for the CFR-PEEK tibial insert, there was no problem with a varus malalignment greater than that of the UHMWPE tibial insert; however, the valgus malalignment should be avoided.

The precise restoration of the mechanical axis and correct implant positioning are major contributors to the improvement of implant longevity and the clinical outcomes of UKR. There is still no general agreement in terms of the optimal position of the tibial component [43].

This study aimed to evaluate the optimal tibial alignment for UKR with UHMWPE and CFR-PEEK tibial inserts, and the potential aberrant performances due to the malalignment of the tibial components. An FE model was used to analyze and compare different combinations of several biomechanical outputs. In addition, the FE model was impractical in the experimental evaluation of progressive OA in the other compartments and tibia bone stress problems, with respect to different insert materials under the varus/valgus conditions. Furthermore, the advantage of computational simulations that use a single subject is that the effects of tibial component alignment and the differences in insert materials, within the same subject, can be determined, except for variables, such as weight, height, bone geometry, differences in ethnicity and sex, ligament properties, and component size [44]. The intact knee model underwent a series of validation steps. The results showed good agreement with previous experimental data, in terms of kinematics and contact area, as demonstrated by the FE analysis for the same subject. In addition, an intact and a UKR model were both validated by using experimental and kinematics data. Therefore, the UKR model developed in the current study, along with the following analysis, can be considered to be reasonable.

As mentioned above, the UHMWPE insert led to result variation in the coronal positioning of the tibial tray. Sawatari et al. [45] analyzed the orientation influence of the unicompartmental tibial component on cancellous bone stresses in the coronal and sagittal planes, and correlated these findings to clinical data. They suggested that a slight valgus inclination of a UKR tibial component is better than a varus or square inclination in the coronal plane. In addition, Isekawa et al. [46] analyzed the inclination influence of the UKR tibial component on stress, in the proximal tibia, and the influence of contact pressure on the metal–bone interface, in the identical femorotibial alignment. They suggested that a slight valgus inclination of the tibial component might be better than varus or even a 0° (square) inclination, as the stress distribution is related. Therefore, a slight valgus inclination is preferable for both. Simpson et al. [47] found that the inclination angles had a minimal effect on the bone strain in the Oxford UKR, with the exclusion of the 2° varus inclination. However, there is a limitation in the three models that are mentioned above, as they only model tibia and not femur or other bony structure and soft tissues such as cartilage and ligament. Recently, Zhu et al. [48] developed a UKR model with entirely bony structure and soft tissue. They investigated the coronal inclination angles of the tibial tray ranging from 10° varus to 10° valgus. They suggested a range from 4° varus to 4° valgus for the inclination of the tibial component in the mobile-bearing UKR. In addition, Innocenti et al. [49] evaluated the biomechanical effects of different varus/valgus alignment tibial component positions in UKR. They proposed that a neutral mechanical or 3 varus alignment exhibits similar biomechanical outputs in the bone, collateral ligament strain, and polyethylene insert. A 6° varus alignment or changes in the valgus alignment were always associated with more detrimental effects. The two studies mentioned above also showed limitations, as they only evaluated the biomechanical effect under static conditions. However, UKR is a surgical treatment for younger patients; therefore, it requires analysis under dynamic loading conditions, such as gait cycles.

We studied the contact stress on other compartments, the stress on the tibial bone and the force on the collateral ligament under a gait cycle. Our results showed that alignment influences the development of OA in other compartments. Previous studies that have attempted to evaluate the influence of alignment were limited due to their short follow-up and absence of accurate knee alignment measurements [10,11,50]. In addition, a previous clinical study only used a radiography parameter (joint space narrowing) for the development of OA in the opposite compartment. This narrowing of joint space shows the articular cartilage loss in the joint and it is considered to be a more reliable marker of OA than the osteophytes or subchondral sclerosis. However, the radiography parameter might cause results to vary, owing to scanning inaccuracies and human error. We evaluated contact stress to investigate the progressive OA in other compartments because the contact parameters are known to be closely related to the degenerative OA of the knee joint [18,51]. An intriguing finding was that the effect of tibial malalignment was different for the different tibial insert materials. In UHMWPE, the contact stress on other compartments decreased in valgus and slightly increased under varus conditions [52]. This trend proved to be in fine agreement with a previous study. The contact force on the other compartment decreased under the valgus condition using UHMWPE and in the cadaveric experiment [52]. However, the CFR-PEEK model it increased in valgus and decreased in varus. Additionally, the difference between contact stresses on other compartments, in both the UHMWPE and CFR-PEEK model, was found during the stance phase. This proved that the contact stress was mainly influenced by the axial force.

The cortical bone always exerted the majority of the load transferred by the tibial baseplate, as its elastic modulus is much larger than that of the cancellous bone. An abnormally high stress of the proximal medial cortical bone was used to understand the cause of persistent pain after UKR [47]. Additionally, the aseptic loosening of prosthetic components, and especially that of the tibial component, is one of the major failure modes in UKR [53]. Excessive stress in both the cortical and cancellous bone cause it, and it leads to stress shielding. The major reason of the latter is the significant difference in the Young's modulus between the bone and tibial baseplate material. In contrast to TKR, the interface between the tibial baseplate and the tibia is significantly smaller. This leads to bone stresses being more sensitive to malalignment and malpositioning of component.

This UHMWPE model showed higher stress in the cortical bone region and lower stress in the cancellous bone region, in comparison to the CFR-PEEK model. The tibial insert material was only changed to CFR-PEEK; however, the stress-shielding effect was reduced because the material properties of CFR-PEEK were similar to the bone's material properties. The increase of bone stresses in the cortical bone and the decrease of bone stresses in the cancellous bone around the tibial baseplate may cause pain, which is induced by a loosening of the tibial baseplate [54–57]. Stress in the cortical bone increased, while, in the cancellous bone, it decreased under the valgus condition for both UHMWPE and CFR-PEEK, in comparison to the neutral position. In other words, the valgus malalignment should be avoided in both UHMWPE and CFR-PEEK.

After medial UKR was implanted, the valgus deformity was induced, even though the neutral knee model had a normal alignment (valgus rotation 0°) [49,58]. This phenomenon can be explained by the different stiffness between the medial and lateral compartments of the UKR knee. On the lateral side, the cartilage of both the femur and tibia had an elastic modulus of 15 MPa. In contrast to the medial side elastic moduli of the tibial insert materials UHMWPE and CFR-PEEK, the elastic modulus was much higher than that of the cartilage. Consequently, the Young's Modulus of the medial and lateral compartments differed by more than one order of magnitude; therefore, the deformation of materials in each compartment depended on their elastic modulus [54]. In a previous study, the valgus deformity that was induced by the strain loading, in the medial-collateral ligament, increased, while the strain in the lateral collateral ligament decreased [54]. Hence, whilst a surgeon balances a knee during UKR in an unloaded state, the knee will no longer be balanced once it is loaded [54].

Our study confirmed this result. The force on the medial-collateral ligament also increased for the UHMWPE and CFR-PEEK models under the valgus condition. This trend was particularly observed in CFR-PEEK. The reason was that CFR-PEEK has a higher elastic modulus than UHMWPE, as mentioned previously. Therefore, the difference in material properties became greater here than in other areas. Our results showed that progressive OA could occur in other compartments under the valgus condition. Additionally, valgus should be avoided because the MCL force rapidly increases in the CFR-PEEK model.

There are several strengths to this study. First, the FE model included the femur, tibia, and related soft tissues in the present study [31,45–47]. Second, gait cycle loading, and complex vertical static loading condition was applied in this study [31,45–49,54]. Third, this study validated not just the initial FE model, but also achieved kinematic validation of the UKR FE models with experimental data [31,45–49,54].

Nevertheless, there are three limitations. First, the FE model represented a fixed bearing UKR, and it cannot apply other implant designs, such as the mobile bearing UKR. Second, a single coefficient of friction value was used, when there is in fact a variety in the coefficients of friction for different materials. The effect of different values will be investigated in future studies.

Third, patient satisfaction and clinical results could not be assessed by the results from FE analysis. However, contact stress on the other compartments, force exerted on ligaments, and bone stresses are important factors that should be investigated for the evaluation of biomechanical effects in computational biomechanics [18–21,31,45–49].

5. Conclusions

The biomechanical justifications for the tibial insert materials UHMWPE and CFR PEEK were evaluated to confirm the suitability of various tibial component alignment positions while using an FE model. We performed a simulation for other compartments to investigate progressive OA. Contact stress on other compartments increased in varus and decreased in valgus for UHMWPE. In CFR-PEEK, an opposite trend was observed, by which the stress-shielding effect was less than that of UHMWPE, because its elastic modulus was closer to that of bone. However, in the CFR-PEEK model, a significant negative biomechanical effect was observed, owing to the valgus condition, in comparison to UHMWPE. In this model, the stress on the cortical and cancellous bone increased and decreased rapidly under the valgus and varus condition, respectively, in comparison to the neutral position. This trend was also observed in UHMWPE; however, the negative biomechanical effects were more pronounced in CFR PEEK; here, the varus allowance was wider than in UHMWPE, as there was less difference in the biomechanical effects from the neutral position to varus 6°. Such a trend could be found in the medial collateral ligament. The force on the medial collateral ligament became greater under the valgus condition of the CFR-PEEK model, in comparison to the UHMWPE model. The UHMPWE model, with a neutral position or minor varus (3°) alignment, exhibits similar biomechanical outputs in terms of the contact stress on other compartments, the stress on the bone, and the collateral ligament force. Therefore, the neutral position and minor varus conditions are recommended in the UHMWPE model. In addition, a greater varus condition of up to 6° is recommended in the CFR-PEEK model, as it showed similar biomechanical output. However, the valgus condition should be avoided in the CFR-PEEK model.

Author Contributions: Y.-G.K. and H.-T.H. contributed equally to the current study and they should be considered as co-first authors. K.-T.K.—Conceptualization; Validation; Writing—reviewing & editing; Methodology.

References

1. Berger, R.A.; Meneghini, R.M.; Jacobs, J.J.; Sheinkop, M.B.; Della Valle, C.J.; Rosenberg, A.G.; Galante, J.O. Results of unicompartmental knee arthroplasty at a minimum of ten years of follow-up. *J. Bone Joint Surg. Am.* **2005**, *87*, 999–1006. [CrossRef] [PubMed]
2. Riddle, D.L.; Jiranek, W.A.; McGlynn, F.J. Yearly incidence of unicompartmental knee arthroplasty in the United States. *J. Arthroplast.* **2008**, *23*, 408–412. [CrossRef] [PubMed]
3. Mochizuki, T.; Sato, T.; Tanifuji, O.; Kobayashi, K.; Koga, Y.; Yamagiwa, H.; Omori, G.; Endo, N. In vivo pre- and postoperative three-dimensional knee kinematics in unicompartmental knee arthroplasty. *J. Orthop. Sci.* **2013**, *18*, 54–60. [CrossRef] [PubMed]
4. Pandit, H.; Jenkins, C.; Gill, H.S.; Barker, K.; Dodd, C.A.; Murray, D.W. Minimally invasive Oxford phase 3 unicompartmental knee replacement: Results of 1000 cases. *J. Bone Joint Surg. Br.* **2011**, *93*, 198–204. [CrossRef] [PubMed]
5. McAuley, J.P.; Engh, G.A.; Ammeen, D.J. Revision of failed unicompartmental knee arthroplasty. *Clin. Orthop. Relat. Res.* **2001**, 279–282. [CrossRef] [PubMed]
6. Weinstein, J.N.; Andriacchi, T.P.; Galante, J. Factors influencing walking and stairclimbing following unicompartmental knee arthroplasty. *J. Arthroplast.* **1986**, *1*, 109–115. [CrossRef]
7. Wilcox, P.G.; Jackson, D.W. Unicompartmental knee arthroplasty. *Orthop. Rev.* **1986**, *15*, 490–495.
8. Goodfellow, J.W.; Kershaw, C.J.; Benson, M.K.; O'Connor, J.J. The Oxford Knee for unicompartmental osteoarthritis. The first 103 cases. *J. Bone Joint Surg. Br.* **1988**, *70*, 692–701. [CrossRef]
9. Klemme, W.R.; Galvin, E.G.; Petersen, S.A. Unicompartmental knee arthroplasty. Sequential radiographic and scintigraphic imaging with an average five-year follow-up. *Clin. Orthop. Relat. Res.* **1994**, *301*, 233–238.
10. Weale, A.E.; Murray, D.W.; Baines, J.; Newman, J.H. Radiological changes five years after unicompartmental knee replacement. *J. Bone Joint Surg. Br.* **2000**, *82*, 996–1000. [CrossRef]
11. Kennedy, W.R.; White, R.P. Unicompartmental arthroplasty of the knee. Postoperative alignment and its influence on overall results. *Clin. Orthop. Relat. Res.* **1987**, *221*, 278–285.
12. Blunn, G.W.; Joshi, A.B.; Minns, R.J.; Lidgren, L.; Lilley, P.; Ryd, L.; Engelbrecht, E.; Walker, P.S. Wear in retrieved condylar knee arthroplasties. A comparison of wear in different designs of 280 retrieved condylar knee prostheses. *J. Arthroplast.* **1997**, *12*, 281–290. [CrossRef]
13. Brockett, C.L.; Carbone, S.; Fisher, J.; Jennings, L.M. *PEEK and CFR PEEK as an Alternative to UHMWPE in Total Knee Replacement*; ORS Annual Meeting Las Vegas: Las Vegas, NV, USA, 2015.

14. Brockett, C.L.; Carbone, S.; Fisher, J.; Jennings, L.M. PEEK and CFR-PEEK as alternative bearing materials to UHMWPE in a fixed bearing total knee replacement: An experimental wear study. *Wear* **2017**, *374–375*, 86–91. [CrossRef] [PubMed]
15. Scholes, S.C.; Unsworth, A. Pitch-based carbon-fibre-reinforced poly (ether-ether-ketone) OPTIMA assessed as a bearing material in a mobile bearing unicondylar knee joint. *Proc. Inst. Mech. Eng. H* **2009**, *223*, 13–25. [CrossRef] [PubMed]
16. Cartier, P.; Sanouiller, J.L.; Grelsamer, R.P. Unicompartmental knee arthroplasty surgery. 10-year minimum follow-up period. *J. Arthroplast.* **1996**, *11*, 782–788. [CrossRef]
17. Thornhill, T.S.; Scott, R.D. Unicompartmental total knee arthroplasty. *Orthop. Clin. N. Am.* **1989**, *20*, 245–256.
18. Kim, Y.S.; Kang, K.T.; Son, J.; Kwon, O.R.; Choi, Y.J.; Jo, S.B.; Choi, Y.W.; Koh, Y.G. Graft extrusion related to the position of allograft in lateral meniscal allograft transplantation: Biomechanical comparison between parapatellar and transpatellar approaches using finite element analysis. *Arthroscopy* **2015**, *31*, 2380–2391. [CrossRef]
19. Kang, K.T.; Kim, S.H.; Son, J.; Lee, Y.H.; Chun, H.J. Computational model-based probabilistic analysis of in vivo material properties for ligament stiffness using the laxity test and computed tomography. *J. Mater. Sci. Mater. Med.* **2016**, *27*, 183. [CrossRef]
20. Kwon, O.R.; Kang, K.T.; Son, J.; Suh, D.S.; Baek, C.; Koh, Y.G. Importance of joint line preservation in unicompartmental knee arthroplasty: Finite element analysis. *J. Orthop. Res.* **2017**, *35*, 347–352. [CrossRef]
21. Kang, K.T.; Kim, S.H.; Son, J.; Lee, Y.H.; Kim, S.; Chun, H.J. Probabilistic evaluation of the material properties of the in vivo subject-specific articular surface using a computational model. *J. Biomed. Mater. Res. B Appl. Biomater.* **2017**, *105*, 1390–1400. [CrossRef]
22. Pena, E.; Calvo, B.; Martinez, M.A.; Palanca, D.; Doblare, M. Why lateral meniscectomy is more dangerous than medial meniscectomy. A finite element study. *J. Orthop. Res.* **2006**, *24*, 1001–1010. [CrossRef] [PubMed]
23. Kayabasi, O.; Ekici, B. The effects of static, dynamic and fatigue behavior on three-dimensional shape optimization of hip prosthesis by finite element method. *Mater. Des.* **2007**, *28*, 2269–2277. [CrossRef]
24. Hoffler, C.E.; Moore, K.E.; Kozloff, K.; Zysset, P.K.; Goldstein, S.A. Age, gender, and bone lamellae elastic moduli. *J. Orthop. Res.* **2000**, *18*, 432–437. [CrossRef] [PubMed]
25. Shepherd, D.E.; Seedhom, B.B. The 'instantaneous' compressive modulus of human articular cartilage in joints of the lower limb. *Rheumatology* **1999**, *38*, 124–132. [CrossRef]
26. Haut Donahue, T.L.; Hull, M.L.; Rashid, M.M.; Jacobs, C.R. How the stiffness of meniscal attachments and meniscal material properties affect tibio-femoral contact pressure computed using a validated finite element model of the human knee joint. *J. Biomech.* **2003**, *36*, 19–34. [CrossRef]
27. Guess, T.M.; Thiagarajan, G.; Kia, M.; Mishra, M. A subject specific multibody model of the knee with menisci. *Med. Eng. Phys.* **2010**, *32*, 505–515. [CrossRef] [PubMed]
28. Takeda, Y.; Xerogeanes, J.W.; Livesay, G.A.; Fu, F.H.; Woo, S.L. Biomechanical function of the human anterior cruciate ligament. *Arthroscopy* **1994**, *10*, 140–147. [CrossRef]
29. Blankevoort, L.; Huiskes, R. Validation of a three-dimensional model of the knee. *J. Biomech.* **1996**, *29*, 955–961. [CrossRef]
30. Zimmer, I. *Zimmer Unicompartmental High Flex Knee: Intramedullary, Spacer Block Option and Extramedullary Minimally Invasive Surgical Techniques*; Zimmer Biomet: Warsaw, IN, USA, 2005.
31. Inoue, S.; Akagi, M.; Asada, S.; Mori, S.; Zaima, H.; Hashida, M. The Valgus Inclination of the Tibial Component Increases the Risk of Medial Tibial Condylar Fractures in Unicompartmental Knee Arthroplasty. *J. Arthroplast.* **2016**, *31*, 2025–2030. [CrossRef]
32. Pegg, E.C.; Walter, J.; Mellon, S.J.; Pandit, H.G.; Murray, D.W.; D'Lima, D.D.; Fregly, B.J.; Gill, H.S. Evaluation of factors affecting tibial bone strain after unicompartmental knee replacement. *J. Orthop. Res.* **2013**, *31*, 821–828. [CrossRef]
33. Godest, A.C.; Beaugonin, M.; Haug, E.; Taylor, M.; Gregson, P.J. Simulation of a knee joint replacement during a gait cycle using explicit finite element analysis. *J. Biomech.* **2002**, *35*, 267–275. [CrossRef]
34. Innocenti, B.; Truyens, E.; Labey, L.; Wong, P.; Victor, J.; Bellemans, J. Can medio-lateral baseplate position and load sharing induce asymptomatic local bone resorption of the proximal tibia? A finite element study. *J. Orthop. Surg. Res.* **2009**, *4*, 26. [CrossRef] [PubMed]

35. Kang, K.-T.; Koh, Y.-G.; Son, J.; Yeom, J.S.; Park, J.-H.; Kim, H.-J. Biomechanical evaluation of pedicle screw fixation system in spinal adjacent levels using polyetheretherketone, carbon-fiber-reinforced polyetheretherketone, and traditional titanium as rod materials. *Compos. Part B Eng.* **2017**, *130*, 248–256. [CrossRef]
36. Knight, L.A.; Pal, S.; Coleman, J.C.; Bronson, F.; Haider, H.; Levine, D.L.; Taylor, M.; Rullkoetter, P.J. Comparison of long-term numerical and experimental total knee replacement wear during simulated gait loading. *J. Biomech.* **2007**, *40*, 1550–1558. [CrossRef] [PubMed]
37. Greco, A.C.; Erck, R.; Ajayi, O.; Fenske, G. Effect of reinforcement morphology on high-speed sliding friction and wear of PEEK polymers. *Wear* **2011**, *271*, 2222–2229. [CrossRef]
38. Suggs, J.F.; Li, G.; Park, S.E.; Steffensmeier, S.; Rubash, H.E.; Freiberg, A.A. Function of the anterior cruciate ligament after unicompartmental knee arthroplasty: An in vitro robotic study. *J. Arthroplast.* **2004**, *19*, 224–229. [CrossRef] [PubMed]
39. Standardization, I.O. f. *ISO 14243-1: Implants for Surgery—Wear of Total Knee-Joint Prostheses—Part 1: Loading and Displacement Parameters for Wear-Testing Machines with Load Control and Corresponding Environmental Conditions for Test*; International Organization for Standardization: Geneva, Switzerland, 2002.
40. Halloran, J.P.; Clary, C.W.; Maletsky, L.P.; Taylor, M.; Petrella, A.J.; Rullkoetter, P.J. Verification of predicted knee replacement kinematics during simulated gait in the Kansas knee simulator. *J. Biomech. Eng.* **2010**, *132*, 081010. [CrossRef]
41. Kutzner, I.; Heinlein, B.; Graichen, F.; Bender, A.; Rohlmann, A.; Halder, A.; Beier, A.; Bergmann, G. Loading of the knee joint during activities of daily living measured in vivo in five subjects. *J. Biomech.* **2010**, *43*, 2164–2173. [CrossRef]
42. Kang, K.T.; Koh, Y.G.; Son, J.; Kwon, O.R.; Baek, C.; Jung, S.H.; Park, K.K. Measuring the effect of femoral malrotation on knee joint biomechanics for total knee arthroplasty using computational simulation. *Bone Joint Res.* **2016**, *5*, 552–559. [CrossRef]
43. Keene, G.; Simpson, D.; Kalairajah, Y. Limb alignment in computer-assisted minimally-invasive unicompartmental knee replacement. *J. Bone Joint Surg. Br.* **2006**, *88*, 44–48. [CrossRef]
44. Thompson, J.A.; Hast, M.W.; Granger, J.F.; Piazza, S.J.; Siston, R.A. Biomechanical effects of total knee arthroplasty component malrotation: A computational simulation. *J. Orthop. Res.* **2011**, *29*, 969–975. [CrossRef] [PubMed]
45. Sawatari, T.; Tsumura, H.; Iesaka, K.; Furushiro, Y.; Torisu, T. Three-dimensional finite element analysis of unicompartmental knee arthroplasty—The influence of tibial component inclination. *J. Orthop. Res.* **2005**, *23*, 549–554. [CrossRef] [PubMed]
46. Iesaka, K.; Tsumura, H.; Sonoda, H.; Sawatari, T.; Takasita, M.; Torisu, T. The effects of tibial component inclination on bone stress after unicompartmental knee arthroplasty. *J. Biomech.* **2002**, *35*, 969–974. [CrossRef]
47. Simpson, D.J.; Price, A.J.; Gulati, A.; Murray, D.W.; Gill, H.S. Elevated proximal tibial strains following unicompartmental knee replacement—A possible cause of pain. *Med. Eng. Phys.* **2009**, *31*, 752–757. [CrossRef] [PubMed]
48. Zhu, G.D.; Guo, W.S.; Zhang, Q.D.; Liu, Z.H.; Cheng, L.M. Finite Element Analysis of Mobile-bearing Unicompartmental Knee Arthroplasty: The Influence of Tibial Component Coronal Alignment. *Chin. Med. J.* **2015**, *128*, 2873–2878. [CrossRef] [PubMed]
49. Innocenti, B.; Pianigiani, S.; Ramundo, G.; Thienpont, E. Biomechanical Effects of Different Varus and Valgus Alignments in Medial Unicompartmental Knee Arthroplasty. *J. Arthroplast.* **2016**, *31*, 2685–2691. [CrossRef]
50. Hernigou, P.; Deschamps, G. Alignment influences wear in the knee after medial unicompartmental arthroplasty. *Clin. Orthop. Relat. Res.* **2004**, *423*, 161–165. [CrossRef]
51. Segal, N.A.; Anderson, D.D.; Iyer, K.S.; Baker, J.; Torner, J.C.; Lynch, J.A.; Felson, D.T.; Lewis, C.E.; Brown, T.D. Baseline articular contact stress levels predict incident symptomatic knee osteoarthritis development in the MOST cohort. *J. Orthop. Res.* **2009**, *27*, 1562–1568. [CrossRef]
52. Heyse, T.J.; El-Zayat, B.F.; De Corte, R.; Scheys, L.; Chevalier, Y.; Fuchs-Winkelmann, S.; Labey, L. Balancing UKA: Overstuffing leads to high medial collateral ligament strains. *Knee Surg. Sports Traumatol. Arthrosc.* **2016**, *24*, 3218–3228. [CrossRef]
53. Berger, R.A.; Nedeff, D.D.; Barden, R.M.; Sheinkop, M.M.; Jacobs, J.J.; Rosenberg, A.G.; Galante, J.O. Unicompartmental knee arthroplasty. Clinical experience at 6- to 10-year followup. *Clin. Orthop. Relat. Res.* **1999**, *367*, 50–60.

54. Innocenti, B.; Bilgen, O.F.; Labey, L.; van Lenthe, G.H.; Sloten, J.V.; Catani, F. Load sharing and ligament strains in balanced, overstuffed and understuffed UKA. A validated finite element analysis. *J. Arthroplast.* **2014**, *29*, 1491–1498. [CrossRef] [PubMed]
55. Bartel, D.L.; Burstein, A.H.; Santavicca, E.A.; Insall, J.N. Performance of the tibial component in total knee replacement. *J. Bone Joint. Surg. Am.* **1982**, *64*, 1026–1033. [CrossRef] [PubMed]
56. Bourne, R.B.; Finlay, J.B. The influence of tibial component intramedullary stems and implant-cortex contact on the strain distribution of the proximal tibia following total knee arthroplasty. An in vitro study. *Clin. Orthop. Relat. Res.* **1986**, *208*, 95–99. [CrossRef]
57. Taylor, M.; Tanner, K.E.; Freeman, M.A. Finite element analysis of the implanted proximal tibia: A relationship between the initial cancellous bone stresses and implant migration. *J. Biomech.* **1998**, *31*, 303–310. [CrossRef]
58. Au, A.G.; Raso, V.J.; Liggins, A.B.; Otto, D.D.; Amirfazli, A. A three-dimensional finite element stress analysis for tunnel placement and buttons in anterior cruciate ligament reconstructions. *J. Biomech.* **2005**, *38*, 827–832. [CrossRef]

10

3D Printing of Bioceramics for Bone Tissue Engineering

Muhammad Jamshaid Zafar, Dongbin Zhu * and Zhengyan Zhang *

School of Mechanical Engineering, Hebei University of Technology, Tianjin 300130, China; jamshaid.zafer@yahoo.com

* Correspondence: zhudongbin@hebut.edu.cn (D.Z.); zzy@hebut.edu.cn (Z.Z.)

Abstract: Bioceramics have frequent use in functional restoration of hard tissues to improve human well-being. Additive manufacturing (AM) also known as 3D printing is an innovative material processing technique extensively applied to produce bioceramic parts or scaffolds in a layered perspicacious manner. Moreover, the applications of additive manufacturing in bioceramics have the capability to reliably fabricate the commercialized scaffolds tailored for practical clinical applications, and the potential to survive in the new era of effective hard tissue fabrication. The similarity of the materials with human bone histomorphometry makes them conducive to use in hard tissue engineering scheme. The key objective of this manuscript is to explore the applications of bioceramics-based AM in bone tissue engineering. Furthermore, the article comprehensively and categorically summarizes some novel bioceramics based AM techniques for the restoration of bones. At prior stages of this article, different ceramics processing AM techniques have been categorized, subsequently, processing of frequently used materials for bone implants and complexities associated with these materials have been elaborated. At the end, some novel applications of bioceramics in orthopedic implants and some future directions are also highlighted to explore it further. This review article will help the new researchers to understand the basic mechanism and current challenges in neophyte techniques and the applications of bioceramics in the orthopedic prosthesis.

Keywords: bioceramics; additive manufacturing; scaffolds; bone tissue engineering

---

1. Introduction

Additive manufacturing or 3D printing has got attention in scaffold design and manufacturing for tissue engineering applications. Initially, this technique was developed by Sachs et al., to create the ink-jet freestyle printing towards the latter part of the 20th century [1]. Later on, it was extended in tailoring the perfect scaffolds on its user-friendly capabilities, which considered the transformation of computer aided design (CAD) information to a rapid and reliable production line of constructs with the coveted material, porosity, and measurements [2,3]. Moreover, it showed a time and cost-efficient potential coupled with interconnected structures, specifically hard tissue deformity regeneration.

Recently, clinical preliminaries and contextual analyses revealed its resounding accomplishments in the field of orthopedic bioengineering. While this procedure has shown significant potential, specific difficulties tend to enhance patient-particular scaffolds for standard acknowledgment in regenerative medicine [4–6].

During the past few decades, many advanced biomaterials were introduced in the biomedical field including different ceramic materials for the skeletal repair and reconstruction. These materials in the field of medical implants are often referred to as "bioceramics" [7]. Bioceramics are peculiar in nature due to their exceptional biological and osteoinduction properties. These materials are specific for scaffolds due to capability to create propagation, self-adhesion, distinction and bone tissues regeneration [8]. Furthermore, excellent chemical and mechanical properties such as better osteoconductivity, superior wear resistant and biocompatibility enabled them as a substitute for bone restoration, [9,10]. It can anticipate that bioceramics have a future due to increasing bone replacement operation per year due to increasing aging population [11].

The clinical importance of AM ceramic scaffold design and implantation envelops an invaluable method for quick and reliable production of hard tissue substitution replica of the biological context of natural bone [12]. In view of the way that customized scaffold can be prepared that suits an individual patient's skeletal imperfection, layer-by-layer sintering is regarded as a lucrative discipline for the utilization of ceramic-based bone substitutes in regenerative medicine [13]. Besides, utilizing AM ceramic scaffolds as medication conveyance systems, it is becoming more attractive and relevant to the bioengineering environment [14–16].

This article is divided into six sections; Section 1 details the bioceramics potential, Section 2 offers an overview of the AM techniques used to fabricate ceramic parts. Section 3 presents achievements in the production of hydroxyapatite (HA); Section 4 depicts about tricalcium phosphate (TCP) and Section 5 describes about bioactive glass (BG) using different AM techniques. Section 6 concludes some important findings with some current challenges and future opportunities in this field.

2. Additive Manufacturing Technologies to Produce Ceramic Parts

Additive manufacturing has been classified into two major classes such as acellular and cellular techniques for biomaterials. The cellular category includes the printing of live cells, while the acellular category does not consider any type of live cells in printing. Figure 1 shows different acellular AM techniques for biomaterials that have been classified as per recommendations of American Society for Testing of Materials (ASTM) [17]. The major AM techniques employed in the processing of bioceramics have been discussed in the following section.

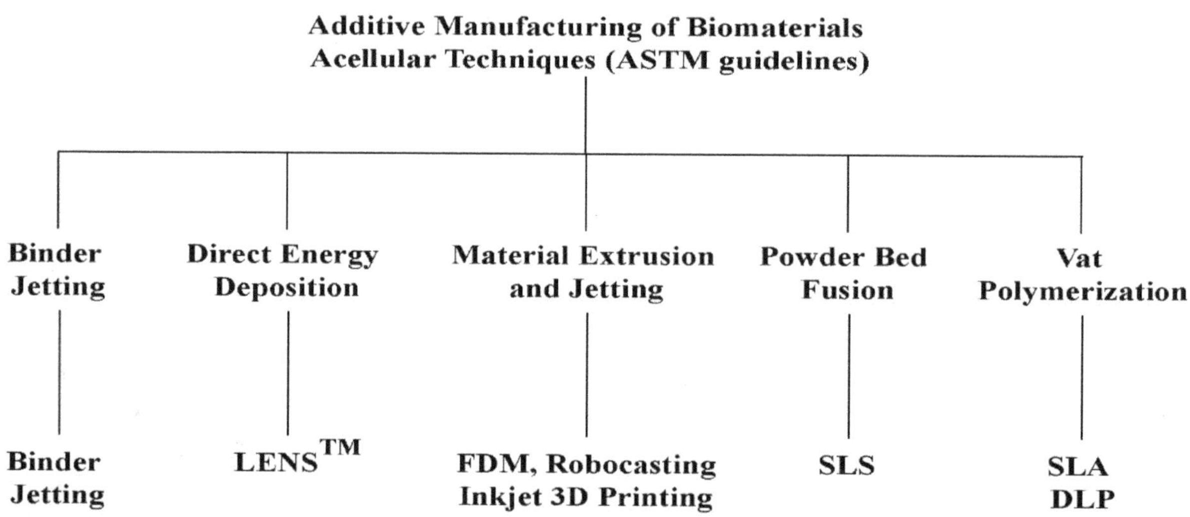

Figure 1. Different types of acellular techniques for biomaterials additive manufacturing (AM).

2.1. Binder Jetting

Binder jetting technique was developed in the early 1990s at Massachusetts Institute of Technology (MIT) [18]. Figure 2 depicts the schematic of binder jetting. In this technique, the binder is selectively used from powder bed to create 3D objects. Binder jetting is a valuable technique for printing powder materials [19,20]. The particle size of the powder has a key influence on powder flowability in binder jetting.

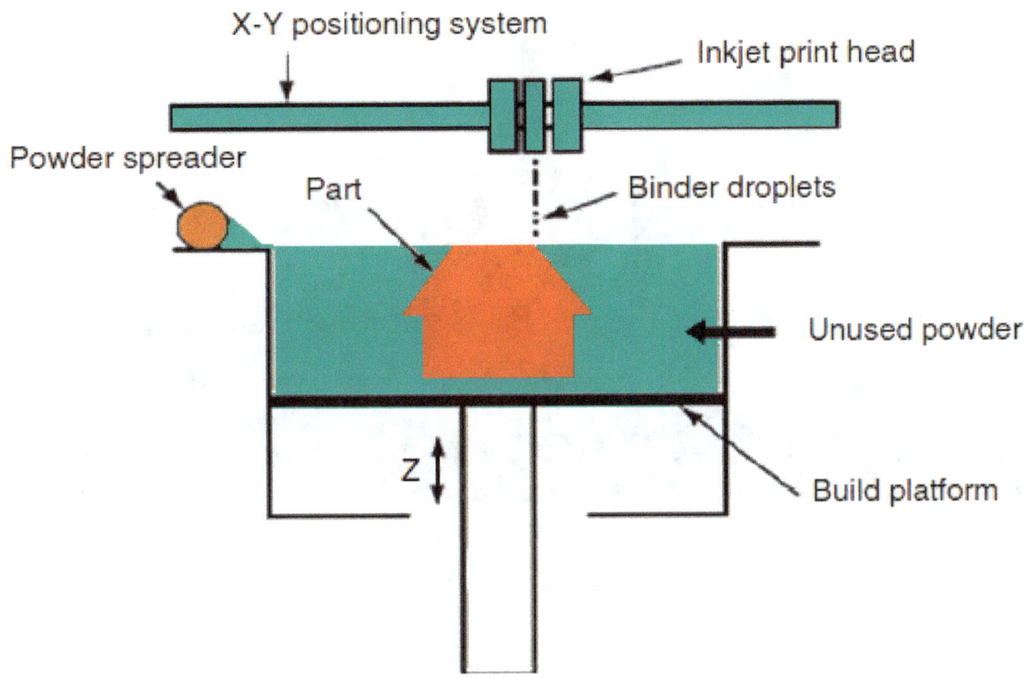

Figure 2. Schematic diagram of binder jetting mechanism [18].

For dry binder jetting, large size particles are preferred due to its outstanding flowability and less surface area. The powder size not only affects the flowability but also significantly affects the quality of the final product. Numerous researchers have reported less surface roughness using fine powder in the binder jetting. The effect of the powder shape is less, as compared to the powder size. However, spherical shape powders have better flowability and lesser friction compared to faceted powders [21–23].

2.2. *Direct Energy Deposition (DED)*

Direct energy deposition-based AM techniques uses energy into a small region to simultaneously deposit, melt and solidify the material such as wire or powder [24]. The direct energy source can be electrical, or laser beam can be used to melt the metal, ceramics or composite materials. Laser assisted Direct Deposition techniques such as laser cladding, laser engineered net shaping (LENS™), and laser melt injection are common examples of this technique.

In ceramic Direct Energy Deposition (DED), the printing head of the apparatus contains a nozzle that feeds ceramic powder particles to the focal point of the laser beam. The ceramic powder melts and solidifies in layer-wise fashion on a substrate [25]. Figure 3 is the schematic illustration of LENS [26].

The major advantages of DED are better compatibility with a wide range of biomaterial viscosities, higher resolution and greater cell density that provide higher control of cell-to-cell adhesions [27]. Besides these advantages, DED has many challenges such as, low speed, cost, high complexity and limited capability to manufacture heterogeneous tissue parts [28]. Due to these challenges, the usage of DED is very limited as compared to other AM techniques particularly in bone tissue engineering. The DED technology needs more research to enhance its productivity.

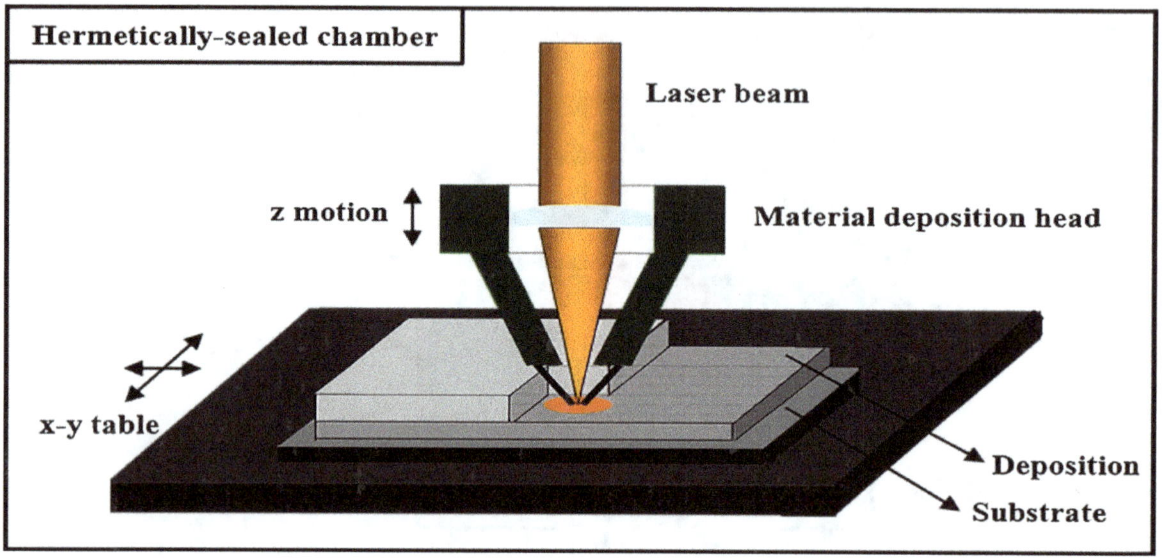

Figure 3. Typical Schematic representation of laser engineered net shaping (LENS) [26].

2.3. Material Extrusion and Jetting

Extrusion assisted additive manufacturing deposits a continuous layer by layer deposition of ceramic loaded paste to create 3D objects. Various terms are used to refer to this technology for instance, Fused Deposition of Ceramics (FDC), Robocasting, Extrusion Freeform Fabrication (EFF), Direct Ink Writing (DIW), Slurry Deposition, and Dispense Plotting [29].

In Fused Deposition, dense ceramic particles (up to 60 vol%) are spread into a wax or thermoplastic filament after which the flexible filament is partly melted and extruded from a moving deposition head onto a fixed worktable layer-by-layer. However, in robocasting, ceramic slurry is ejected from a precise nozzle to form a filament that is directly deposited in a designed pattern to create complex 3D objects in a layer-by-layer fashion [30].

In another research work, an indirect Fused Deposition Modeling (FDM) method was applied to prepare ceramic parts. At the preliminary stage, FDM was used to prepare a honeycomb shaped polymer structural mold. Secondly, the ceramic slurry was permeated into the polymer mold-sintering to remove the mold. The porous ceramics made a correct pore size and porosity through this technique [31].

Another technique named Extrusion-based bioprinting has also a greater potential in perspective of deposition and printing speed compared to other AM techniques. This technique is also beneficial to achieve better scalability in a shorter time [32], wide range flexibility of bioinks selection [33]. This is because developing new bioinks is a critical procedure for quick, sustainable and safe delivery of cells in a biomimetic microenvironment [32]. Besides many advantages, some complexities are also associated with this technology such as low resolution and shear stress effect on cells. The schematic of the process with part microstructure was shown in Figure 4.

The material jetting techniques are the "AM processes in which droplets of build material are selectively deposited" [17], that can be used to manufacture different kinds of ceramic parts. Inkjet 3D printing technology was among the first material jetting AM techniques that were employed for additive manufacturing of ceramic parts. It was developed by Sachs et al. in 1992 at MIT and defined as a process for the manufacturing of ceramic casting cores and shells using inkjet 3D printing [1]. Figure 5 shows the Schematic of ink-jet 3D printing [34].

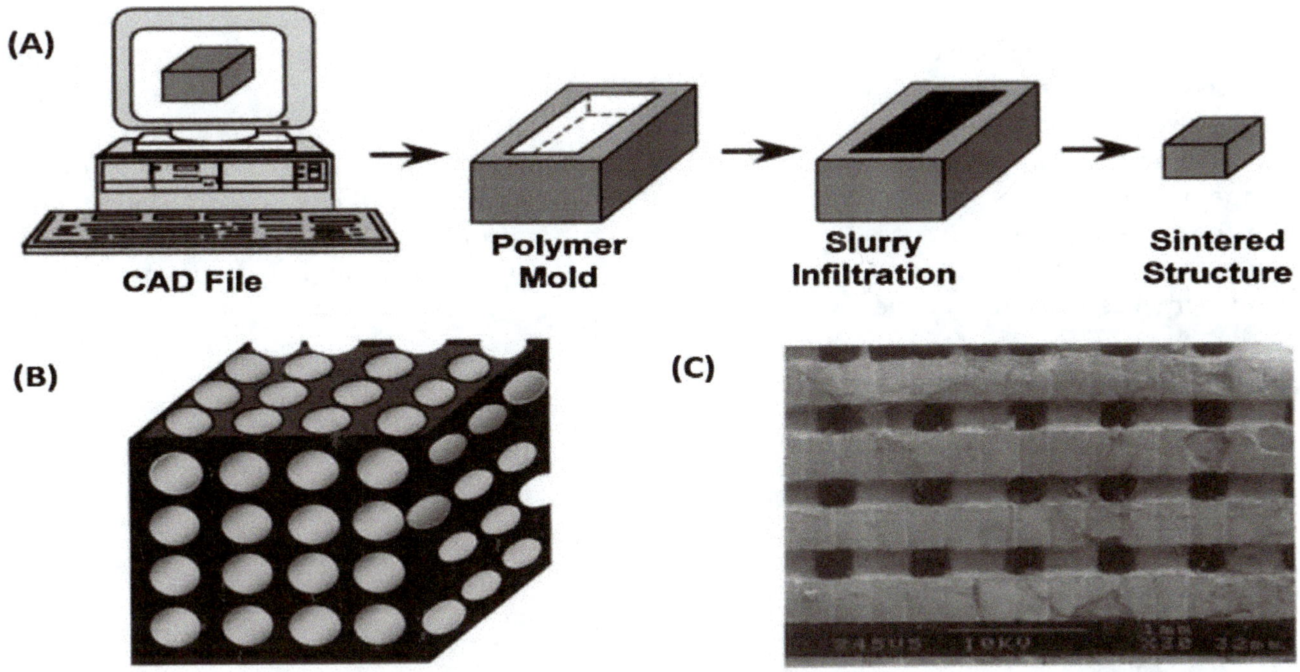

Figure 4. (**A**) Schematic of indirect Fused Deposition Modeling (FDM) processing of ceramic parts (**B**) Straight channels (**C**) Top view of sintered porous ceramic part [31].

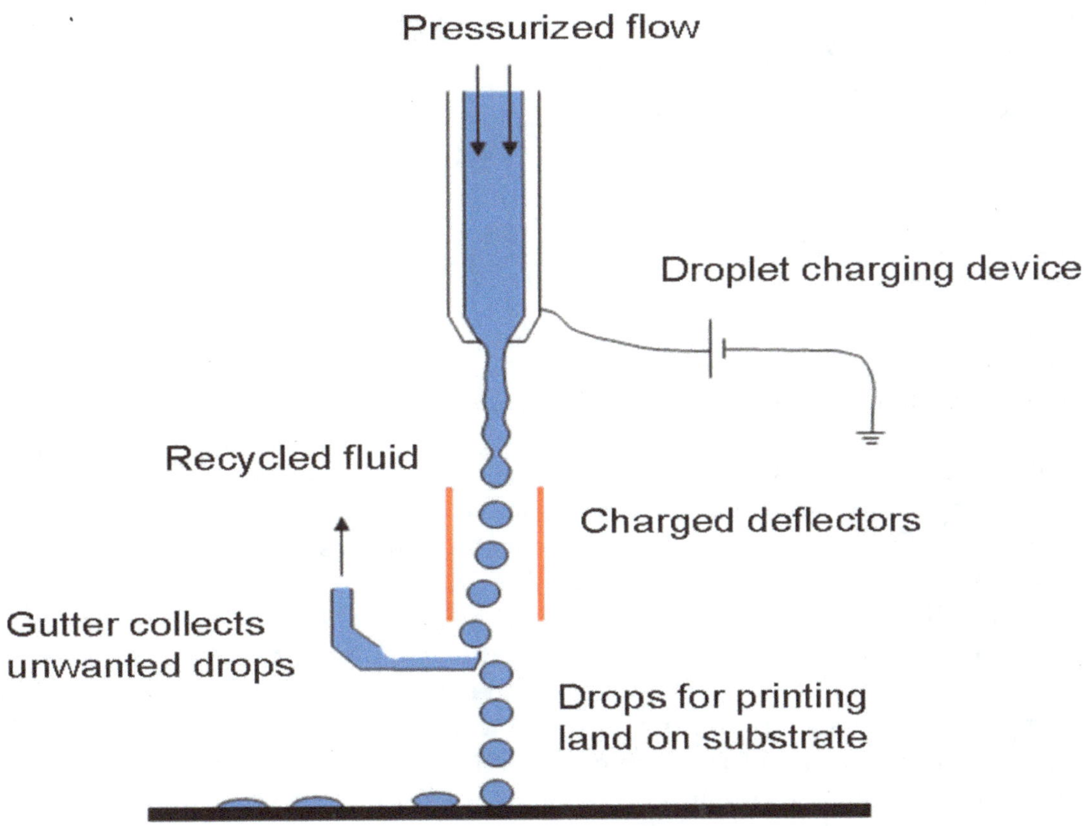

Figure 5. Schematic diagram depicts the basic working principle of ink-jet 3D printing [34].

2.4. Powder Bed Fusion

Powder bed fusion (PBF) technologies are among pioneer commercially used AM techniques created by the University of Texas USA. Selective laser sintering (SLS) based PBF technique [18], which melts the ceramic powder by laser energy source. The laser sintered the powder nearly to the melting point of the material to make each layer according to the given 3D design. The laser beam scans each new single layer of free-packed powder particles and consolidates them by sintering this process and proceeds in a layer-wise fashion to complete the final 3D object [35–37]. SLS is a powder bed fusion process have numerous applications in the bioengineering field such as to prepare customized products, biomedical implants as well as orthopedic implants [38]. The major disadvantage of SLS is the usage of higher temperatures that limits the insertion of biomaterial and cells into SLS scaffolds during the manufacturing process [39]. A schematic diagram illustrates the underlying operating system [40] of the powder bed fusion provided in Figure 6. While SLS technology is amended, the PBF method to increase machine efficiency.

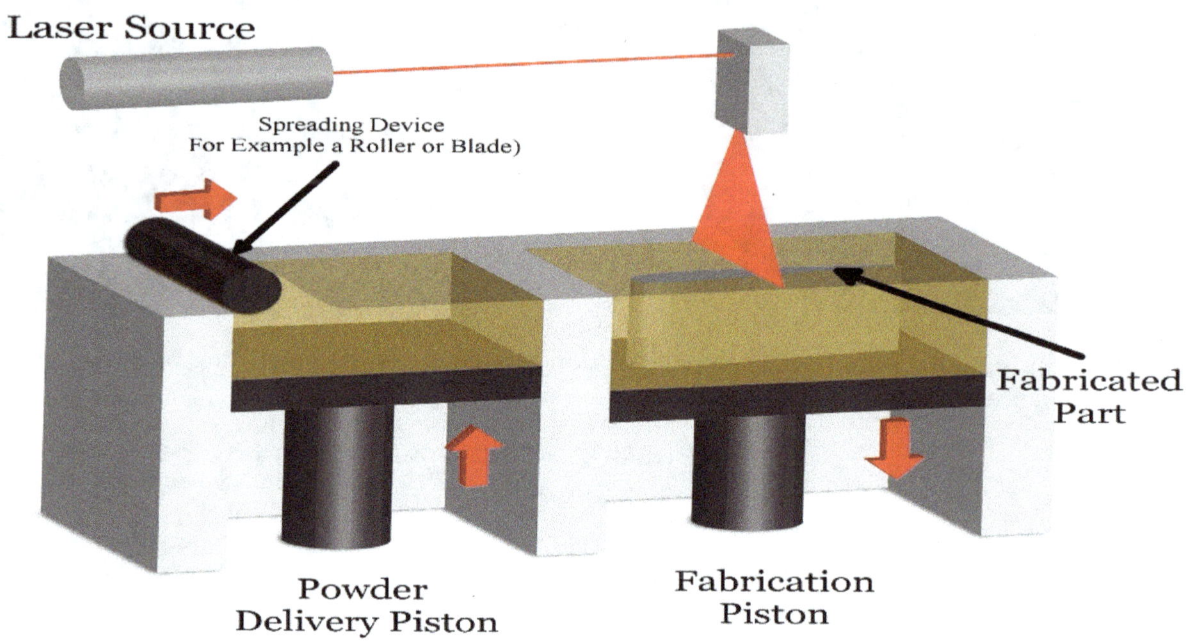

Figure 6. Schematic showing the working principle of powder bed fusion technique [40].

2.5. Vat Polymerization (SLA)

Vat Polymerization also known as stereolithography (SLA) is a promising AM technique to fabricate tissue scaffolds in the field of regenerative medicine. The SLA technique has exceptional control over porosity of scaffolds, pore sizes, design flexibility, and interconnectivity [41]. Despite excellent advantages, numerous researchers have highlighted several challenges in scaffold manufacturing such as, difficult in creating micron-sized scaffold due to over curing and layer thickness. In addition, some of the frequently used biomaterials in bone tissue engineering have shown compatibility with SLA due to limitations in viscosity, refractive index and stability [42].

Some other problems such as some SLA processes light pixels restrict in-plane microstructure construction. Although indirect SLA have overcome this problem, it is a costly, time and material consuming process [43]. Li et al. have used indirect stereolithography to manufacture microporous β-TCP. The resin molds were prepared through this technique and filled with filled with aqueous thermosetting ceramic suspension for ceramic gel casting. The heat treatment process was used to remove the molds. Results have concluded that TCP scaffolds after sintering have shown desired porosity, shape and higher strength were obtained [44].

Some other researchers have mentioned preparation of 3D objects by photo-curing a liquid resin through ultraviolet (UV) laser in a layerwise fashion [45,46]. The major advantage of this process includes better surface finish and accuracy [47]. A schematic of three different light sources used in stereolithography provided in Figure 7 [18]. Table 1 summarizing some basic bioprinting techniques for bone tissue engineering.

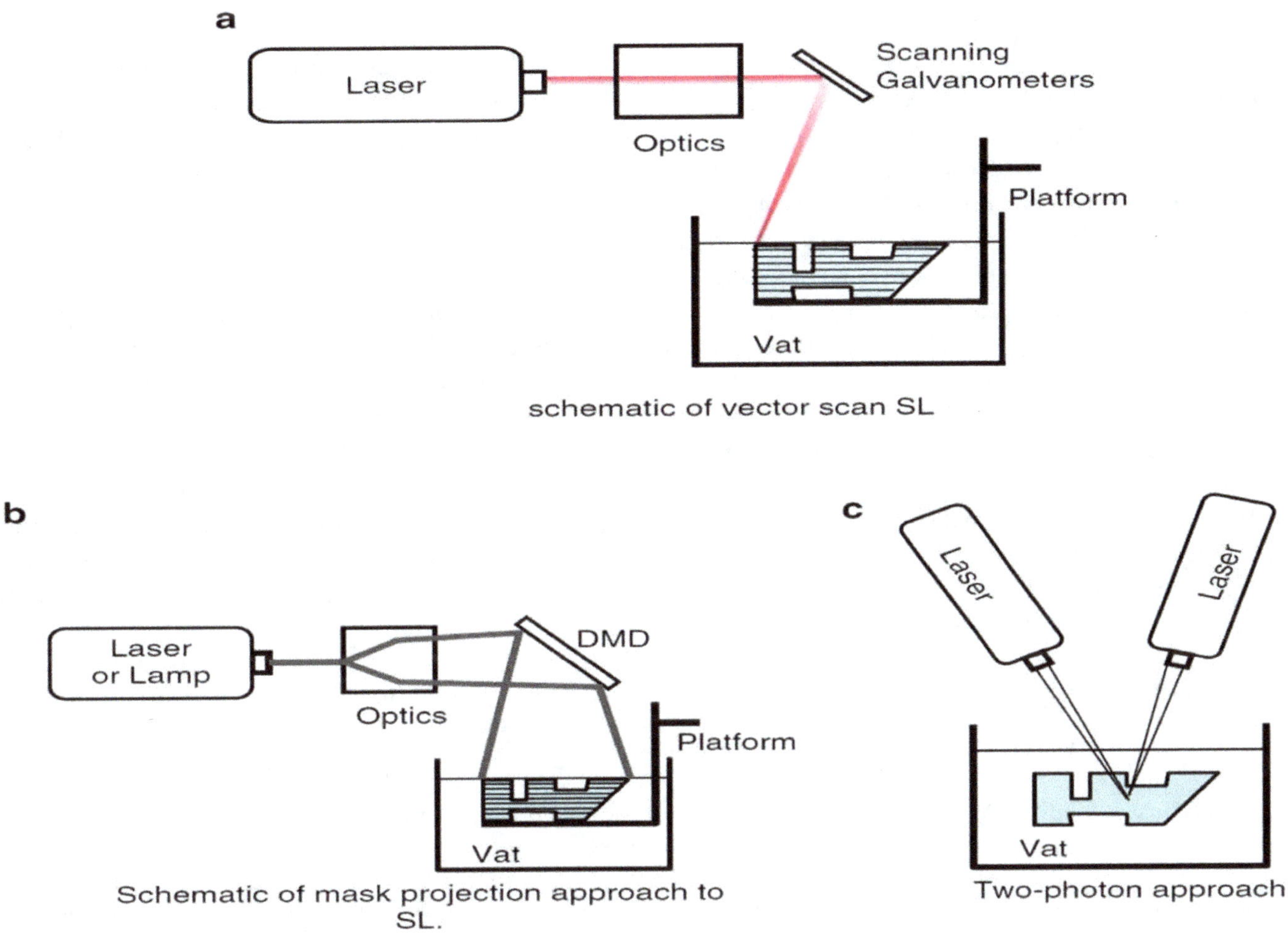

Figure 7. Schematic diagrams of three different techniques of photopolymerization [18].

Table 1. Summary of major 3D-bioprinting techniques for bone tissue engineering.

Technique	Principle	Advantages	Drawbacks
Inkjet	A liquid binding material is selectively deposited in layer-wise fashion into the powder bed to create three dimensional objects.	Ability to print biomaterials with low viscosity, high resolution, fast manufacturing speed, low cast	Intrinsic inability to deliver a continuous flow, low cell densities, lack of functionality for vertical objects
Extrusion	This process involves extruding the material in viscous form to create 3D objects	Capability to print variety of biomaterials, Capable of printing high cell densities	Applicable to viscous liquids only
Laser-assisted	In this technique, a laser beam stimulates a specified area of target to fabricate 3D objects	High resolution, capable of printing both solid and liquid phase biomaterials	High cost, low speed, high complexity, thermal damage due laser irritation
Stereolithography (SLA)	In this method an ultraviolet (UV) laser beam selectively hardens the photo-polymer resin to construct 3D models in layer-wise fashion	Nozzle free method, high cell viability, high accuracy, Printing time independent of complexity, high cell viability, high accuracy	UV light can cause toxicity to cells, during photo curing damage to cells, Applicable to photopolymers only

3. Additive Manufacturing of Bioceramics

In the last few decades, bioceramics have frequently been used in the restoration and replacements of injured tissues due to numerous advantages such as precise chemical composition, which has a vital role in the integration of hard and soft tissues [48,49]. Hydroxyapatite (HA) $Ca_{10}(PO_4)_6(OH)_2$ is one bioceramic to have frequently been employed as a scaffold material for bone tissue engineering owing to its exceptional biocompatibility and resemblance to natural bone material [50–52]. It is often combined with a biopolymer or bioceramics to enhance binding interaction and mechanical properties of the material during the AM process [53,54].

Beta tri-calcium phosphate (β-TCP) is a suitable material for craniofacial defects owing to its excellent biodegradability, wear resistance and chemical bonding with the bone tissues under all load bearing conditions [55,56]. The critical challenge for β-TCP is to maintain the sintering temperature of 1100 °C. Above this temperature, beta tri-calcium phosphate (β-TCP) transforms to alpha tri-calcium phosphate (α-TCP) that is soluble and chemically unstable, as compared to β-TCP [57,58].

In addition, bioglasses are also extensively used in hard tissue implants due to their excellent bonding capability with hard and soft both tissues. Bioglasess are also extremely helpful in upregulating the osteogenesis, however, their application in load bearing bone defects are very limited due to their high brittleness, low fracture toughness and mechanical strength [59–61]. Properties of some frequently used ceramic material for bone tissue engineering illustrated in Table 2.

Table 2. A brief review of ceramic materials and its properties used in 3D printing of Scaffolds.

Materials	Precursors	Properties
Hydroxyapatite (HA)	Poly (acrylic acid), photo-curable resin, polycaprolactone, poly (lactic acid) etc.	Higher biocompatibility, differentiation and proliferation, better cell adhesion
Tricalcium Phosphate (TCP)	Hydroxypropyl methylcellulose, polyethylenimine, polymethacrylate, etc.	In physiological environment better biocompatibility and degradation, lower compressive strength
Bioactive glasses alkali-free bioactive glass, 45S5 BG,13-93 bioactive glass, 6P53B glass	Polycaprolactone, methylcellulose, poly (lactic acid)	Improved bioactivity in vitro and in vivo for the bone tissue growth

The key factor affecting the performance of bioceramics is Ca to P ratio that affects the dissolution property. Calcium phosphates with lower Ca to P ratio (β-TCP) have higher solubility and acidic nature as compared to calcium-phosphate having high Ca to P ratio (HA) [62]. Table 3 shows that lower the Ca/P ratio higher the CaP dissolution [63]. Different bioceramics have been discussed in the following section such as hydroxyapatite, beta tri-calcium phosphate (β-TCP) and bioactive glass (BG) using different AM techniques. Figure 8 [64] shows complete process of bone tissue engineering.

Table 3. Characteristics of main CaPs used as bone substitutes and cements [63].

Name	Formula	Ca/P Ratio	Water Solubility at 25 °C, g/L
	Monocalcium Phosphate		
Monohydrate (MCPM)	$Ca(H_2PO_4)_2$, H_2O	0.50	~18
Anhydrous (MCPA)	$Ca(H_2PO_4)_2$		~17
	Dicalcium phosphate		
Dihydrate (DCPD)	$CaHPO_4$, H_2O	1.00	~0.088
Anhydrous (DCPA)	$CaHP_4$		~0.048
	Tricalcium Phosphate		
Alpha α-TCP	(α) $Ca_3(PO_4)_2$	1.50	~0.0025
Beta β-TCP	(β) $Ca_3(PO_4)_2$		~0.0005
Hydroxyapatite (HA)	$Ca_5(PO_4)_3OH$	1.67	~0.0003

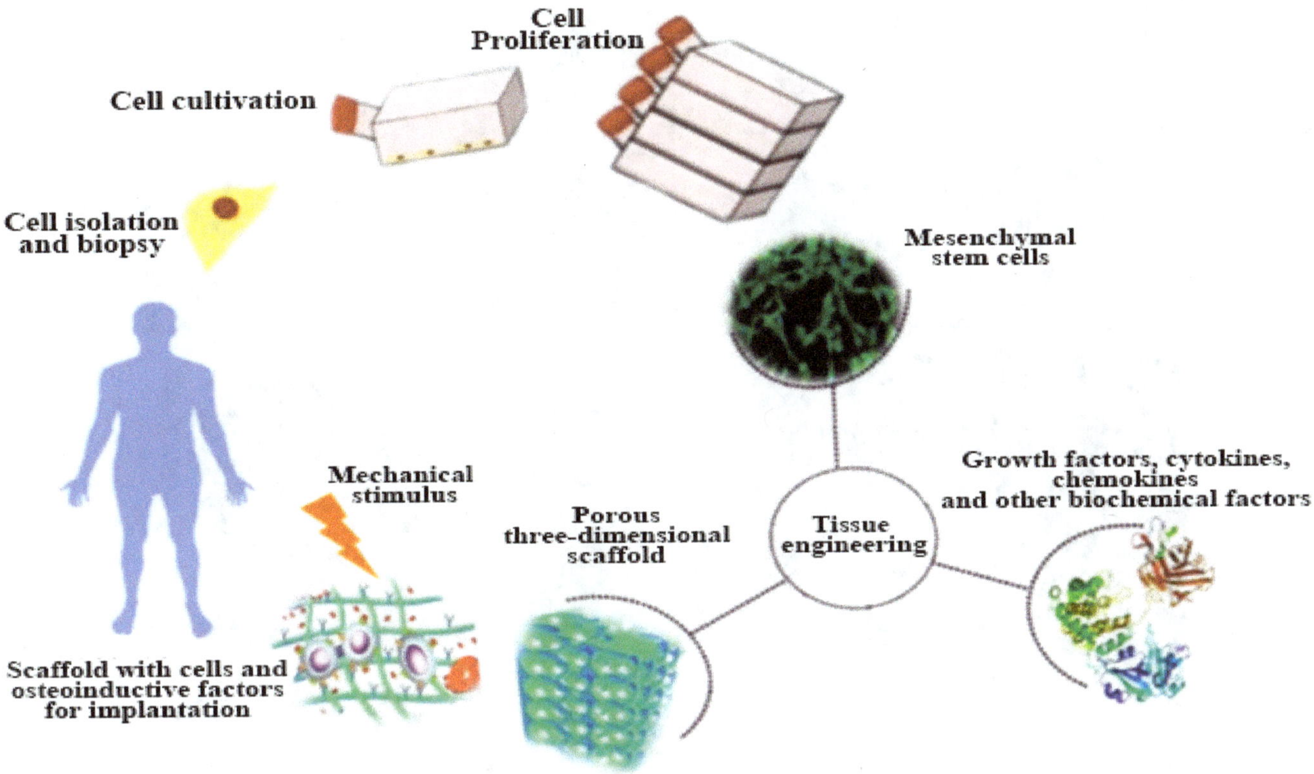

Figure 8. Schematic representation of bone tissue engineering [64].

3.1. Hydroxyapatite (HA)

Hydroxyapatite (HA) portrayed as $Ca_{10}(PO_4)_6(OH)_2$, encompasses almost 65% of the entire bone mass. It is less toxic and more stable, as compared to other calcium-phosphate due to their desirable Ca to P ratio of 1.67. The hydroxyapatite has major inorganic part of human bone and teeth to develop the properties and novel applications of bioceramics for hard tissue replacements [65–68]. Numerous researchers have reported HA scaffolds in the bone and teeth transplants [69–77].

Laser Stereolithography has been identified as one of the most effective and frequently used AM techniques to produce complex HA parts. Barry et al. have prepared HA-based oligocarbonate dimethacrylate (OCM-2) composite scaffolds using helium-cadmium (HeCd) based laser technology. The outcomes referred the laser-based HA scaffolds provided fortified cell attachment inside the scaffold. Through laser machining, toxic leftovers were removed effectively through supercritical carbon dioxide ($scCO_2$) to make scaffolds biocompatible. The HA based composite materials treated by $scCO_2$ showed better attachment of cells in both vivo and vitro studies [78]. In a very recent study, a bio-ink was prepared for 3D printing by dispersing two different types of hydroxyapatites, nano hydroxyapatite (nHA) and deproteinized bovine bone (DBB) into collagen. Thereby, a porous structure was created by 3D printing. The chemical and physical properties of the materials, including biocompatibility and effect on the osteogenic differentiation of the human bone marrow-derived mesenchyme stem cells (hBMSCs) were investigated. Both nHA/CoL and DBB/CoL Bio-inks were used to print biomimic 3D scaffolds effectively. The outcomes from this study showed that the two types of hydroxyapatite composites which help hBMSCs proliferation and differentiation proved to be a promising candidate for a 3D scaffold bio-ink [79].

Woeszn et al. fabricated microporous HA scaffolds having a pore size of 450 μm through stereolithography coupled with ceramic gelcating. A photosensitive liquid resin filled with water based thermosetting slurry was used in the mold. The mold resin and sintering were burnt to achieve the desired features. The final Scaffolds were seeded on MC3T3-E1 cells for 14 days under deep penetration of cells to achieve outstanding osteogenesis as shown in Figure 9 [80].

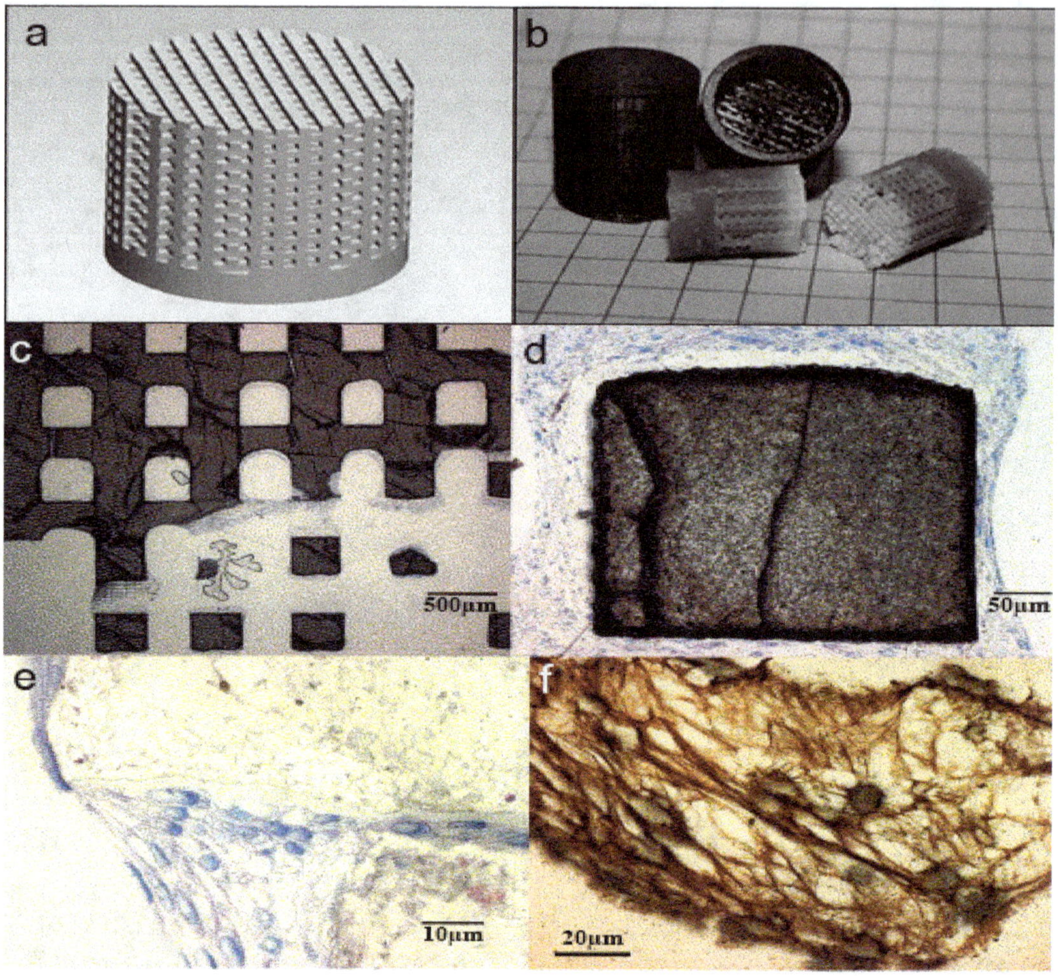

Figure 9. (**a**) Computer aided design (CAD) designed virtual structure of casting mold; (**b**) Resin casting molds manufactured by stereolithography and sintered hydroxyapatite (HA) structures; (**c**) SEM image of HA scaffold after culturing with MC3T3-E1 cells for 2 weeks, scaffold is visible in (dark grey) and cells (blue); (**d**) SEM image of strut of HA scaffold (grey), entirely attached with cells (blue/pink); (**e**) SEM image of microstructure of a crack between two struts, which was totally covered by MC3T3 cells (blue) and matrix created by the cells(pink); (**f**) SEM images of collagen produced by the cells (the microtome sectioning eliminates the mineral scaffold) [80].

The AM based extrusion process is also very common to manufacture HA scaffolds. The robocasting based extrusion process contains ceramic ink in the form of water-based viscous slurry deposited on a robotic nozzle in layer-wise fashion based on computer-aided design. The process contains high loading of HA particles to minimize the cracks and distortion during sintering. Saiz et al. have fabricated HA scaffolds with controlled pore sizes through robocasting extrusion to find the optimum sintering temperature. The hydroxyapatite slurry was prepared by mixing 40–50 vol.% of HA powder in distilled water, 1.5 wt% of Darvan C dispersant, (~7 mg/mL of solution) hydroxypropyl methylcellulose, an adequate amoqunt of polyethyleneimine (PEI) and at the end HNO_3 or HN_4OH to balance the pH level of the slurry. Results concluded that porous HA scaffolds manufactured with robocasting showed the sintering temperature should remain between 1100 °C~1200 °C and no phase change was observed for firing 1300 °C for 3 h. The characteristics of printed scaffolds through this technique have been presented in Figure 10 [81].

Keriquel et al. have successfully printed the nano-HA scaffold in the mouse calvaria defect model in vivo using laser-assisted additive manufacturing. The printed cells showed the existence of vivacious blood vessels after bone defect treatment. The outcomes of this study demonstrated that laser-assisted bioprinting have perfectly treated bone defects. Through literature numerous authors have mentioned potential of this technology could offer new perspectives to additive manufacturing for the practical applications of bone tissue engineering [82].

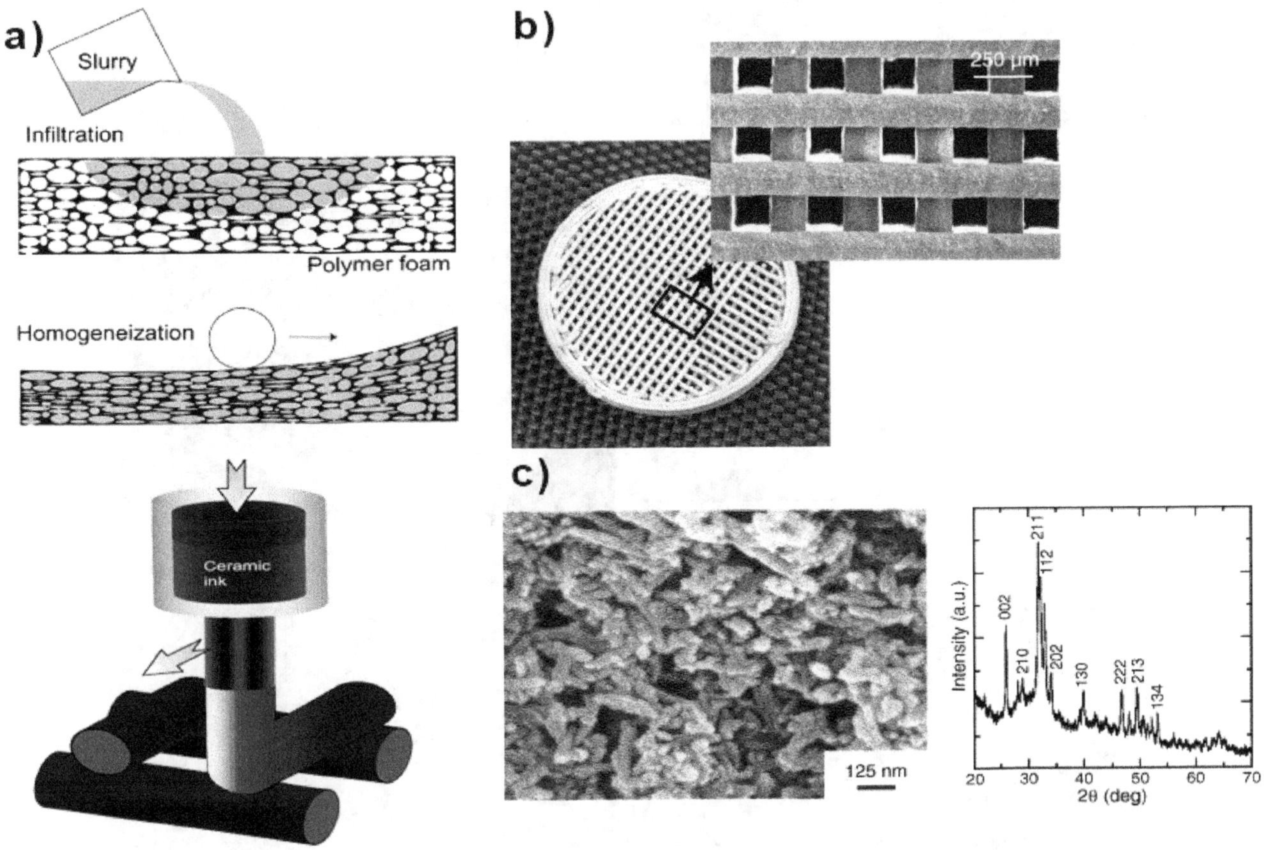

Figure 10. (**a**) Graphical representation of methods used in the manufacturing of porous ceramic scaffolds (**b**) Microstructure of HA scaffolds fabricated by robocasting (**c**) SEM micrograph and XRD of HA powders used in this process [81].

3.2. *Tricalcium Phosphate (TCP)*

Since the last two decades, beta tri-calcium phosphate (β-TCP) ceramic-based scaffolds have clinically accepted the bone graft replacement materials in several orthopedic and dental applications [83–89]. The TCP contains α, $\alpha\prime$ and $\beta\prime$ phases and Ca to P ratio is about 1.5. Cao et al. manufactured sphingosine 1-phosphate (S1P) coated β-TCP scaffold. Immunoregulation capability was tested on macrophages and rat bone marrow stromal cells of the coated scaffold was used to test osteogenic capability. The scaffold exhibit improved osteogenesis, better cell compatibility and also helpful to regulate the immune response as compared to traditionally manufactured scaffold. Figure 11 is the representation of 3D printed scaffold and its cell viability [90].

Bian et al. introduced a novel stereolithographic method to produce osteochondral beta-tricalcium phosphate/collagen scaffold. This bio-inspired scaffold manufactured by a combination of ceramic stereolithography (CSL) and gel casting using (β-TCP) and type-I collagen. Histological examination was performed to investigate the morphological properties between cartilage and bone. The obtained information from this examination were used to design biomimetic biphasic scaffolds. The pores size of β-TCP scaffolds varied between 700–900 μm with 50–65% porosity and compressive strength of 12 MPa. Physical locking formed by biomimetic transitional structure was used to achieve an adequate binding force among cartilage phase and a ceramic phase. The results concluded that CSL performed well in comparison with traditional techniques to get an ideal scaffold for bone tissue engineering applications [91].

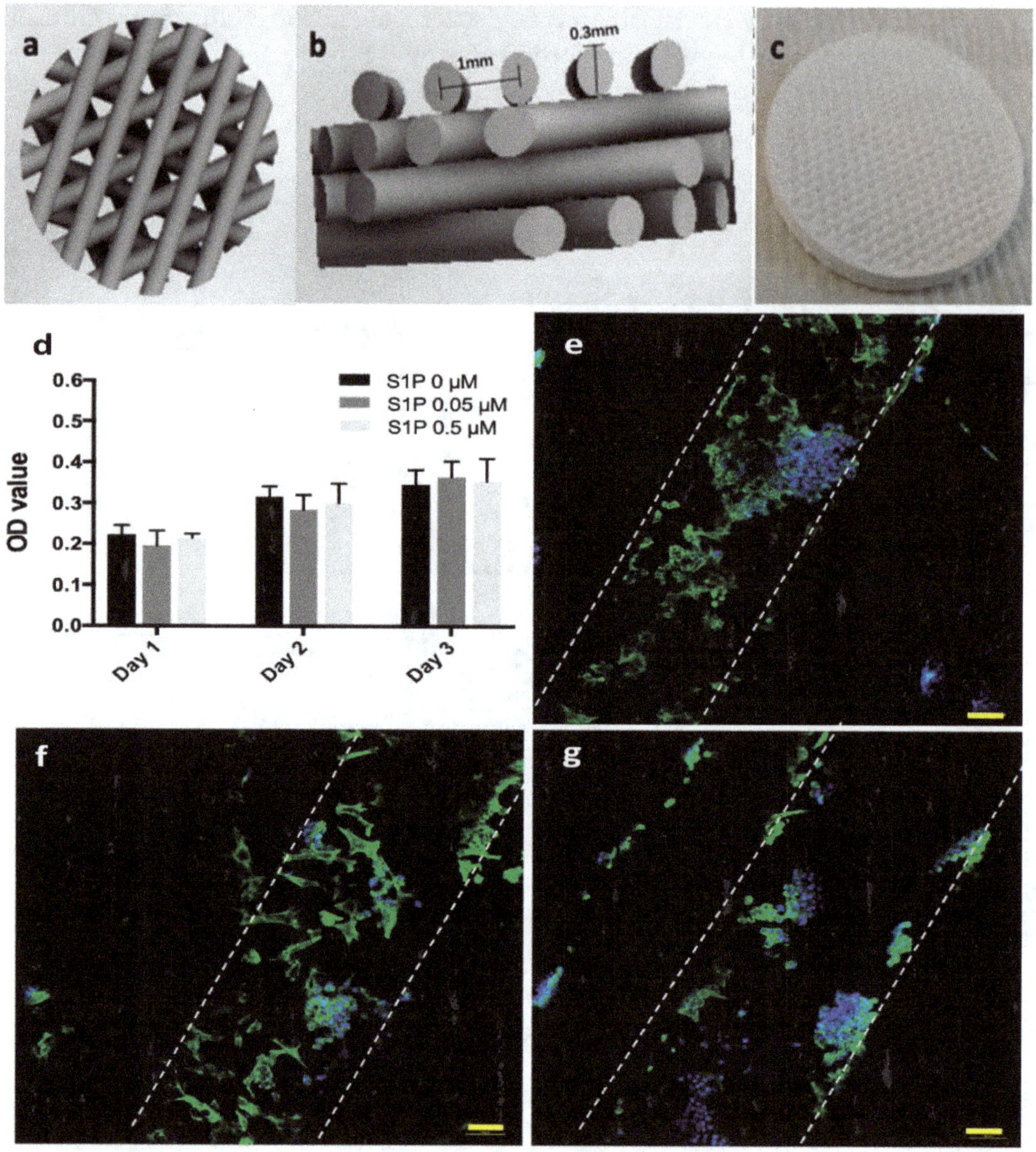

Figure 11. (**a–c**) Illustrates the schematic of 3D printed scaffold. (**d**) showing that there is no noticeable difference on viability of bone marrow-derived mesenchyme stem cells (BMSC) cells on additively manufactured scaffolds coated with S1P among the control group (S1P 0 mM) and other groups after 3 days. (**e**) S1P 0 mM group, (**f**) S1P 0.05 mM group, (**g**) S1P 0.5 mM group. Dyed blue area representing the cell nuclei and green area showing cytoskeletons. Edge of filaments showed by dotted lines [90].

In a recent study, Bose et al. have investigated the effect of Fe^{3+} and Si^{4+} dopants on the bio-mechanical properties of 3D printed β-TCP scaffold in a rat distal-femur for the period of 4, 8 and 12 weeks. The scaffold was fabricated by binder jetting technique using synthesized β-TCP powder. The outcomes from this analysis demonstrated that the addition of Fe^{3+} to TCP scaffold speed up the early stage bone restoration boosting type I collagen production. Si^{4+} doped TCP scaffold showed neovascularization after 12 weeks as shown in Figure 12. The finding from this study proved that ceramic powder-based scaffolds with improved chemistry has a promising future in bone defect restoration [92]. Tarafder et al. manufactured β-TCP scaffolds with 27%, 35% and 41% designed macroporosity with pore sizes of 500 μm, 75 μm and 1000 μm, respectively by 3D printing method. After that the scaffolds were sintered at the temperature of 1150 °C to 1200 °C in conventional and microwave furnaces to achieve mechanical strength. Microwave sintering heated scaffolds showed higher mechanical strength, as compared to conventional sintering.

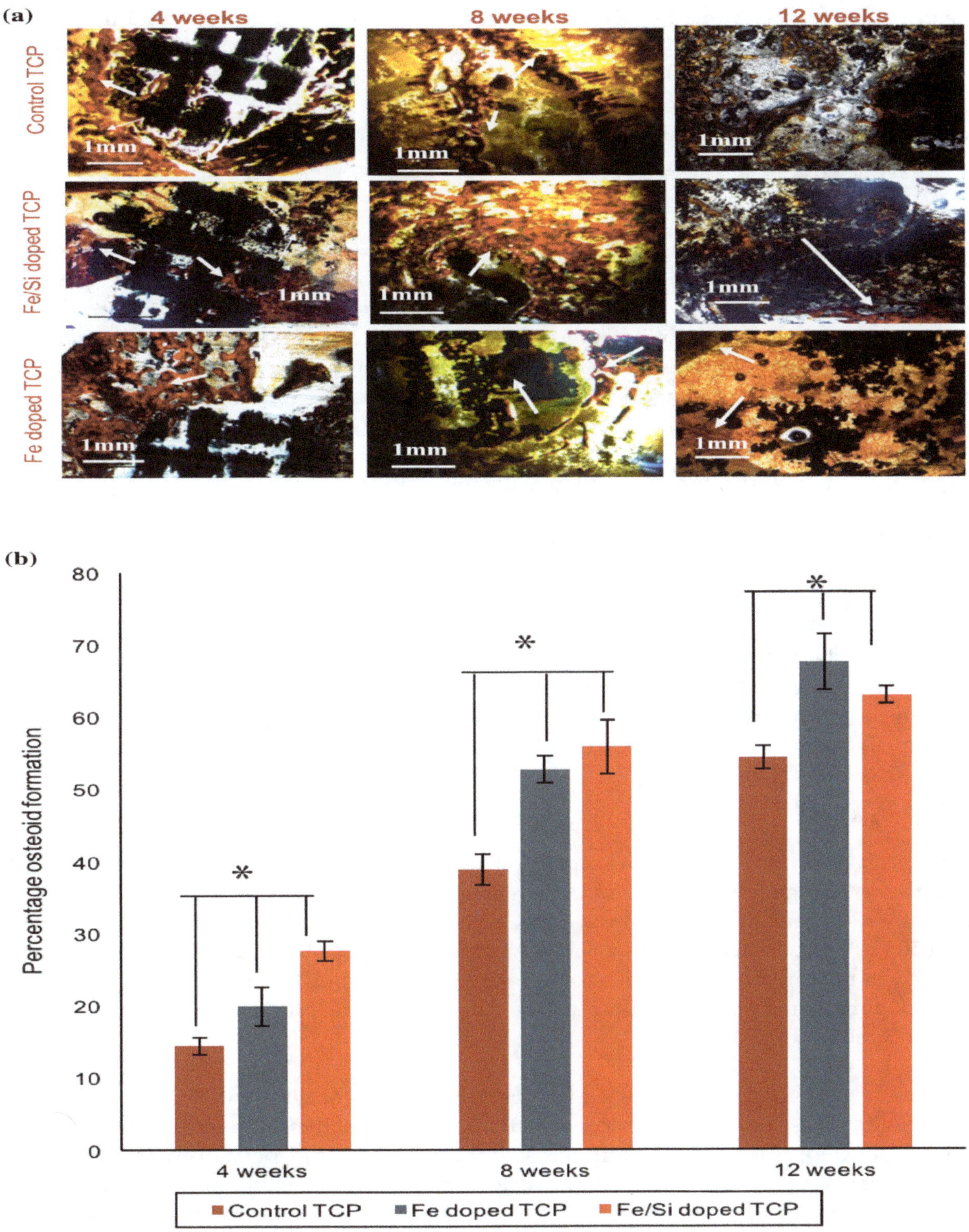

Figure 12. (**a**) Osteoid formation in pure and doped tricalcium phosphate (TCP) scaffolds after Modified Masson-Goldner trichrome staining after 4, 8, and 12 weeks. Black: prosthesis, orange and red: osteoid, bluish green: mineralized bone. Reddish-orange colors indicated by arrows showing new bone formation. Fe doping showed more bone mineralization as compared to others. (**b**) Histomorphic analysis showed Fe-Si doped TCP boosted initial stage osteoid formation for the period of 8 weeks and Fe doped TCP shows better mineralization of bone for 12 weeks of implantation [92].

The pore size was examined by Human osteoblast cells. This study showed that a decline in pore size from 1000 to 750 and 500 μm has increased the cell density. Histomorphology tests in femoral defects of Sprague-Dawley rats revealed that the existence of both micro and macro pores accelerated the new bone construction. It was concluded that additive manufactured TCP scaffolds have outstanding potential in hard tissue engineering applications [93].

3.3. *Bioactive Glass (BG)*

Bioactive glasses (BG) are the type of bioceramics that exist in both nonporous and solid forms. The bio glass contains silicon dioxide, sodium oxide, calcium oxide and phosphorous. Different types of bioglass have been created by varying the vol.% of these components [94]. Silicate part plays have an essential role in the biocompatibility of bioactive glasses. The bio glass with 45–52 vol.% silicate has ideal bone-graft bonding [95]. The 45S5-bioglass is a well-known commercially available extensively used in bone replacement [96]. However, bioglasses have also some limitations due to poor mechanical properties and brittleness that makes them unsuitable for load-bearing applications, internally brittle and deficient mechanical strength. However, several researchers have reported different additives, such as metal, polymer and ceramic to enhance the mechanical properties [97–101].

Recently, Nommeots-Nomn et al. robocasted bioglass scaffolds with a 150 μm interconnected pore size (41–43% porosity) and measured compressive strengths were 32–48 MPa. The network connectivity (NC) of these scaffolds is like the 45S5 bioglass. In this process, ICIE16 and PSrBG compositions were used comprising < 50 mol% SiO_2 to maintain the amorphous structure and to achieve the required NC closer to 45S5 bioglass. The manufactured scaffolds were compared with 13–93 vol.% composition bioglass. The comparison highlighted that 3D porous scaffolds have similar NC values with 45S5 bioglass using two low silica contents. In addition, Pluronic F-127 binder could be accepted as a universal binder for bioactive glasses regardless of their composition and reactivity. Results also showed that ICIE16 and PSrBG based scaffolds are highly reactive and significantly enhanced the bone regeneration speed [102].

Padilla et al. used calcined bioglass suspension to fabricate porous scaffolds through integrating the stereolithography and gel-casting method. A polymeric negative mold was used via stereolithography to cast bioglass suspension with Darvan-811 (sodium polyacrylate) as a dispersant. The slurry containing 50 vol% was heated at 1100 °C for 55 s and later it was polymerized. The negative mold was removed by heat treatment. The scaffolds containing interconnected 3D channels of 400–470 μm length and 1.4 μm of pore diameter. The results illustrated that the entire interconnected porous scaffold was created by this method [103].

Westhauser et al. inspected the osteo-inductive properties of different polymer coated 3D-45S5 bioglass scaffolds. These scaffolds are seeded with human mesenchymal stem cells (hMSC) implanted into immunodeficient mice. The gelatin, cross-linked gelatin, and poly (3-hydroxybutyrate-co-3-hydroxyvalerate) type coatings were used. histomorphometry and micro-computed topography analysis were performed to evaluate the new formation after eight weeks of implantation. Although, every bioglass scaffolds showed noticeable bone regeneration. However, gelatin-coated bioglass scaffolds showed highest cell formation in comparison with other coated-bioglasses, as shown in Figure 13 [104]. Some latest researches on 3D printing of bioceramics have been compiled in Table 4.

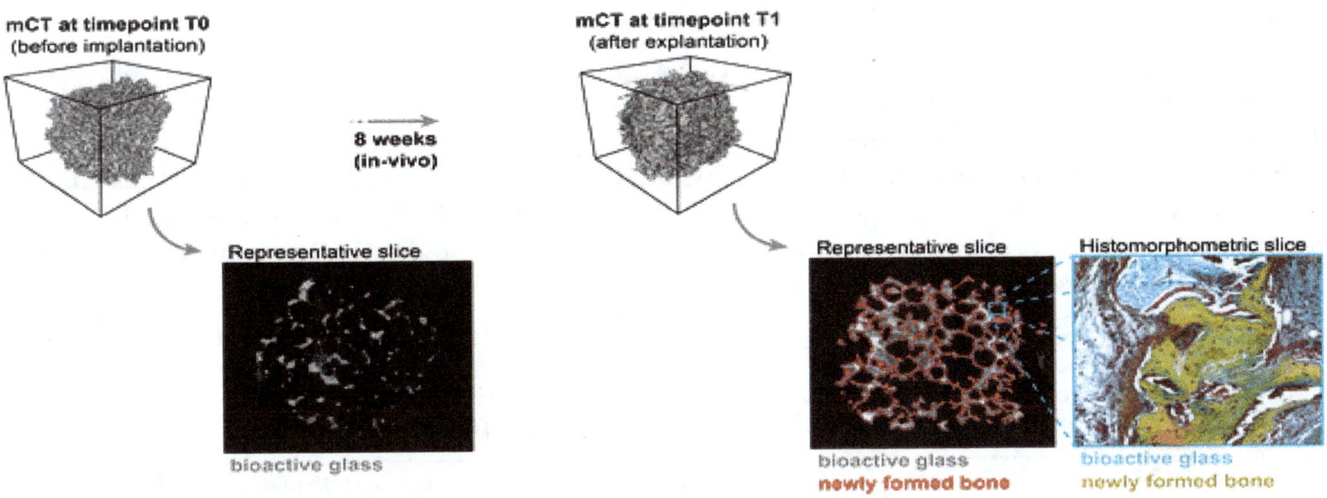

Figure 13. Histomorphometric and micro-CT analysis showing new bone development in polymer coated Bioglass (BG) scaffolds inserted in mice for eight weeks [104].

Table 4. Overview of 3D printed bioceramics for bone tissue engineering.

Material	Process	In Vivo/In Vitro Model	Key Findings	Ref.
HA + liquid sodium polyacrylate + photopolymer	A ball crusher was used to milled all the materials for 12 h to make a slurry with solid content of 10~60 wt%. The ceramic scaffold was fabricated by using digital light processing (DLP) technique	Mouse osteoblast precursor cells (MC3T3.E1) were cultured in the condition of α-MEM (10% fetal bovine serum 4% penicillin-streptomycin)	3D printed scaffold showed better biocompatibility, adhesion, differentiation and also able to promote osteoblast proliferation	[105]
Biphasic calcium phosphate (HA/β-TCP = 60:40) + HMPC+ polyethylenimine + ZrO_2	Extruded at pressure of 600 kPa with printing speed of 100 mm/min. Constructs were sintered at 1100 °C	Investigated on osteoblast like sarcoma cells for cytotoxicity and for differentiation potential of the scaffolds hMSCs cells were used	Better mechanical properties of scaffolds at 10% (w/w) of ZrO_2 was observed with improved BMP-2 expression.	[106]
β−TCP/polycaprolactone	β-TCP powder with 550 nm particle size were used to fabricate 350 µm pore size cylindrical scaffolds.	Composite scaffolds were tested using human fetal osteoblast cells (hFOB) for 3, 7 and 11 days of incubation period	Enhanced early bone formation and effective for controlled alendronate release	[107]
β−TCP/sphingosine 1-phosphate (SIP)	The scaffolds were printed in four layers and in different sizes to fit in 6-well and 12-well plates. Printed scaffolds were sintered at 1100 °C for 3 h.	Immunoregulation capability was investigated on macrophages and the osteogenic capability was tested on rat bone marrow stromal cells of the coated scaffolds.	Good biocompatibility, improved bone regeneration process	[90]
Bioactive glass/alginate	Composite scaffolds of type 13-93 bioactive glass (13-93 BG) and sodium alginate (SA) were prepared with mass ratio of 0:4, 1:4, 2:4 and 4:4 under mild conditions for bone regeneration.	The apatite mineralization abilities of the 13-93 BG/SA scaffolds were tested by soaking scaffolds in simulated body fluid (SBF), using 200 mL g^{-1} of scaffold mass, at 37 °C for 0 and 10 days.	Improved porosity and reduced shrinkage ratios	[108]
Bioglass (BG)/gelatin/cross linked-gelatin/ploy (3-hydroxybutyrate-co-3-hydroxyvalerate)	Three different types of 3D-polymer coated BG (45S5-type) scaffolds were fabricated by the well-established foam replica method and coated with the biopolymers.	Osteo-inductive properties of 3D-45S5 bioglass scaffolds were investigated by seeding human mesenchymal stem cells (hMSC) implanted into immunodeficient mice for the period of 8 weeks.	Under standard conditions biopolymer coated 3D 45S5 BG scaffolds have ability to induce bone formation. Gelation coated scaffolds showed the best results.	[104]

4. Application of Bioceramics in Orthopedic Implants

Natural bone has self-repair capability after the damage. The smaller fractures heal itself correctly, however segmental bone defects (SBDs) lead to permanent paralysis [109,110]. SBDs fractures treated with autologous bone graft technique requires harvesting of non-vital bone, such as, the iliac crest.

However, some complexities are also associated with bone grafting such as bone availability, the mismatch between harvested bone and affected site, morbidity of donor site results in poor integration [111]. Over the past three decades, a variety of synthetic materials have been introduced to overcome the complexities such as calcium phosphates (bioactive glasses) and hybrid bioceramics-polymer materials [112–115]. Table 5 showing different materials for bone tissue engineering.

Table 5. Additive manufacturing (AM) materials for bone prostheses.

Material	Binder	Layer Thickness	References
TCP	Aqueous based	20 μm	[93]
HA	-	100 μm	[116]
α/β-TCP modified with 5 wt% hydroxypropymethylcellulose	Water	100 μm	[117]
β-TCP, SiO_2-ZnO-dope β-TCP	Water based binder	20 μm (β-TCP) 30 μm (SiO_2-ZnO-doped β-TCP)	[118]
HA	α-n-butyl cyanoacrylate (NBCA)	-	[119]
TCP	20% (v/v) phosphoric acid	125 μm	[120]
TTCP/β-TCP	25% citric acid	100 μm	[121]
α-TCP	10 wt.% phosphoric acid	50 μm	[122]
HA/Maltrodextrin	Water based	175 μm	[123]
HA & Maltrodextrin/ apatite-wollastonite glass	Water based	100 μm	[124]

Roohani-Esfahani et al. fabricated glass-ceramic scaffolds with hexagonal pore structure via extrusion-based AM method shown in Figure 14. The fabricated scaffolds have 150 times greater strength compared to polymeric-composite scaffolds and five times greater than ceramic-glass scaffolds having same porosity. The study has shown that these scaffolds have excellent capability to load-bearing and segmental bone defects treatment [125].

Fierz et al. prepared HA based cylindrical scaffolds ranging from nanometer to millimeter with straight channels and micro-pores through n-HA granules, ink-jet 3D printing AM technique. The structure of 3D-printed scaffolds is almost similar to human cortical and cancellous bone. The histological analysis has confirmed that osteogenic-stimulated progenitor-based 3D-printed scaffolds are suitable for clinical use [126].

In another study, a robocasting technique was utilized to transport bone morphogenic protein 2 (BMP-2). HA slurry and polymethylmethacrylate (PMMA) microspheres were mixed together to achieve controlled microporosity. Resins were eliminated by sintering the scaffolds at 1300 °C for 2 h. Thereafter, 10 μg of bone morphogenic protein 2 was added to the microporous scaffolds in goat bone for in vivo characterization for 4 and 8 weeks. Outcomes from this study showed great potential for manufacturing HA scaffolds containing interconnected porosity. Furthermore, the existence of bone morphogenic protein 2 and micro porosity upgraded scaffold osteogenesis ability as illustrated in Figure 15 [127].

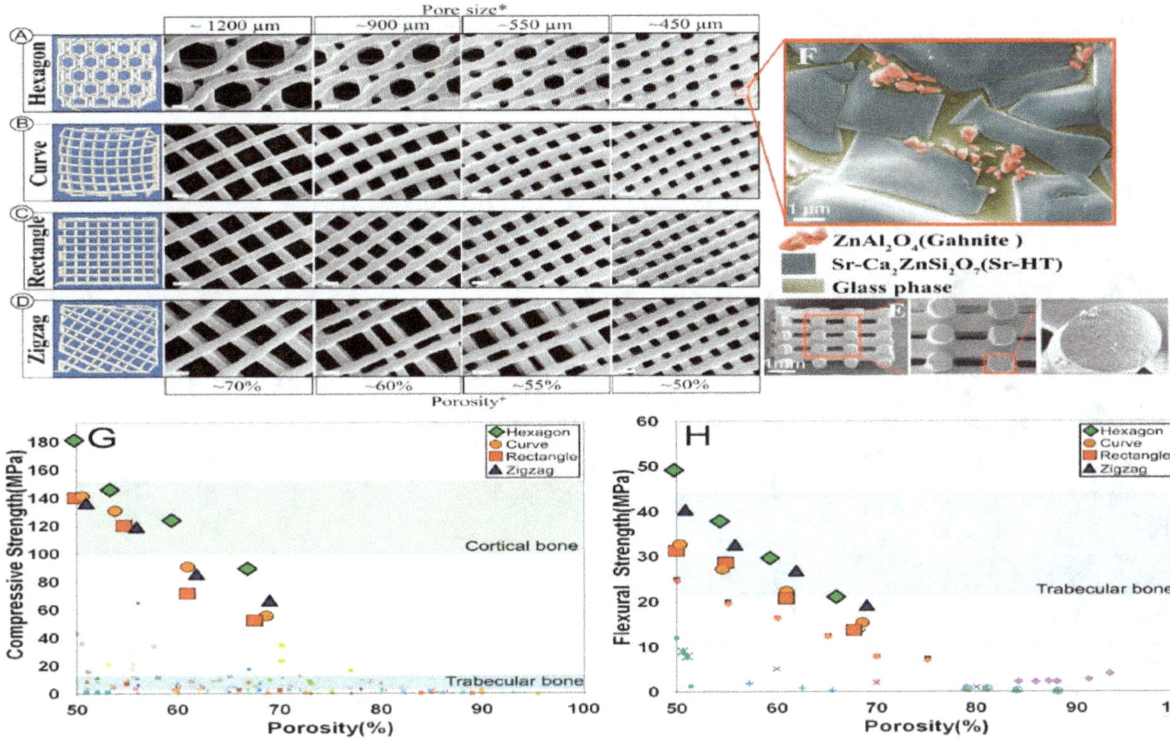

Figure 14. Models (left column) and SEM images of inspected scaffolds (scale bars: 500 μm unless stated otherwise); (**A**) Hexagonal; (**B**) curved; (**C**) rectangular and; (**D**) zigzag shape; (**E**) SEM images of fracture surface of a Sr-HT-Gahnite scaffold fabricated by robocasting; (**F,G**) the microstructure of Sr-HT-Gahnite scaffolds with distinct pore geometries vs porosity, and (**H**) flexural strength of Sr-HT-Gahnite scaffolds with hydroxyapatite and BG scaffolds [125].

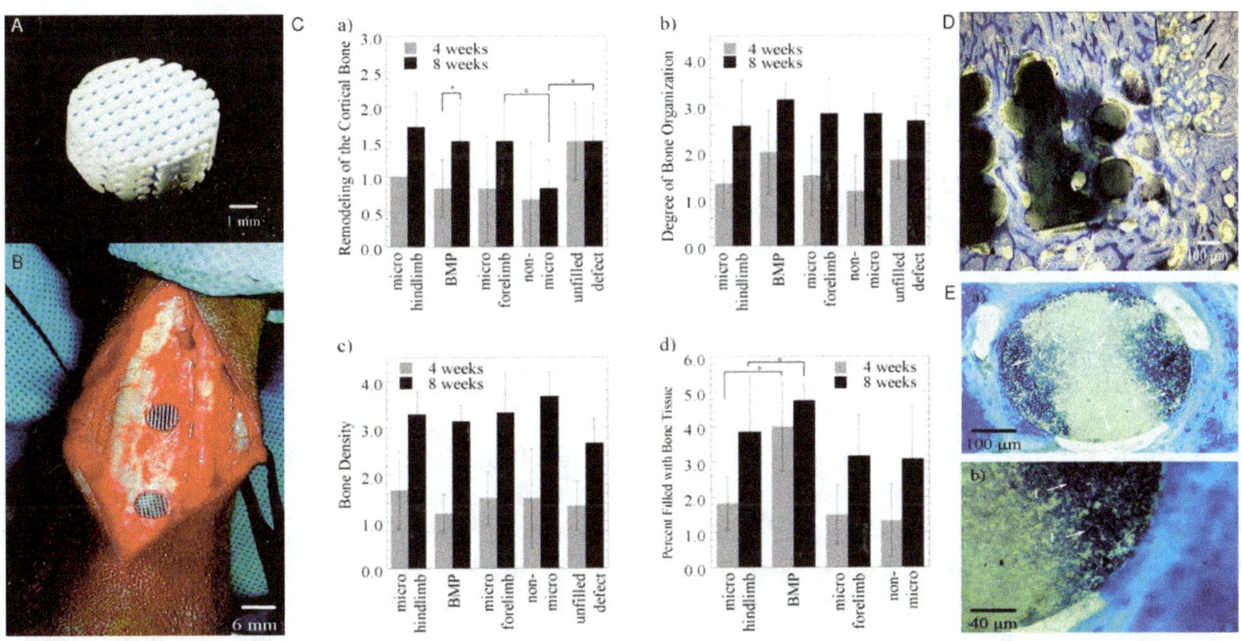

Figure 15. (**A**) Scaffold fabricated by directed deposition method. (**B**) The image of HA scaffold implantation in the metacarpal bone of goat. (**C**) BMP-2 and microporosity on cortical bone. (**D**) Image of BMP scaffold after 8 weeks representing the remodeling of the host bone, indicated by arrows. (**E-a**) and (**E-b**) are the images of histological section of micro hindlimb after 4 weeks indicating the staining of the microporous scaffolds at (**a**) low magnification and at (**b**) high magnification. Arrows indicate (1) stained and (2) unstained and (3) regions where staining extends into the scaffold [127].

Fielding et al. introduced (SiO_2/ZnO) doped three-dimensional composite TCP scaffolds with a pore size of 300 µm using binder jetting technique. The pure and (SiO_2/ZnO) doped 3D-printed TCP scaffolds implanted into a rat femur bone for the period of 6, 8 and 12 weeks to analyze the histomorphometry and Immunohistochemistry. Results have proved that combining SiO_2-ZnO dopants in TCP are best alternative to achieve osteoinductive properties of calcium phosphates (CaPs) for the clinical application of bone implants as shown in Figure 16 [118].

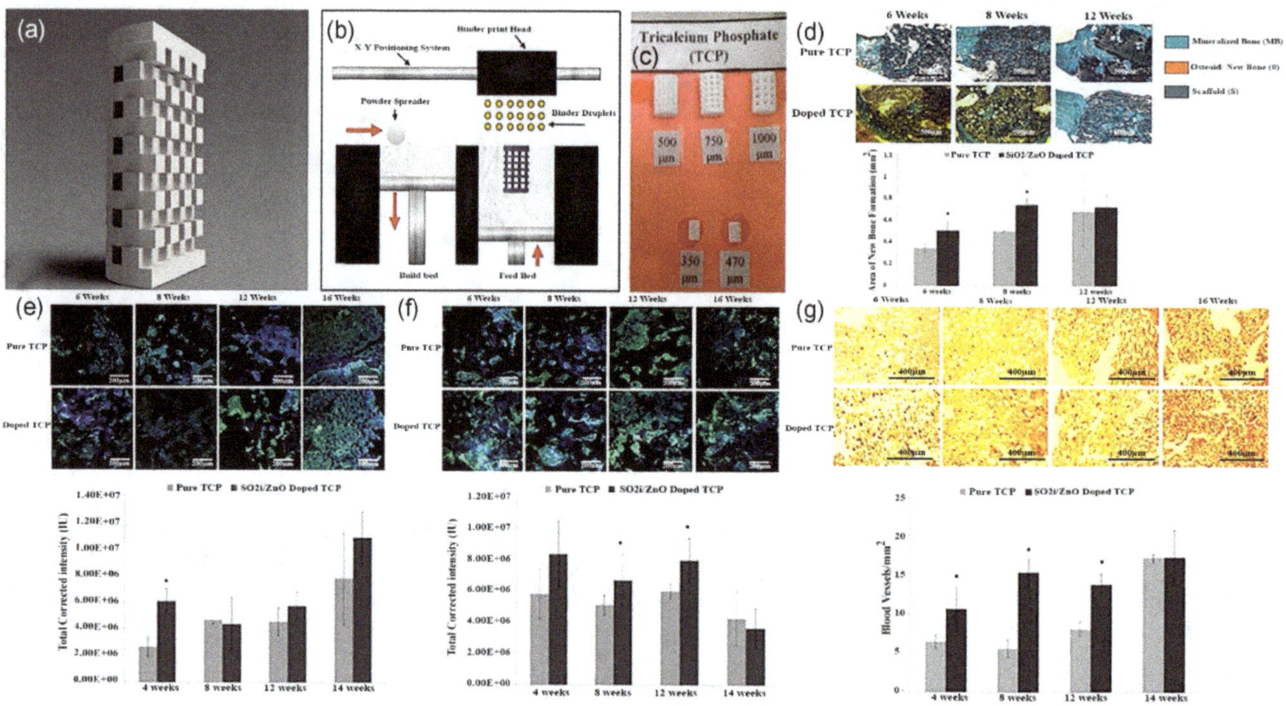

Figure 16. (**a**) CAD design used for 3D printing of porous scaffolds; (**b**) Schematic diagram illustration of 3D printing process (binder jetting); (**c**) Real 3D printed scaffolds, numbers indicating the pore size of scaffolds; (**d**) Staining of implant section via Goldner's trichrome. Gray/brown color shows CaP implants, blue is mineralized implants and osteoid formation can be seen by orange color. Histomorphometry has done on trichrome sections ($P < 0.1$, where $n = 3$); (**e**) Confocal micrographs of collagen I formation (green) over the period of 16 weeks; (**f**) Confocal micrographs of osteocalcin (green). While blue color indicates counterstain for cell nuclei; (**g**) Light micrographs showing vWF staining (the dark red spots) [118].

5. Challenges and Future Perspective

Despite all the achievements made in the past in 3D printing of tissue engineering, several challenges still exist. Challenges can be divided into two major categories: (1) 3D printing of biomaterials including live cells and (2) Post-implantation integration and functionality in vivo model. One of the most common problems during manufacturing is nozzle clogging in nozzle-based 3D printing techniques. To overcome nozzle clogging, printing precursor should have proper viscosity and need to be homogenous. Another problem is that the 3D printed constructs need to be adequately stable and mechanically stiff to ensure effective prosthesis. For instance, in hard tissue transplant, the scaffolds elastic modulus should be high enough to sustain its designed porosity and structure to help natural cell growth [128].

3D printed constructs for bone tissue engineering, being eventually implanted in a body, so these constructs also need to support vascularization to deliver sufficient amount of oxygen and nutrition to the cells in vivo to enhance the growth of newly implanted bone [129]. Vascularization plays a pivotal role in a successful bone tissue implant. However, it remains a daunting challenge in bone tissue engineering, particularly, in clinical application of large bone defects. Development of vascularized and clinically applicable bone substitutes with adequate blood supply, capable of inducing angiogenesis and sustaining implant viability remains a critical challenge. Since oxygen is only accessible to those cells through diffusion that are 100–200 μm from blood vessels, bioprinted constructs thicker than 400 μm face oxygenation problem. Therefore, it is a critical task to provide ideal conditions to help vascularization in implanted bone constructs. There is a need for some extensive research to completely understand the mechanism of the biological system of bone. Thus, manufacturing a biomimetic vascularized bone that mimics the native bone can be helpful to overcome these hurdles. Due to the ability of bioprinters utilizing several print-heads loaded with different cell types, introducing vasculature was made possible to a 3D printed construct [130–132].

Recently, nozzle-based 3D-printers enabled the printing of endothelial cells using multiple bioinks for the development of thick vascularized [133,134]. Especially, digital light processing (DLP) based 3D bioprinting can offer extraordinary speed, scalability and resolution for printing complex 3D structures with micrometer resolution [135,136]. For instance, Zhu et al. printed well-designed vascular channels without using perfusion or sacrificial materials by utilizing a rapid microscale continuous optical bioprinter (μCOB). In this method, glycidyl methacrylate-hyaluronic acid (GM-HA) and GelMA-cell laden bioinks were used to create channels and channel adjacent regions. From the outcomes of this study, researchers were able to demonstrate the progressive formation of endothelial network and formation of the lumen-like structures in vivo/vitro model. Anastomosis between the bioprinted endothelial network and circulation was observed with functional blood vessels featuring red blood cells [137]. Moreover, hypoxia is also having an important role in vascularization and bone regeneration process. Hypoxia belongs to the family of Hypoxia-Inducible Transcription Factors (HIFs) [138]. Kuss et al. utilized short-term hypoxic conditions to endorse vascularization in a hybrid 3D printed scaffold of polycaprolactone/hydroxyapatite (PCL/HAp) and stromal vascular fraction (SVF) derived cell laden bioink [139].

Another type of challenge is regulatory hurdles, customized 3D printing technology entails series of difficulties in the regulatory approval field. Though, it is urgent for the managing authorities to establish appropriate laws and regulations to ensure sustainable progress of 3D printing technology. At present, 3D-printed scaffolds and tissues are used for evaluation and screening purposes in animal models.

6. Conclusions

In summary, this review outlined the latest researches on development of 3D printing of bioceramics for bone tissue engineering, current state of the art is also discussed. Extensive amount of research on 3D bioprinting over the past 10 years highlighted its wide range of applications and potentials in bone tissue engineering. Although, plethora of goals have been accomplished in 3D printing of bioceramics, but it is still in its emerging stage.

However, to deal with challenges such as vascularization, and printing related problems, further research on development of bioinks, integration of different 3D bioprinting technologies, improvement of the mechanical properties of existing bioceramics, development of composites with excellent biocompatibility and better understanding of bonding mechanism between bone mineral and collagen are some primary areas of concern that can help to improve the applications of 3D printing in bone tissue engineering.

Recently, a very limited number of bio-printed products have been commercially available. Due to the rapid expansion of this industry in the last few years, it is foreseeable that more bio-printed constructs will ultimately become commercially available to help wide range of patients suffering from different kind of diseases. The technical problems related to clinical requirements and materials selection are mentioned above, multidisciplinary research will be required to tackle those problems and to comprehensively understand the potential of bioprinting in bone tissue engineering.

Author Contributions: Conceptualization, Methodology, Original draft preparation and data curation; M.J.Z. and D.Z. contributed equally; formal analysis, revision and supervision done by D.Z. and Z.Z.

References

1. Sachs, E.; Cima, M.; Williams, P.; Brancazio, D.; Cornie, J. Three-Dimensional Printing: Rapid Tooling and Prototypes Directly from a CAD Model. *J. Eng. Ind.* **1992**, *114*, 481–488. [CrossRef]
2. Malik, H.H.; Darwood, A.R.J.; Shaunak, S.; Kulatilake, P.; El-Hilly, A.A.; Mulki, O.; Baskaradas, A. Three-dimensional printing in surgery: A review of current surgical applications. *J. Surg. Res.* **2015**, *199*, 512–522. [CrossRef] [PubMed]
3. An, J.; Teoh, J.E.M.; Suntornnond, R.; Chua, C.K. Design and 3D Printing of Scaffolds and Tissues. *Engineering* **2015**, *1*, 261–268. [CrossRef]
4. Ma, H.; Feng, C.; Chang, J.; Wu, C. 3D-printed bioceramic scaffolds: From bone tissue engineering to tumor therapy. *Acta Biomater.* **2018**′ *79*, 37–59. [CrossRef]
5. Derby, B. Printing and Prototyping of Tissues and Scaffolds. *Science* **2012**′ *338*, 921–926. [CrossRef]
6. Turnbull, G.; Clarke, J.; Picard, F.; Riches, P.; Jia, L.; Han, F.; Li, B.; Shu, W. 3D bioactive composite scaffolds for bone tissue engineering. *Bioact. Mater.* **2018**, *3*, 278–314. [CrossRef]
7. Best, S.M.; Porter, A.E.; Thian, E.S.; Huang, J. Bioceramics: Past, present and for the future. *J. Eur. Ceram. Soc.* **2008**, *28*, 1319–1327. [CrossRef]
8. Blokhuis, T.J.; Arts, J.J.C. Bioactive and osteoinductive bone graft substitutes: Definitions, facts and myths. *Injury* **2011**, *42*, 26–29. [CrossRef]
9. Jones, J.R.; Hench, L.L. Regeneration of trabecular bone using porous ceramics. *Curr. Opin. Solid State Mater. Sci.* **2003**, *7*, 301–307. [CrossRef]
10. Schieker, M.; Seitz, H.; Drosse, I.; Seitz, S.; Mutschler, W.J.E.J.O.T. Biomaterials as Scaffold for Bone Tissue Engineering. *Eur. J. Trauma* **2006**, *32*, 114–124. [CrossRef]
11. Bose, S.; Tarafder, S. Calcium phosphate ceramic systems in growth factor and drug delivery for bone tissue engineering: A review. *Acta Biomater.* **2012**, *8*, 1401–1421. [CrossRef] [PubMed]
12. Wu, S.; Liu, X.; Yeung, K.W.K.; Liu, C.; Yang, X. Biomimetic porous scaffolds for bone tissue engineering. *Mater. Sci. Eng. R Rep.* **2014**, *80*, 1–36. [CrossRef]
13. Brie, J.; Chartier, T.; Chaput, C.; Delage, C.; Pradeau, B.; Caire, F.; Boncoeur, M.-P.; Moreau, J.-J. A new custom made bioceramic implant for the repair of large and complex craniofacial bone defects. *J. Cranio Maxillofac. Surg.* **2013**, *41*, 403–407. [CrossRef] [PubMed]
14. Tang, D.; Tare, R.S.; Yang, L.-Y.; Williams, D.F.; Ou, K.-L.; Oreffo, R.O.C. Biofabrication of bone tissue: Approaches, challenges and translation for bone regeneration. *Biomaterials* **2016**, *83*, 363–382. [CrossRef] [PubMed]
15. Brunello, G.; Sivolella, S.; Meneghello, R.; Ferroni, L.; Gardin, C.; Piattelli, A.; Zavan, B.; Bressan, E. Powder-based 3D printing for bone tissue engineering. *Biotechnol. Adv.* **2016**, *34*, 740–753. [CrossRef] [PubMed]
16. Murphy, S.V.; Atala, A. 3D bioprinting of tissues and organs. *Nat. Biotechnol.* **2014**, *32*, 773. [CrossRef] [PubMed]
17. *ASTM F2792-12a*; Standard Terminology for Additive Manufacturing Technologies, (Withdrawn 2015); ASTM International: West Conshohocken, PA, USA, 2012.
18. Gibson, I.; Rosen, D.; Stucker, B. *Additive Manufacturing Technologies: 3D Printing, Rapid Prototyping, and Direct Digital Manufacturing*; Springer: New York, NY, USA, 2015.
19. Miyanaji, H.; Orth, M.; Akbar, J.M.; Yang, L.J.F.O.M.E. Process development for green part printing using binder jetting additive manufacturing. *Front. Mech. Eng.* **2018**, *13*, 504–512. [CrossRef]
20. Snelling, D.A.; Williams, C.B.; Suchicital, C.T.; Druschitz, A.P. Binder jetting advanced ceramics for metal-ceramic composite structures. *Int. J. Adv. Manuf. Technol.* **2017**, *92*, 531–545. [CrossRef]
21. Cima, L.G.; Cima, M.J. Massachusetts Institute of Technology, Assignee. Preparation of Medical Devices by Solid Free-Form Fabrication. U.S. Patent Application No. 08138345, 13 February 1996.
22. Sachs, E.M.; Haggerty, J.S.; Cima, M.J.; Williams, P.A. Three-Dimensional Printing Techniques. U.S. Patent Application No. 5387380A, 7 February 1995.

23. Lu, K.; Hiser, M.; Wu, W. Effect of particle size on three-dimensional printed mesh structures. *Powder Technol.* **2009**, *192*, 178–183. [CrossRef]
24. Lee, J.-Y.; An, J.; Chua, C.K. Fundamentals and applications of 3D printing for novel materials. *Appl. Mater. Today* **2017**, *7*, 120–133. [CrossRef]
25. Balla, V.K.; Bose, S.; Bandyopadhyay, A. Processing of Bulk Alumina Ceramics Using Laser Engineered Net Shaping. *Int. J. Appl. Ceram. Technol.* **2008**, *5*, 234–242. [CrossRef]
26. Zhai, Y.; Lados, D.A.; Brown, E.J.; Vigilante, G.N. Fatigue crack growth behavior and microstructural mechanisms in Ti-6Al-4V manufactured by laser engineered net shaping. *Int. J. Fatigue* **2016**, *93*, 51–63. [CrossRef]
27. Schiele, N.; Chrisey, D.; Corr, D. Gelatin-Based Laser Direct-Write Technique for the Precise Spatial Patterning of Cells. *Tissue Eng. Part C Methods* **2011**, *17*, 289–298. [CrossRef] [PubMed]
28. Ozbolat, I.T.; Yu, Y. Bioprinting Toward Organ Fabrication: Challenges and Future Trends. *IEEE Trans. Biomed. Eng.* **2013**, *60*, 691–699. [CrossRef] [PubMed]
29. Ghazanfari, A.; Li, W.; Leu, M.; Hilmas, G. A Novel Extrusion-Based Additive Manufacturing Process for Ceramic Parts. In Proceedings of the 27th Annual International Solid Freeform Fabrication Symposium, Austin, TX, USA, 8–10 August 2016; pp. 1509–1529.
30. Deckers, J.; Vleugels, J.; Kruth, J.P. Additive Manufacturing of Ceramics: A Review. *J. Ceram. Sci. Technol.* **2014**, *5*, 245–260.
31. Bose, S.; Suguira, S.; Bandyopadhyay, A. Processing of controlled porosity ceramic structures via fused deposition. *Scr. Mater.* **1999**, *41*, 1009–1014. [CrossRef]
32. Ozbolat, I.T.; Hospodiuk, M. Current advances and future perspectives in extrusion-based bioprinting. *Biomaterials* **2016**, *76*, 321–343. [CrossRef]
33. Ji, S.; Guvendiren, M. Recent Advances in Bioink Design for 3D Bioprinting of Tissues and Organs. *Front. Bioeng. Biotechnol.* **2017**, *5*, 23. [CrossRef]
34. Derby, B. Additive Manufacture of Ceramics Components by Inkjet Printing. *Engineering* **2015**, *1*, 113–123. [CrossRef]
35. Sing, S.L.; Yeong, W.Y.; Wiria, F.E.; Tay, B.Y.; Zhao, Z.; Zhao, L.; Tian, Z.; Yang, S. Direct selective laser sintering and melting of ceramics: A review. *Rapid Prototyp. J.* **2017**, *23*, 611–623. [CrossRef]
36. Qian, B.; Shen, Z. Laser sintering of ceramics. *J. Asian Ceram. Soc.* **2013**, *1*, 315–321. [CrossRef]
37. Kruth, J.P.; Mercelis, P.; Van Vaerenbergh, J.; Froyen, L.; Rombouts, M. Binding mechanisms in selective laser sintering and selective laser melting. *Rapid Prototyp. J.* **2005**, *11*, 26–36. [CrossRef]
38. Bertrand, P.; Bayle, F.; Combe, C.; Goeuriot, P.; Smurov, I. Ceramic components manufacturing by selective laser sintering. *Appl. Surf. Sci.* **2007**, *254*, 989–992. [CrossRef]
39. Mazzoli, A. Selective laser sintering in biomedical engineering. *Med. Biol. Eng. Comput.* **2013**, *51*, 245–256. [CrossRef] [PubMed]
40. Haeri, S. Optimisation of blade type spreaders for powder bed preparation in Additive Manufacturing using DEM simulations. *Powder Technol.* **2017**, *321*, 94–104. [CrossRef]
41. Chartrain, N.A.; Williams, C.B.; Whittington, A.R. A review on fabricating tissue scaffolds using vat photopolymerization. *Acta Biomater.* **2018**, *74*, 90–111. [CrossRef] [PubMed]
42. Melchels, F.P.W.; Feijen, J.; Grijpma, D.W. A review on stereolithography and its applications in biomedical engineering. *Biomaterials* **2010**, *31*, 6121–6130. [CrossRef]
43. Stevens, A.G.; Oliver, C.R.; Kirchmeyer, M.; Wu, J.; Chin, L.; Polsen, E.S.; Archer, C.; Boyle, C.; Garber, J.; Hart, A.J. Conformal Robotic Stereolithography. *3D Print. Addit. Manuf.* **2016**, *3*, 226–235. [CrossRef]
44. Li, X.; Li, D.; Lu, B.; Wang, C. Fabrication of bioceramic scaffolds with pre-designed internal architecture by gel casting and indirect stereolithography techniques. *J. Porous Mater.* **2008**, *15*, 667–671. [CrossRef]
45. Wu, H.; Liu, W.; He, R.; Wu, Z.; Jiang, Q.; Song, X.; Chen, Y.; Cheng, L.; Wu, S. Fabrication of dense zirconia-toughened alumina ceramics through a stereolithography-based additive manufacturing. *Ceram. Int.* **2017**, *43*, 968–972. [CrossRef]
46. Islam, M.N.; Gomer, H.; Sacks, S. Comparison of dimensional accuracies of stereolithography and powder binder printing. *Int. J. Adv. Manuf. Technol.* **2017**, *88*, 3077–3087. [CrossRef]
47. He, L.; Song, X.J.J. Supportability of a High-Yield-Stress Slurry in a New Stereolithography-Based Ceramic Fabrication Process. *JOM* **2018**, *70*, 407–412. [CrossRef]
48. Hench, L.L. Bioceramics and the origin of life. *J. Biomed. Mater. Res.* **1989**, *23*, 685–703. [CrossRef] [PubMed]

49. Habraken, W.; Habibovic, P.; Epple, M.; Bohner, M. Calcium phosphates in biomedical applications: Materials for the future? *Mater. Today* **2016**, *19*, 69–87. [CrossRef]
50. Oonishi, H. Orthopaedic applications of hydroxyapatite. *Biomaterials* **1991**, *12*, 171–178. [CrossRef]
51. Petit, R. The use of hydroxyapatite in orthopaedic surgery: A ten-year review. *Eur. J. Orthop. Surg. Traumatol.* **1999**, *9*, 71–74. [CrossRef]
52. Zeng, Y.; Yan, Y.; Yan, H.; Liu, C.; Li, P.; Dong, P.; Zhao, Y.; Chen, J. 3D printing of hydroxyapatite scaffolds with good mechanical and biocompatible properties by digital light processing. *J. Mater. Sci.* **2018**, *53*, 6291–6301. [CrossRef]
53. Szcześ, A.; Hołysz, L.; Chibowski, E. Synthesis of hydroxyapatite for biomedical applications. *Adv. Colloid Interface Sci.* **2017**, *249*, 321–330. [CrossRef]
54. Zhou, H.; Lee, J. Nanoscale hydroxyapatite particles for bone tissue engineering. *Acta Biomater.* **2011**, *7*, 2769–2781. [CrossRef]
55. Bouler, J.M.; Pilet, P.; Gauthier, O.; Verron, E. Biphasic calcium phosphate ceramics for bone reconstruction: A review of biological response. *Acta Biomater.* **2017**, *53*, 1–12. [CrossRef]
56. Busuttil Naudi, K.; Ayoub, A.; McMahon, J.; Di Silvio, L.; Lappin, D.; Hunter, K.D.; Barbenel, J. Mandibular reconstruction in the rabbit using beta-tricalcium phosphate (β-TCP) scaffolding and recombinant bone morphogenetic protein 7 (rhBMP-7)—Histological, radiographic and mechanical evaluations. *J. Cranio Maxillofac. Surg.* **2012**, *40*, 461–469. [CrossRef] [PubMed]
57. Ryu, H.-S.; Youn, H.-J.; Sun Hong, K.; Chang, B.-S.; Lee, C.-K.; Chung, S.-S. An improvement in sintering property of β-tricalcium phosphate by adition of calcium pyrophosphate. *Biomaterials* **2002**, *23*, 909–914. [CrossRef]
58. Brazete, D.; Torres, P.M.C.; Abrantes, J.C.C.; Ferreira, J.M.F. Influence of the Ca/P ratio and cooling rate on the allotropic α β-tricalcium phosphate phase transformations. *Ceram. Int.* **2018**, *44*, 8249–8256.
59. Fernandes, J.S.; Gentile, P.; Pires, R.A.; Reis, R.L.; Hatton, P.V. Multifunctional bioactive glass and glass-ceramic biomaterials with antibacterial properties for repair and regeneration of bone tissue. *Acta Biomater.* **2017**, *59*, 2–11. [CrossRef]
60. Baino, F.; Fiorilli, S.; Vitale-Brovarone, C. Bioactive glass-based materials with hierarchical porosity for medical applications: Review of recent advances. *Acta Biomater.* **2016**, *42*, 18–32. [CrossRef]
61. Rahaman, M.N.; Day, D.E.; Sonny Bal, B.; Fu, Q.; Jung, S.B.; Bonewald, L.F.; Tomsia, A.P. Bioactive glass in tissue engineering. *Acta Biomater.* **2011**, *7*, 2355–2373. [CrossRef]
62. Liu, H.; Yazici, H.; Ergun, C.; Webster, T.J.; Bermek, H. An in vitro evaluation of the Ca/P ratio for the cytocompatibility of nano-to-micron particulate calcium phosphates for bone regeneration. *Acta Biomater.* **2008**, *4*, 1472–1479. [CrossRef]
63. Parent, M.; Baradari, H.; Champion, E.; Damia, C.; Viana-Trecant, M. Design of calcium phosphate ceramics for drug delivery applications in bone diseases: A review of the parameters affecting the loading and release of the therapeutic substance. *J. Control. Release* **2017**, *252*, 1–17. [CrossRef]
64. Ahmad, O.; Soodeh, A. Application of Bioceramics in Orthopedics and Bone Tissue Engineering. Available online: https://www.researchgate.net/publication/321939283_Application_of_Bioceramics_in_Orthopedics_and_Bone_Tissue_Engineering (accessed on 11 October 2019).
65. Hench, L.L. Bioceramics: From Concept to Clinic. *J. Am. Ceram. Soc.* **1991**, *74*, 1487–1510. [CrossRef]
66. Chevalier, J.; Gremillard, L. Ceramics for medical applications: A picture for the next 20 years. *J. Eur. Ceram. Soc.* **2009**, *29*, 1245–1255. [CrossRef]
67. Dorozhkin, S.V. Calcium orthophosphate bioceramics. *Ceram. Int.* **2015**, *41*, 13913–13966. [CrossRef]
68. Oonishi, H.; Oonishi, H.; Ohashi, H.; Kawahara, I.; Hanaoka, Y.; Iwata, R.; Hench, L.L. Clinical Applications of Hydroxyapatite in Orthopedics. In *Advances in Calcium Phosphate Biomaterials*; Ben-Nissan, B., Ed.; Springer Berlin Heidelberg: Berlin/Heidelberg, Germany, 2014; pp. 19–49. [CrossRef]
69. Asri, R.I.M.; Harun, W.S.W.; Hassan, M.A.; Ghani, S.A.C.; Buyong, Z. A review of hydroxyapatite-based coating techniques: Sol-gel and electrochemical depositions on biocompatible metals. *J. Mech. Behav. Biomed. Mater.* **2016**, *57*, 95–108. [CrossRef] [PubMed]
70. Cox, S.C.; Thornby, J.A.; Gibbons, G.J.; Williams, M.A.; Mallick, K.K. 3D printing of porous hydroxyapatite scaffolds intended for use in bone tissue engineering applications. *Mater. Sci. Eng. C* **2015**, *47*, 237–247. [CrossRef] [PubMed]

71. Ayoub, G.; Veljovic, D.; Zebic, M.L.; Miletic, V.; Palcevskis, E.; Petrovic, R.; Janackovic, D. Composite nanostructured hydroxyapatite/yttrium stabilized zirconia dental inserts—The processing and application as dentin substitutes. *Ceram. Int.* **2018**, *44*, 18200–18208. [CrossRef]
72. Hung, K.-Y.; Lo, S.-C.; Shih, C.-S.; Yang, Y.-C.; Feng, H.-P.; Lin, Y.-C. Titanium surface modified by hydroxyapatite coating for dental implants. *Surf. Coat. Technol.* **2013**, *231*, 337–345. [CrossRef]
73. Ciobanu, G.; Harja, M. Cerium-doped hydroxyapatite/collagen coatings on titanium for bone implants. *Ceram. Int.* **2019**, *45*, 2852–2857. [CrossRef]
74. Shi, P.; Liu, M.; Fan, F.; Yu, C.; Lu, W.; Du, M. Characterization of natural hydroxyapatite originated from fish bone and its biocompatibility with osteoblasts. *Mater. Sci. Eng. C* **2018**, *90*, 706–712. [CrossRef]
75. Carfi Pavia, F.; Conoscenti, G.; Greco, S.; La Carrubba, V.; Ghersi, G.; Brucato, V. Preparation, characterization and in vitro test of composites poly-lactic acid/hydroxyapatite scaffolds for bone tissue engineering. *Int. J. Biol. Macromol.* **2018**, *119*, 945–953. [CrossRef]
76. He, X.; Fan, X.; Feng, W.; Chen, Y.; Guo, T.; Wang, F.; Liu, J.; Tang, K. Incorporation of microfibrillated cellulose into collagen-hydroxyapatite scaffold for bone tissue engineering. *Int. J. Biol. Macromol.* **2018**, *115*, 385–392. [CrossRef]
77. Sposito Corcione, C.; Gervaso, F.; Scalera, F.; Padmanabhan, S.K.; Madaghiele, M.; Montagna, F.; Sannino, A.; Licciulli, A.; Maffezzoli, A. Highly loaded hydroxyapatite microsphere/ PLA porous scaffolds obtained by fused deposition modelling. *Ceram. Int.* **2019**, *45*, 2803–2810. [CrossRef]
78. Barry, J.J.A.; Evseev, A.V.; Markov, M.A.; Upton, C.E.; Scotchford, C.A.; Popov, V.K.; Howdle, S.M. In vitro study of hydroxyapatite-based photocurable polymer composites prepared by laser stereolithography and supercritical fluid extraction. *Acta Biomater.* **2008**, *4*, 1603–1610. [CrossRef] [PubMed]
79. Li, Q.; Lei, X.; Wang, X.; Cai, Z.; Lyu, P.; Zhang, G. Hydroxyapatite/Collagen Three-Dimensional Printed Scaffolds and Their Osteogenic Effects on Human Bone Marrow-Derived Mesenchymal Stem Cells. *Tissue Eng. Part A* **2019**, *25*, 1261–1271. [CrossRef] [PubMed]
80. Woesz, A.; Rumpler, M.; Stampfl, J.; Varga, F.; Fratzl-Zelman, N.; Roschger, P.; Klaushofer, K.; Fratzl, P. Towards bone replacement materials from calcium phosphates via rapid prototyping and ceramic gelcasting. *Mater. Sci. Eng. C* **2005**, *25*, 181–186. [CrossRef]
81. Saiz, E.; Gremillard, L.; Menendez, G.; Miranda, P.; Gryn, K.; Tomsia, A.P. Preparation of porous hydroxyapatite scaffolds. *Mater. Sci. Eng. C* **2007**, *27*, 546–550. [CrossRef]
82. Virginie, K.; Fabien, G.; Isabelle, A.; Bertrand, G.; Sylvain, M.; Joëlle, A.; Jean-Christophe, F.; Sylvain, C. In vivo bioprinting for computer- and robotic-assisted medical intervention: preliminary study in mice. *Biofabrication* **2010**, *2*, 014101.
83. Tian, Y.; Lu, T.; He, F.; Xu, Y.; Shi, H.; Shi, X.; Zuo, F.; Wu, S.; Ye, J. β-tricalcium phosphate composite ceramics with high compressive strength, enhanced osteogenesis and inhibited osteoclastic activities. *Colloids Surf. B Biointerfaces* **2018**, *167*, 318–327. [CrossRef]
84. Hirakawa, Y.; Manaka, T.; Orita, K.; Ito, Y.; Ichikawa, K.; Nakamura, H. The accelerated effect of recombinant human bone morphogenetic protein 2 delivered by β-tricalcium phosphate on tendon-to-bone repair process in rabbit models. *J. Shoulder Elb. Surg.* **2018**, *27*, 894–902. [CrossRef]
85. Cheng, L.; Duan, X.; Xiang, Z.; Shi, Y.; Lu, X.; Ye, F.; Bu, H. Ectopic bone formation cannot occur by hydroxyapatite/β-tricalcium phosphate bioceramics in green fluorescent protein chimeric mice. *Appl. Surf. Sci.* **2012**, *262*, 200–206. [CrossRef]
86. Stähli, C.; Bohner, M.; Bashoor-Zadeh, M.; Doebelin, N.; Baroud, G. Aqueous impregnation of porous β-tricalcium phosphate scaffolds. *Acta Biomater.* **2010**, *6*, 2760–2772. [CrossRef]
87. Horch, H.H.; Sader, R.; Pautke, C.; Neff, A.; Deppe, H.; Kolk, A. Synthetic, pure-phase beta-tricalcium phosphate ceramic granules for bone regeneration in the reconstructive surgery of the jaws. *Int. J. Oral Maxillofac. Surg.* **2006**, *35*, 708–713. [CrossRef]
88. Zerbo, I.R.; Bronckers, A.L.J.J.; De Lange, G.L.; Burger, E.H.; Van Beek, G.J. Histology of human alveolar bone regeneration with a porous tricalcium phosphate. *Clin. Oral Implant. Res.* **2001**, *12*, 379–384. [CrossRef]
89. Li, B.; Liu, Z.; Yang, J.; Yi, Z.; Xiao, W.; Liu, X.; Yang, X.; Xu, W.; Liao, X. Preparation of bioactive β-tricalcium phosphate microspheres as bone graft substitute materials. *Mater. Sci. Eng. C* **2017**, *70*, 1200–1205. [CrossRef] [PubMed]

90. Cao, Y.; Xiao, L.; Cao, Y.; Nanda, A.; Xu, C.; Ye, Q. 3D printed β-TCP scaffold with sphingosine 1-phosphate coating promotes osteogenesis and inhibits inflammation. *Biochem. Biophys. Res. Commun.* **2019**, *512*, 889–895. [CrossRef] [PubMed]
91. Bian, W.; Li, D.; Lian, Q.; Li, X.; Zhang, W.; Wang, K.; Jin, Z. Fabrication of a bio-inspired beta-Tricalcium phosphate/collagen scaffold based on ceramic stereolithography and gel casting for osteochondral tissue engineering. *Rapid Prototyp. J.* **2012**, *18*, 68–80. [CrossRef]
92. Bose, S.; Banerjee, D.; Robertson, S.; Vahabzadeh, S. Enhanced In Vivo Bone and Blood Vessel Formation by Iron Oxide and Silica Doped 3D Printed Tricalcium Phosphate Scaffolds. *Ann. Biomed. Eng.* **2018**, *46*, 1241–1253. [CrossRef]
93. Tarafder, S.; Balla, V.K.; Davies, N.M.; Bandyopadhyay, A.; Bose, S. Microwave-sintered 3D printed tricalcium phosphate scaffolds for bone tissue engineering. *J. Tissue Eng. Regen. Med.* **2013**, *7*, 631–641. [CrossRef]
94. Giannoudis, P.V.; Dinopoulos, H.; Tsiridis, E. Bone substitutes: An update. *Injury* **2005**, *36*, 20–27. [CrossRef]
95. Välimäki, V.-V.; Aro, H. Molecular basis for action of bioactive glasses as bone graft substitute. *Scand. J. Surg.* **2006**, *95*, 95–102. [CrossRef]
96. Eqtesadi, S.; Motealleh, A.; Miranda, P.; Pajares, A.; Lemos, A.; Ferreira, J.M.F. Robocasting of 45S5 bioactive glass scaffolds for bone tissue engineering. *J. Eur. Ceram. Soc.* **2014**, *34*, 107–118. [CrossRef]
97. Xynos, I.D.; Edgar, A.J.; Buttery, L.D.K.; Hench, L.L.; Polak, J.M. Gene-expression profiling of human osteoblasts following treatment with the ionic products of Bioglass® 45S5 dissolution. *J. Biomed. Mater. Res.* **2001**, *55*, 151–157. [CrossRef]
98. Wu, C.; Luo, Y.; Cuniberti, G.; Xiao, Y.; Gelinsky, M. Three-dimensional printing of hierarchical and tough mesoporous bioactive glass scaffolds with a controllable pore architecture, excellent mechanical strength and mineralization ability. *Acta Biomater.* **2011**, *7*, 2644–2650. [CrossRef] [PubMed]
99. Pei, P.; Tian, Z.; Zhu, Y. 3D printed mesoporous bioactive glass/metal-organic framework scaffolds with antitubercular drug delivery. *Microporous Mesoporous Mater.* **2018**, *272*, 24–30. [CrossRef]
100. Baino, F. Bioactive glasses—When glass science and technology meet regenerative medicine. *Ceram. Int.* **2018**, *44*, 14953–14966. [CrossRef]
101. Hsu, F.-Y.; Hsu, H.-W.; Chang, Y.-H.; Yu, J.-L.; Rau, L.-R.; Tsai, S.-W. Macroporous microbeads containing apatite-modified mesoporous bioactive glass nanofibres for bone tissue engineering applications. *Mater. Sci. Eng. C* **2018**, *89*, 346–354. [CrossRef]
102. Nommeots-Nomm, A.; Lee, P.D.; Jones, J.R. Direct ink writing of highly bioactive glasses. *J. Eur. Ceram. Soc.* **2018**, *38*, 837–844. [CrossRef]
103. Padilla, S.; Sánchez-Salcedo, S.; Vallet-Regí, M. Bioactive glass as precursor of designed-architecture scaffolds for tissue engineering. *J. Biomed. Mater. Res. Part A* **2007**, *81*, 224–232. [CrossRef]
104. Westhauser, F.; Weis, C.; Prokscha, M.; Bittrich, L.A.; Li, W.; Xiao, K.; Kneser, U.; Kauczor, H.-U.; Schmidmaier, G.; Boccaccini, A.R.; et al. Three-dimensional polymer coated 45S5-type bioactive glass scaffolds seeded with human mesenchymal stem cells show bone formation in vivo. *J. Mater. Sci. Mater. Med.* **2016**, *27*, 119. [CrossRef]
105. Liu, Z.; Liang, H.; Shi, T.; Xie, D.; Chen, R.; Han, X.; Shen, L.; Wang, C.; Tian, Z. Additive manufacturing of hydroxyapatite bone scaffolds via digital light processing and in vitro compatibility. *Ceram. Int.* **2019**, *45*, 11079–11086. [CrossRef]
106. Wang, Y.; Wang, K.; Li, X.; Wei, Q.; Chai, W.; Wang, S.; Che, Y.; Lu, T.; Zhang, B. 3D fabrication and characterization of phosphoric acid scaffold with a HA/beta-TCP weight ratio of 60:40 for bone tissue engineering applications. *PLoS ONE* **2017**, *12*, e0174870.
107. Tarafder, S.; Bose, S. Polycaprolactone-Coated 3D Printed Tricalcium Phosphate Scaffolds for Bone Tissue Engineering: In Vitro Alendronate Release Behavior and Local Delivery Effect on In Vivo Osteogenesis. *ACS Appl. Mater. Interfaces* **2014**, *6*, 9955–9965. [CrossRef]
108. Luo, G.; Ma, Y.; Cui, X.; Jiang, L.; Wu, M.; Hu, Y.; Luo, Y.; Pan, H.; Ruan, C. 13-93 bioactive glass/alginate composite scaffolds 3D printed under mild conditions for bone regeneration. *RSC Adv.* **2017**, *7*, 11880–11889. [CrossRef]
109. Dimitriou, R.; Jones, E.; McGonagle, D.; Giannoudis, P. Bone regeneration: current concepts and future directions. *BMC Med.* **2011**, *9*, 66. [CrossRef] [PubMed]
110. Pilia, M.; Guda, T.; Appleford, M. Development of Composite Scaffolds for Load-Bearing Segmental Bone Defects. *BioMed Res. Int.* **2013**, *2013*, 458253. [CrossRef] [PubMed]

111. Reichert, J.C.; Wullschleger, M.E.; Cipitria, A.; Lienau, J.; Cheng, T.K.; Schütz, M.A.; Duda, G.N.; Nöth, U.; Eulert, J.; Hutmacher, D. Custom-made composite scaffolds for segmental defect repair in long bones. *Int. Orthop.* **2011**, *35*, 1229–1236. [CrossRef]
112. Wagoner Johnson, A.J.; Herschler, B.A. A review of the mechanical behavior of CaP and CaP/polymer composites for applications in bone replacement and repair. *Acta Biomater.* **2011**, *7*, 16–30. [CrossRef]
113. Chengtie, W.; Jiang, C. A review of bioactive silicate ceramics. *Biomed. Mater.* **2013**, *8*, 032001.
114. Fu, Q.; Saiz, E.; Rahaman, M.N.; Tomsia, A.P. Bioactive glass scaffolds for bone tissue engineering: state of the art and future perspectives. *Mater. Sci. Eng. C* **2011**, *31*, 1245–1256. [CrossRef]
115. Rezwan, K.; Chen, Q.Z.; Blaker, J.J.; Boccaccini, A.R. Biodegradable and bioactive porous polymer/inorganic composite scaffolds for bone tissue engineering. *Biomaterials* **2006**, *27*, 3413–3431. [CrossRef]
116. Vorndran, E.; Klarner, M.; Klammert, U.; Grover, L.M.; Patel, S.; Barralet, J.E.; Gbureck, U. 3D Powder Printing of β-Tricalcium Phosphate Ceramics Using Different Strategies. *Adv. Eng. Mater.* **2008**, *10*, 67–71. [CrossRef]
117. Detsch, R.; Schaefer, S.; Deisinger, U.; Ziegler, G.; Seitz, H.; Leukers, B. In vitro -Osteoclastic Activity Studies on Surfaces of 3D Printed Calcium Phosphate Scaffolds. *J. Biomater. Appl.* **2011**, *26*, 359–380. [CrossRef]
118. Fielding, G.; Bose, S. SiO_2 and ZnO dopants in three-dimensionally printed tricalcium phosphate bone tissue engineering scaffolds enhance osteogenesis and angiogenesis in vivo. *Acta Biomater.* **2013**, *9*, 9137–9148. [CrossRef] [PubMed]
119. Wang, Y.; Li, X.; Wei, Q.; Yang, M.; Wei, S. Study on the Mechanical Properties of Three-Dimensional Directly Binding Hydroxyapatite Powder. *Cell Biochem. Biophys.* **2015**, *72*, 289–295. [CrossRef] [PubMed]
120. Miguel, C.; Marta, D.; Elke, V.; Uwe, G.; Paulo, F.; Inês, P.; Barbara, G.; Henrique, A.; Eduardo, P.; Jorge, R. Application of a 3D printed customized implant for canine cruciate ligament treatment by tibial tuberosity advancement. *Biofabrication* **2014**, *6*, 025005.
121. Butscher, A.; Bohner, M.; Doebelin, N.; Hofmann, S.; Müller, R. New depowdering-friendly designs for three-dimensional printing of calcium phosphate bone substitutes. *Acta Biomater.* **2013**, *9*, 9149–9158. [CrossRef] [PubMed]
122. Chumnanklang, R.; Panyathanmaporn, T.; Sitthiseripratip, K.; Suwanprateeb, J. 3D printing of hydroxyapatite: Effect of binder concentration in pre-coated particle on part strength. *Mater. Sci. Eng. C* **2007**, *27*, 914–921. [CrossRef]
123. Suwanprateeb, J.; Sanngam, R.; Suvannapruk, W.; Panyathanmaporn, T. Mechanical and in vitro performance of apatite—Wollastonite glass ceramic reinforced hydroxyapatite composite fabricated by 3D-printing. *J. Mater. Sci. Mater. Med.* **2009**, *20*, 1281. [CrossRef]
124. Hwa, L.C.; Rajoo, S.; Noor, A.M.; Ahmad, N.; Uday, M.B. Recent advances in 3D printing of porous ceramics: A review. *Curr. Opin. Solid State Mater. Sci.* **2017**, *21*, 323–347. [CrossRef]
125. Roohani-Esfahani, S.-I.; Newman, P.; Zreiqat, H. Design and Fabrication of 3D printed Scaffolds with a Mechanical Strength Comparable to Cortical Bone to Repair Large Bone Defects. *Sci. Rep.* **2016**, *6*, 19468. [CrossRef]
126. Fierz, F.C.; Beckmann, F.; Huser, M.; Irsen, S.H.; Leukers, B.; Witte, F.; Degistirici, Ö.; Andronache, A.; Thie, M.; Müller, B. The morphology of anisotropic 3D-printed hydroxyapatite scaffolds. *Biomaterials* **2008**, *29*, 3799–3806. [CrossRef]
127. Dellinger, J.G.; Eurell, J.A.C.; Jamison, R.D. Bone response to 3D periodic hydroxyapatite scaffolds with and without tailored microporosity to deliver bone morphogenetic protein 2. *J. Biomed. Mater. Res.* **2006**, *76*, 366–376. [CrossRef]
128. Hollinger, J.O.; Brekke, J.; Gruskin, E.; Lee, D. Role of Bone Substitutes. *Clin. Orthop. Relat. Res.* **1996**, *324*, 55–65. [CrossRef] [PubMed]
129. Kaully, T.; Kaufman-Francis, K.; Lesman, A.; Levenberg, S. Vascularization—The Conduit to Viable Engineered Tissues. *Tissue Eng. Part B Rev.* **2009**, *15*, 159–169. [CrossRef] [PubMed]
130. Shahabipour, F.; Ashammakhi, N.; Oskuee, R.K.; Bonakdar, S.; Hoffman, T.; Shokrgozar, M.A.; Khademhosseini, A. Key components of engineering vascularized 3-dimensional bioprinted bone constructs. *Transl. Res.* **2019**. [CrossRef] [PubMed]
131. Jammalamadaka, U.; Tappa, K. Recent Advances in Biomaterials for 3D Printing and Tissue Engineering. *J. Funct. Biomater.* **2018**, *9*, 22. [CrossRef] [PubMed]

132. Tappa, K.; Jammalamadaka, U. Novel Biomaterials Used in Medical 3D Printing Techniques. *J. Funct. Biomater.* **2018**, *9*, 17. [CrossRef]
133. Kolesky, D.B.; Homan, K.A.; Skylar-Scott, M.A.; Lewis, J.A. Three-dimensional bioprinting of thick vascularized tissues. *Proc. Natl. Acad. Sci. USA* **2016**, *113*, 3179–3184. [CrossRef]
134. Bertassoni, L.; Cecconi, M.; Manoharan, V.; Nikkhah, M.; Hjortnaes, J.; Cristino, A.; Barabaschi, G.; Demarchi, D.; Dokmeci, M.; Yang, Y.; et al. Hydrogel Bioprinted Microchannel Networks for Vascularization of Tissue Engineering Constructs. *Lab Chip* **2014**, *14*, 2202–2211. [CrossRef]
135. Zhang, A.P.; Qu, X.; Soman, P.; Hribar, K.C.; Lee, J.W.; Chen, S.; He, S. Rapid Fabrication of Complex 3D Extracellular Microenvironments by Dynamic Optical Projection Stereolithography. *Adv. Mater.* **2012**, *24*, 4266–4270. [CrossRef]
136. Tumbleston, J.; Shirvanyants, D.; Ermoshkin, N.; Janusziewicz, R.; Johnson, A.; Kelly, D.; Chen, K.; Pinschmidt, R.; Rolland, J.; Ermoshkin, A.; et al. Additive manufacturing. Continuous liquid interface production of 3D objects. *Science* **2015**, *347*, 1349–1352. [CrossRef]
137. Zhu, W.; Qu, X.; Zhu, J.; Ma, X.; Patel, S.; Liu, J.; Wang, P.; Lai, C.S.E.; Gou, M.; Xu, Y.; et al. Direct 3D bioprinting of prevascularized tissue constructs with complex microarchitecture. *Biomaterials* **2017**, *124*, 106–115. [CrossRef]
138. Araldi, E.; Schipani, E. Hypoxia, HIFs and bone development. *Bone* **2010**, *47*, 190–196. [CrossRef] [PubMed]
139. Kuss, M.A.; Harms, R.; Wu, S.; Wang, Y.; Untrauer, J.B.; Carlson, M.A.; Duan, B. Short-term hypoxic preconditioning promotes prevascularization in 3D bioprinted bone constructs with stromal vascular fraction derived cells. *RSC Adv.* **2017**, *7*, 29312–29320. [CrossRef] [PubMed]

11

Macrophage Biocompatibility of CoCr Wear Particles Produced under Polarization in Hyaluronic Acid Aqueous Solution

Blanca Teresa Perez-Maceda [1], María Encarnación López-Fernández [1], Iván Díaz [2], Aaron Kavanaugh [3], Fabrizio Billi [3], María Lorenza Escudero [2], María Cristina García-Alonso [2] and Rosa María Lozano [1,*]

1 Cell-Biomaterial Recognition Lab., Department of Cellular and Molecular Biology, Centro de Investigaciones Biológicas (CIB-CSIC), Ramiro de Maeztu 9, 28040 Madrid, Spain; bpm@cib.csic.es (B.T.P.-M.); lfmarien@gmail.com (M.E.L.-F.)

2 Department of Surface Engineering, Corrosion and Durability, Centro Nacional de Investigaciones Metalúrgicas (CENIM-CSIC), Avda. Gregorio del Amo 8, 28040 Madrid, Spain; ivan.diaz@cenim.csic.es (I.D.); escudero@cenim.csic.es (M.L.E.); crisga@cenim.csic.es (M.C.G.-A.)

3 Department of Orthopaedic Surgery, David Geffen School of Medicine, University of California Los Angeles, Orthopaedic Hospital Research Center, 615 Charles E. Young Dr. South, Room 450A, Los Angeles, CA 90095, USA; akavanaugh@mednet.ucla.edu (A.K.); fabrizio.billi@gmail.com (F.B.)

* Correspondence: rlozano@cib.csic.es

Abstract: Macrophages are the main cells involved in inflammatory processes and in the primary response to debris derived from wear of implanted CoCr alloys. The biocompatibility of wear particles from a high carbon CoCr alloy produced under polarization in hyaluronic acid (HA) aqueous solution was evaluated in J774A.1 mouse macrophages cultures. Polarization was applied to mimic the electrical interactions observed in living tissues. Wear tests were performed in a pin-on-disk tribometer integrating an electrochemical cell in phosphate buffer solution (PBS) and in PBS supplemented with 3 g/L HA, an average concentration that is generally found in synovial fluid, used as lubricant solution. Wear particles produced in 3 g/L HA solution showed a higher biocompatibility in J774A.1 macrophages in comparison to those elicited by particles obtained in PBS. A considerable enhancement in macrophages biocompatibility in the presence of 3 g/L of HA was further observed by the application of polarization at potentials having current densities typical of injured tissues suggesting that polarization produces an effect on the surface of the metallic material that leads to the production of wear particles that seem to be macrophage-biocompatible and less cytotoxic. The results showed the convenience of considering the influence of the electric interactions in the chemical composition of debris detached from metallic surfaces under wear corrosion to get a better understanding of the biological effects caused by the wear products.

Keywords: polarization; CoCr alloy; wear particles; hyaluronic acid; macrophages biocompatibility

1. Introduction

Macrophages are cells involved in inflammatory processes [1]. All orthopedic biomaterials may induce a biologic host response to generated wear debris, which is strictly dependent on the nature of the debris. Metal wear particles and metal ions from prosthetic devices may induce a cascade of adverse cellular reactions that may include inflammatory complications, macrophage activation, bone resorption, and, although rarely, neoplasia [2,3]. In this context, macrophages play a decisive role in the hostile inflammatory reactions that can lead to implant loosening and failure.

Implanted metal surfaces in biological environments are exposed to cells and to physiological milieu interacting between them, an interaction that affects both the cells and the metallic surface. Implanted metallic materials, such as CoCr alloys, undergo dissolution and formation of a passive film that is affected by factors such as pH, ions present in the physiological medium, temperature, and biopotentials. Biopotentials are natural electrical properties that control the normal growth and development of different types of cells and tissues [4,5]. When a tissue is injured, its potentials undergo alterations to the normal potential of intact tissue [6,7]. Both biopotentials and injury potentials are found in bone and these potentials induced between injured and intact tissues persist until the tissue heals. Potentials in injured tissue can span over hundreds of microns and are generated by electric fields or ions flowing through the injured tissue [8,9] with a range of 10–100 mV/cm [10]. Assuming the resistivity of soft tissues to be 100 Ω cm [9,11], the resulting current density is in the 1–100 $\mu A/cm^2$ range [8,12]. Fukada and Yasuda had already described in 1957 the piezoelectric nature of the bone tissue [13]. Endogenous electrical properties of bone may play a role in the feedback mechanism of bone remodeling and development [14,15]. In vivo, these electrical signals work in collaboration to provide the correct environment for normal bone growth and development, but can be disrupted or altered by an injury after a trauma and during the healing process. Moreover, the resulting voltage gradients may induce modifications in the electrochemical potential of metallic implants and consequently may affect their surface properties.

Díaz et al. [16] recently characterized the CoCr alloy oxide films in a phosphate buffer solution containing 3 g/L of hyaluronic acid, the approximate concentration found in the synovial fluid of healthy joints [17], and under potentials with current density similar to those reported for injured tissues (1–100 $\mu A/cm^2$). Potentiostatic pulses applied during the growth of the CoCr oxide film produced a modification of the film that affected its chemical composition, thickness, and structure compared to the passive film formed in air [16]. These modifications induced surface heterogeneities at the atomic scale, geometric irregularities, such as nano-roughness, and a variation of the oxide composition [16]. Moreover, application of potentials of 0.7 V vs. Ag/AgCl induced changes in the oxide layer with the formation of 10–50 nm diameter nanopores, uniformly distributed along the surface and an increase in Cr (VI) and Mo (VI) concentration [16].

Despite the presence of the passive film, metals are susceptible to corrosion, particularly in aqueous environments, which may affect the surrounding tissue. Corrosion events generate electrical currents due to electron transfer from ions in the solution to the metallic surface where reactions are occurring. Wear-corrosion phenomena and micromotion or fretting-corrosion mechanically removes material, including the passive film, causing continuous activation/repassivation cycles [18]. These continuous and dynamic processes not only weaken the surface performance but also lead to an increase in the debris around the implant. Wear debris is considered one of the main factors responsible for aseptic loosening of orthopedic endoprostheses [19,20]. Implant failure due to aseptic loosening, or osteolysis, may result from the release of wear debris or electrochemical ions generated during corrosion events [20–22].

From the electrochemical point of view, on the metallic surfaces of implants, the breakdown of the passive film under the wear-corrosion process causes a drastic decrease in the open circuit potential of the metal towards negative potentials, i.e., from the passive to active state. This situation can suppose a polarization of about 500–700 mV with respect to the original open circuit potential. The change from the passive to active state can be induced mechanically under wear and electrochemically applying anodic polarization on the tribological system. Several researchers have studied the wear corrosion processes by application of anodic potentiodynamic polarization under wear processes [23,24].

The object of this paper was to evaluate the biocompatibility of particles produced during wear-corrosion assays of a CoCr alloy at potentiodynamic range to cover a wide polarization window on the samples. The hyaluronic acid, the lubricant component of the synovial liquid, was selected as the electrolyte for the generation of wear particles in conditions that represent more closely the prosthesis environment. Since macrophages are the main cells involved in the primary response to foreign bodies, cytotoxicity and biocompatibility of the wear particles were evaluated using these cells, measuring lactate dehydrogenase and mitochondrial activity, respectively.

2. Results and Discussion

2.1. Wear-Corrosion Tests

The interaction of physiological fluids with the bearing surfaces of hip implants is of great importance in the research of artificial joint lubrication, although this study has been so far little explored.

The effect of sliding of the alumina ball on the HCCoCr alloys is clearly shown in the drastic change in the open circuit potential. As an example, Figure 1 shows the change in the open circuit potential when the HCCoCr surfaces in PBS supplemented with 3 g/L HA (PBS-HA) are subjected to wear. The open circuit potential without wear was around −0.25 V versus Ag/AgCl, decreasing sharply when the alumina ball (pin) started the circular movement under 5 N load at 120 rpm. At this moment, the open circuit potential decreased until achieving values of about −0.55 V vs. Ag/AgCl, i.e., about 300 mV, and remained constant until the end of the test. The reduction in the potential value towards more negative values indicates that the HCCoCr surface becomes electrochemically active. This variation is due to the breakdown of the passive film under sliding, promoting the release of metallic ions and particles.

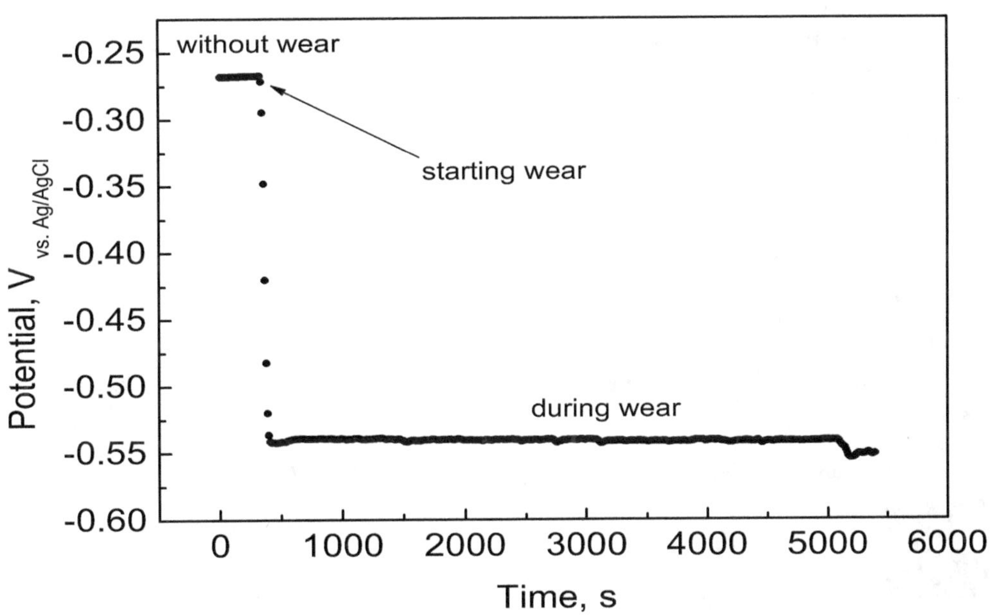

Figure 1. Open circuit potential of HCCoCr disks under wear. Measurement of the open circuit potential before and during the wear corrosion test of HCCoCr in PBS containing 3 g/L HA (PBS-HA).

Figure 2 panels a and b show the coefficient of friction (COF) for HCCoCr/alumina pair in PBS and PBS supplemented with 3 g/L HA (PBS-HA) during anodic potentiodynamic polarization and the anodic polarization curves drawn at 10 mV/min of HCCoCr in PBS and PBS containing 3 g/L HA under wear conditions (between point 1 and 2 in Figure 2a), respectively. The anodic polarization curve of HCCoCr in PBS-HA without wear has been also added in Figure 2b for comparative reasons. It can be seen that under sliding at the corrosion potential (before point 1 in Figure 2a), the COF was significantly higher in PBS than in PBS-HA. This result agrees with the hypothesis that the hyaluronic acid has a known lubricant role in the joint, acting as a shock absorber [25] and thus facilitating smooth joint movement by reducing friction between both surfaces. At the next stage (from point 1 to 2, in Figure 2a), the difference between both COF (in PBS and PBS-HA) remained, but higher fluctuations were detected. The fluctuations could be related to the continuous formation of hard particulate matter that enhances friction between both counterparts and decreases the friction when ejected from the track to surrounding areas where it accumulates (Figure 3). The load applied on the CoCr surfaces while sliding activates mechano-chemical reactions, causing not only the detachment of the passive film [26] but also bulk material resulting in an increase of COF. The hyaluronic acid in PBS maintains the lubricant effect during most of the wear corrosion tests.

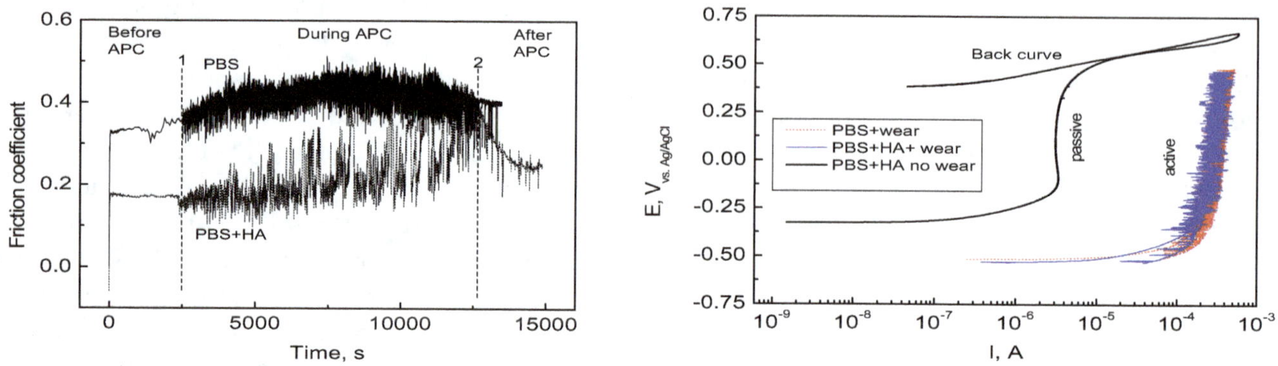

(a) (b)

Figure 2. Friction coefficient of HCCoCr/alumina pair (**a**) and anodic polarization curves (APC) of HCCoCr disks (**b**) during wear corrosion tests in PBS and PBS containing 3 g/L HA (PBS-HA). Measurement of the friction coefficient before, during, and after application of anodic polarization current (APC). Anodic polarization curve for HCCoCr alloy in PBS-HA without wear is added for comparative analysis.

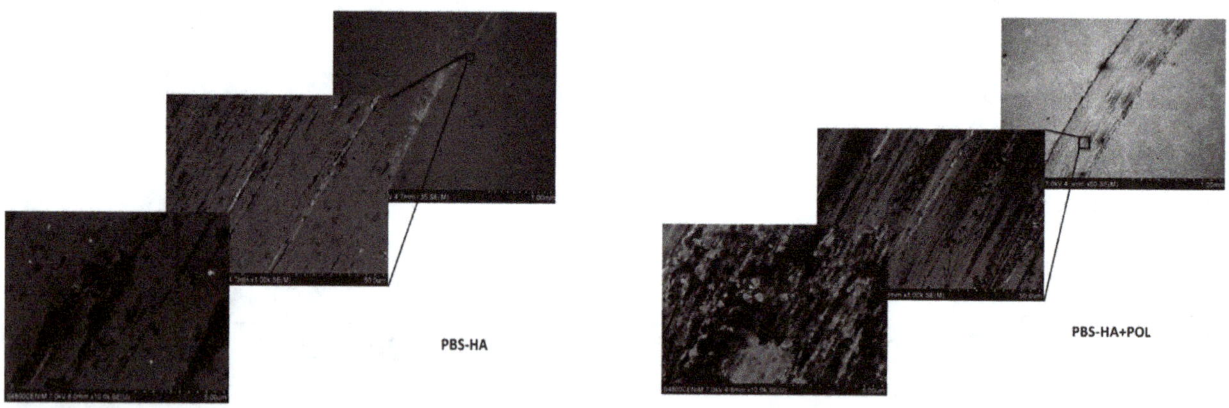

(a) (b)

Figure 3. Secondary electron images of wear tracks on HCCoCr disks. Images by SEM of HCCoCr samples in PBS-HA under wear: (**a**) at the open circuit potential (PBS-HA) and (**b**) applying anodic potentiodynamic polarization (PBS-HA+POL).

As a consequence of mechanically assisted corrosion, the passive film on the HCCoCr surface was rapidly broken in both media, PBS and PBS-HA, producing an increase of approximately 3 orders of magnitude in current (Figure 2b) with respect to the anodic polarization curve without wear. Corrosion progresses on the wear track drawn by the sliding of alumina ball on the HCCoCr disks (Figure 3). Having in mind the wide passive region seen in the anodic polarization curve drawn without wear (Figure 2), the potential applied could be employed in forming rapidly the new oxide film. However, the sliding rate is quick enough to avoid the repassivation and formation of new protective chromium oxides. The constant value of the current density around 1 mA (three orders of magnitude higher than without wear) indicates that under these experimental conditions (5 N load and sliding rate of 120 rpm), the passive film is destroyed and remains in an active state until the end of the test.

Figure 3 shows the secondary electron (SE) images of the tracks of HCCoCr in PBS-HA after wear corrosion tests, at the corrosion potential (PBS-HA) and under anodic potentiodynamic polarization (PBS-HA+POL). In both cases (a) and (b), debris is accumulated in the immediate vicinity of the wear tracks, but the surface inside the track is especially altered when anodic potentiodynamic potential is applied. Figure 4 shows, as an example, the semiquantitative analysis taken by EDS of the three areas of interest in the HCCoCr alloy immersed in PBS-HA after wear corrosion under polarization (PBS-HA-POL): away from the track (spectrum 1), immediate vicinity (spectrum 2), and inside the track (spectrum 3). The most important feature found is the high % C content accumulated in the vicinity of the track. It means that the debris is mainly composed of C and O, the greatest proportion probably coming from the hyaluronic acid.

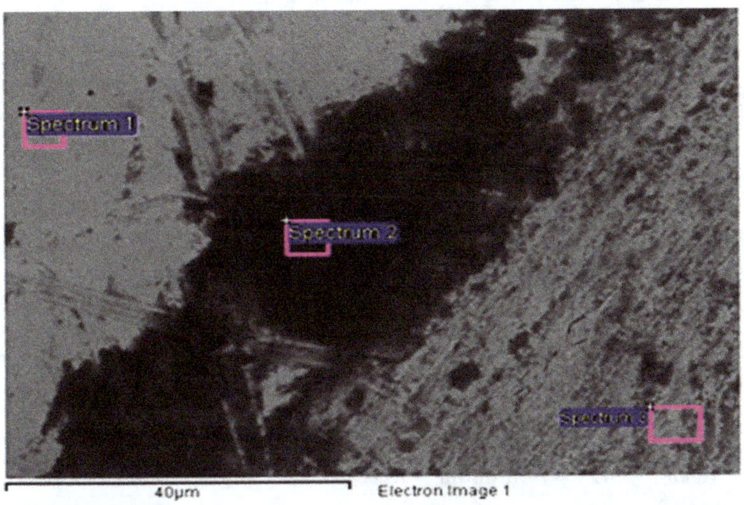

PBS-HA+POL

Element	Spectrum 1	Spectrum 2	Spectrum 3
Co	58.0	14.2	45.7
Cr	31.4	7.7	26.8
Mo	3.7	1.0	3.3
C	6.9	61.9	13.6
O	-	15.2	10.6

Figure 4. HCCoCr surface after wear corrosion applying anodic potentiodynamic polarization. Secondary electron image and EDS analyses away from the track, in the immediate vicinity, and inside the track in the HCCoCr surface in PBS-HA+POL.

The morphology and chemical characterization of the wear particles detached during wear corrosion tests revealed some interesting results. Figure 5 shows, as an example, the secondary electron image of wear particles collected from the tribocorrosion test in PBS containing 3 g/L HA and the semiquantitative analysis of some particles, identified from 1 to 6 and marked in blue color.

The statistical results of the effect of the corrosive medium and polarization applied in the wear corrosion tests on the chemical composition of the wear-detached particles collected appear in Table 1. In this table, three condition numbers assigned to 1, the PBS corrosive medium, 2, the PBS-HA corrosive medium without applying polarization, and 3, the PBS-HA corrosive medium applying polarization (PBS-HA-POL), have been considered. Mean, standard deviation, minimum and maximum value, C25 and C75, and median are shown.

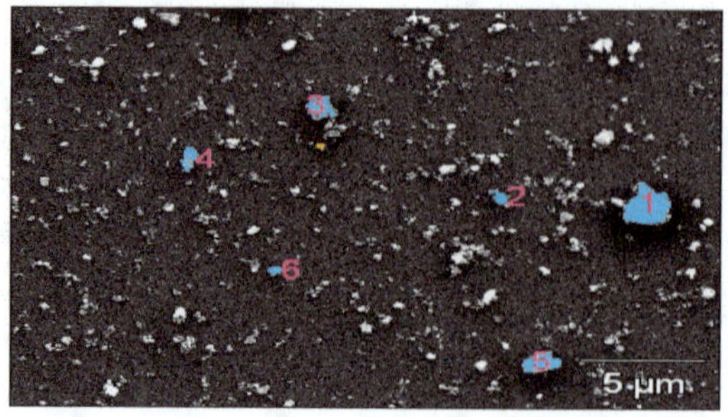

	C	O	Al	P	Cr	Co
	Wt.%	Wt.%	Wt.%	Wt.%	Wt.%	Wt.%
pt1	0	34.02	0	16.87	35.30	13.81
pt2	0	41.31	0	20.24	38.45	0
pt3	0	33.72	0	23.16	43.13	0
pt4	0	41.95	0	15.76	30.75	11.54
pt5	0	23.79	10.62	26.36	34.38	4.85
pt6	0	54.36	0	16.31	29.33	0

Figure 5. Secondary electron images of wear particles. Particles were collected from wear corrosion tests performed in PBS containing 3 g/L HA (PBS-HA) and deposited on silicon wafer to analyze the chemical composition of detached particles. Blue colors represent the particle where EDS has been performed and the particle number shown in pink is correlated to the pt shown in the table attached.

Table 1. Statistical analysis by Kruskal–Wallis test for the chemical composition (wt %) of wear particles detached during wear corrosion tests of CoCr samples in PBS (condition number 1), PBS+ 3 g/L HA (condition number 2) and under anodic potentiodynamic polarization (condition number 3), where *n* is the number of samples, mean is the average value, SD is the standard deviation, C25 is the value of the 25% of the data, C75 is the value of the 75% of the data, and *p* * is the significant difference at 0.95 confidence level.

	Condition Number	*n*	Mean	SD	Minimum	Maximum	C_{25}	Median	C_{75}	*p* *
Cr	1	7	33.28	6.92	21.61	43.13	29.33	34.38	38.45	0.034
	2	24	28.53	8.73	14.06	48.82	21.28	27.52	33.66	
	3	7	39.09	11.02	22.34	57.01	33.65	37.60	47.67	
Co	1	7	4.31	6.02	0.00	13.81	0.00	0.00	11.54	0.001
	2	24	7.73	16.94	0.00	54.07	0.00	0.00	5.99	
	3	7	36.08	17.59	15.14	58.64	17.57	32.12	51.48	
Mo	1	7	0.00	0.00	0.00	0.00	0.00	0.00	0.00	0.006
	2	24	0.45	1.54	0.00	5.63	0.00	0.00	0.00	
	3	7	2.71	2.60	0.00	5.48	0.00	4.00	5.45	
P	1	7	18.59	5.02	11.46	26.36	15.76	16.87	23.16	0.051
	2	24	14.11	5.90	0.96	27.48	11.64	13.24	17.83	
	3	7	9.40	7.30	1.30	19.57	1.89	8.79	16.10	
Al	1	7	1.52	4.01	0.00	10.62	0.00	0.00	0.00	0.123
	2	24	0.18	0.68	0.00	3.17	0.00	0.00	0.00	
	3	7	0.76	1.06	0.00	2.57	0.00	0.00	1.85	
O	1	7	40.10	10.67	23.79	54.36	33.72	41.31	51.57	0.002
	2	24	41.82	17.72	3.52	72.84	34.64	49.54	51.69	
	3	7	10.91	7.03	3.76	23.11	4.83	8.28	16.05	
C	1	7	2.19	5.80	0.00	15.35	0.00	0.00	0.00	0.022
	2	24	6.98	7.49	0.00	19.94	0.00	6.39	14.16	
	3	7	0.00	0.00	0.00	0.00	0.00	0.00	0.00	

* *p*-value in the Kruskal–Wallis test.

It can be seen that the particles are mainly composed of Co, Cr, Mo, P, C and O, with some traces of Al in some isolated particles. The Kruskal–Wallis test indicated that there are significant differences in the levels of Cr, Co, Mo, O and C, comparing the different conditions, i.e., depending on the composition of corrosive medium (PBS-condition 1 or PBS-HA-condition 2) and the application of polarization in wear corrosion tests (PBS-HA-POL, condition 3, and PBS-HA, condition 2). However, no significant differences in P and Al levels were obtained.

The results of the post hoc Mann–Whitney test used to determine which pairs differed among them are shown in Table 2. Cr levels are significantly higher in condition number 3 than 2 ($p = 0.021$). Co and Mo levels are significantly higher in condition number 3 than 1 and 2 ($p = 0.002$ and $p = 0.001$, $p = 0.025$ and $p = 0.002$, respectively). O levels are significantly lower in condition number 3 than 1 and 2 ($p = 0.002$ in both cases). C levels are significantly lower in condition number 3 than 2 ($p = 0.017$).

Table 2. Post hoc Mann–Whitney analysis to determine which pairs differed among them (condition numbers: 1-PBS, 2-PBS-HA, and 3-PBS-HA+POL).

	Comparison between Pairwise		
	p **** 1 vs. 2**	***p*** **** 1 vs. 3**	***p*** **** 2 vs. 3**
Cr	0.119	0.277	0.021
Co	0.556	0.002	0.001
Mo	0.438	0.025	0.008
P	-	-	-
Al	-	-	-
O	0.508	0.002	0.002
C	0.098	0.317	0.017

** *p*-value in the Mann–Whitney test.

In summary, the statistical analysis confirmed that factors such as "composition of the corrosive medium" and "polarization applied" have an influence on the dependent variable chemical composition of the particles that is discussed immediately below.

The main significant effect of the addition of hyaluronic acid in the PBS to the wear particles detached is observed in the increase of the C content in the chemical composition of the particles. In both media (PBS, condition 1, and PBS-HA, condition 2), particles are mainly composed of Cr and O, followed by P and some Co. This chemical composition can be directly linked to the detachment of the native passive film during the wear corrosion test.

It has been proven by XPS (data not shown) that the immersion of the HCCoCr surfaces in PBS-HA causes a decrease in the Co species in the passive film and the enrichment in chromium oxide where phosphorus is included. It has been reported in literature that phosphate is adsorbed upon freshly exposed metal at the same time that ions are released into the solution until the passive layer is formed, whose composition varies significantly depending upon the environment [27]. Lewis et al. established that the corrosion, especially when associated with mechanical wear, is controlled by phosphate anions that absorb or react with the Co and Cr dissolution products. This promotes the formation of a mixed composition of phosphates, hydroxides, and oxides originating from the bulk metal.

This means that most of the particles collected after the wear corrosion tests in PBS and PBS-HA come from the native passive film (whose thickness is about 5–7 nm) and are mainly composed of chromium oxide and phosphate.

With respect to applying polarization during the wear corrosion tests in PBS-HA (condition 3), this factor has an important effect on the chemical composition of the wear particles detached. In this condition, particles are mainly composed of Cr and Co, followed by O, P, and Mo. The main significant effect of the polarization is the significant enrichment in Co, Cr, and Mo in the chemical composition of the detached particles. In this case, the wear particles produced under anodic polarization increased the Co/Cr ratio (with a value of 0.9 in comparison with a value of 0.3 found in PBS-HA without polarization). As wear particles obtained without polarization, these particles also contained P, although in a low proportion (Table 1). It has been reported in the literature [16] that the potential applied on the HCCoCr induces a change in the chemical composition of the passive film. Díaz et al. established that the increase in polarization (from 0.5 to 0.7 V) induced the preferential dissolution of cobalt whereas chromium was concentrated in the surface oxide film [16]. The passive film grown at a potential of 0.5 V vs. Ag/AgCl (into the passive region of the anodic polarization curve) consisted predominantly of Cr_2O_3 and $Cr(OH)_3$. However, the oxidation at a potential of 0.7 V vs. Ag/AgCl caused the appearance of Cr (VI) in the passive film but Co was not increased. In the case of wear corrosion under anodic potentiodynamic polarization, the continuous sliding of the alumina ball on the HCCoCr surface did not allow the regeneration of the oxide film. Instead, an active state stimulated by polarization was induced on the surface where bulk material was directly exposed and detached to the electrolyte. Considering this situation, the results reveal that the anodic polarization on CoCr surfaces under wear-corrosion processes accelerated and induced the release of larger metallic particles with higher Co content coming from the base material.

2.2. *Macrophage Cell Response*

Macrophages are a primary immune cell type and the main cellular type involved in inflammatory processes [1] and in host response [28], so their biologic host response to wear particles generated from the implanted materials is of great interest.

Macrophage response to wear particles derived from the tribocorrosion assays was evaluated by measuring the effect on cell toxicity and respiratory activity.

Cytotoxicity induced by HCCoCr wear particles was analyzed by measuring LDH activity released from cells (Figure 6), whose levels increase upon plasma membrane damage, a sign of cell death [29]. As is shown in Figure 6, exposure of macrophages cultures to wear particles induced a degree of cytotoxicity that was mainly dependent on the conditions used during wear-corrosion assays and particle concentration. As shown in Figure 6 panel A, particles concentration of 0.5 mg/mL obtained in PBS produced almost 58% cytotoxicity, a percentage that was significantly reduced to almost 12% when wear particles were generated from tribocorrosion tests in the presence of 3 g/L of hyaluronic acid (PBS-HA), an effect that could indicate a protective role of the hyaluronic acid on the metallic surface under wear stress conditions (Table 3). Concentrations of 1 mg/mL of wear particles from the PBS test produced an increase in the macrophage cytotoxicity to almost 75%, a value elevated in comparison with the cytotoxicity induced by the wear particles obtained in PBS containing 3 g/L of HA, where cytotoxicity reached 14% (data not shown). No additional increase in the cytotoxicity was observed at higher concentrations of wear particles (2 mg/mL) generated in PBS as macrophages cytotoxicity appeared comparable to the one elicited by exposure to lower concentrations of particles (0.5 and 1 mg/mL), where approximately a 64% cytotoxicity was detected (data not shown).

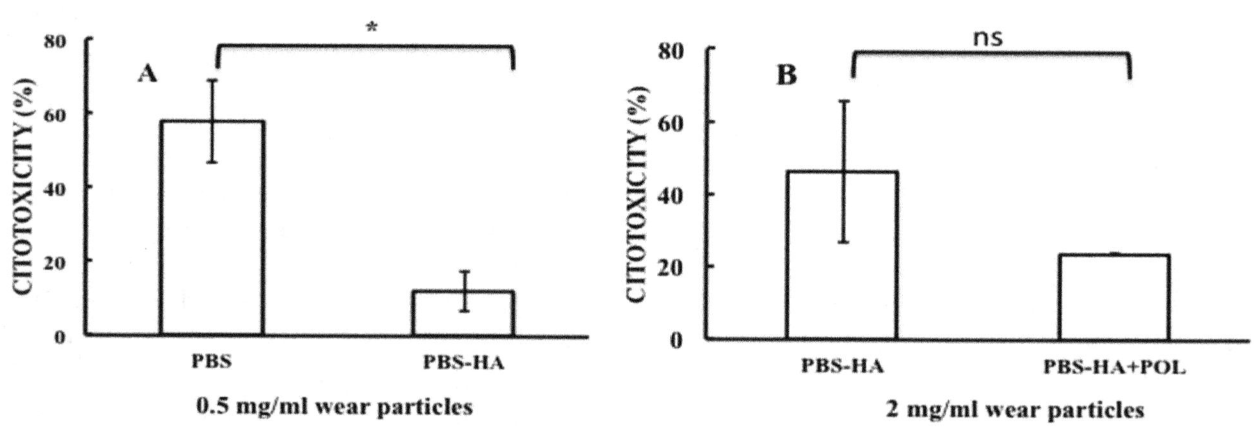

Figure 6. Macrophage cytotoxicity, measured as LDH activity, of cell cultures exposed for 72 h to HCCoCr wear particles. Panel A: Exposure of macrophages culture to 0.5 mg/mL wear particles. Particles were obtained in PBS and in PBS containing 3 g/L HA (PBS-HA). A p value of ≤ 0.05 was considered significant (*); Panel B: Exposure of macrophages culture to 2 mg/mL wear particles obtained in PBS containing 3 g/L HA with and without polarization application, PBS-HA+POL and PBS-HA, respectively. Experimental data were done as independent triplicate. Differences between data analyzed here were not significantly different (labeled as ns).

Table 3. Statistical analyses of cytotoxicity data. Mean differences of cytotoxicity effects between P2 (0.5 mg/mL) vs. P3 (0.5 mg/mL) and P3 (2 mg/mL) vs. P6 (2 mg/mL) were studied with Student's *t* tests ($\alpha = 0.05$), respectively. (**a**) Wear particles obtained in PBS (P2) and in PBS containing 3 g/L HA (P3). (**b**) Wear particles obtained in PBS containing 3 g/L HA (P3) and in PBS containing 3 g/L HA with polarization application (P6).

(a)		
P2 (0.5 mg/mL) vs. P3 (0.5 mg/mL)		
Mean of P2	Mean of P3	*P* Value
57.84	12.24	0.015

(b)		
P3 (2 mg/mL) vs. P6 (2 mg/mL)		
Mean of P3 (2 mg/mL)	Mean of P6 (2 mg/mL)	*P* Value
46.18	23.9	0.248

Particles produced in PBS containing 3 g/L of HA at concentrations of 2 mg/mL elicited an increase in the macrophages cytotoxicity that reached almost 46% (Figure 6, panel B, PBS-HA). Although such an increase was higher than the one produced by particles concentrations of 0.5 and 1 mg/mL, which were 12% and 14%, respectively, it was reduced to 24% when polarization conditions characteristic of damaged tissue were applied (Figure 6, panel B, PBS-HA+POL). Although the statistical analysis of the data from Figure 6 panel B (Table 3) gave no significant differences between results analyzed here, the application of anodic polarization to HA aqueous solution seems to have important observable differences on the mean value of the cytotoxicity. This feature could be relevant and, for this reason, verification by other biocompatibility assays is required. With this purpose, the wear particles collected from the tribocorrosion assays of CoCr alloy in PBS-HA without and applying anodic polarization were tested on macrophages cultures by measuring the mitochondrial activity. It is well known that the mitochondrial activity measurement is directly proportional to the number of metabolically active cells in culture [29] constituting a measure of cell viability and biocompatibility. As it is shown with Figure 7 by white bars, wear particles collected in the PBS-HA produced a gradual and significant reduction in the mitochondrial respiratory response of macrophages. This result seemed to be directly related to the concentration of particles to which macrophages were exposed (Table 4). Nevertheless, no reduction in the mitochondrial respiratory activity was observed in macrophages exposed to wear particles generated when polarization was applied during wear-corrosion tests. No significant effects in respiratory activity were observed in the range of particles concentrations tested (Figure 7, black dotted bars, and Table 5). The results suggest that the polarization conditions in the wear-corrosion assays in PBS containing HA at the approximate concentration found in synovial fluid seem to be beneficial to macrophage viability and biocompatibility.

Table 4. Statistical analyses of mitochondrial respiratory activity. The effects of the particle (P), the concentration, and their interaction on the changes in respiratory activity were analyzed with a two-way analysis of variance. A p value of ≤ 0.05 was considered significant. Mean pairwise comparisons were computed with a Tukey's test ($\alpha = 0.05$). All analyses were performed with the R software version 3.4.2 (R Core Team, Vienna, Austria, 2017).

ANOVA				
	Sum Sq	**Df**	***F* Value**	**Pr (>F)**
P	5745.2	1	266.75	4.64×10^{-9}
conc	2191.39	2	50.87	2.76×10^{-6}
$P \times$ conc	2648.33	2	61.48	1.07×10^{-6}
Residuals	236.91	11	-	-

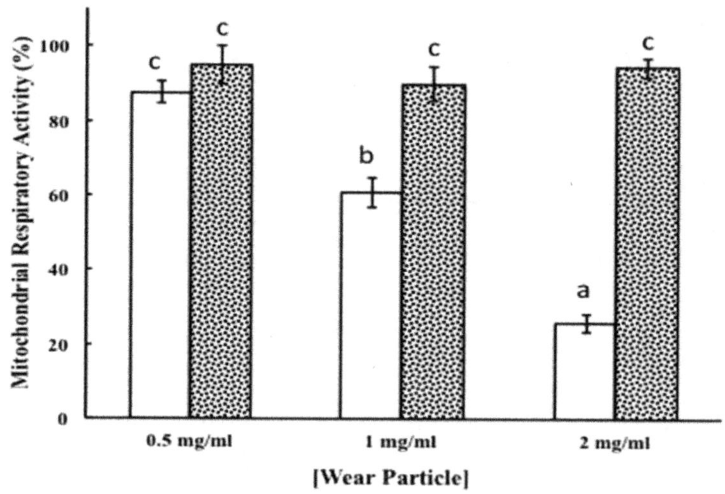

Figure 7. Mitochondrial respiratory activity of macrophages cell cultures exposed for 72 h to different doses of HCCoCr wear particles. Wear particles were obtained in PBS containing 3 g/L HA without (white bars) and with polarization (dotted black bars). Cell cultures were exposed to the following wear particles concentrations: 0.5, 1 and 2 mg/mL. Experiments were done as independent triplicate. Bars labeled with different letters show statistically significant differences and bars labeled with the same letter (c) show nonsignificant differences.

Table 5. As the interaction was significant, simple effects were compared. Means with the same letter are not significantly different.

P	Conc	Mean	Lower.CL	Upper.CL	Group
P3	2	25.7	17.1	34.3	a
P3	1	60.9	52.3	69.4	b
P3	0.5	87.5	77	98	c
P6	1	89.8	81.3	98.4	c
P6	2	94.3	85.8	102.9	c
P6	0.5	95	86.4	103.5	c

The dose-dependence effect on mitochondrial respiratory activity by particles detached in PBS-HA could be explained by the chemical composition of wear particles collected from wear-corrosion tests in this solution as a decrease in Co was observed, as well as an enrichment in chromium oxide, a compound with high toxicity [30] in comparison with the composition of PBS-HA-POL wear particles. The results suggest that polarization conditions applied to an HA aqueous solution at the approximate concentration found in synovial fluid produce changes in material tribocorrosion behavior inducing wear particles that seem to be beneficial to macrophage viability and biocompatibility. Data that could explain the higher biocompatibility of wear particles generated in PBS-HA+POL could be related to the fact that under these conditions, wear processes did not allow the regeneration of the oxide film. This event could determine the creation of an active state where CoCr base material was directly exposed to the electrolyte without enough time to build up the new oxide film that induced the release of metallic particles with higher Co content probably coming from the base material.

3. Materials and Methods

3.1. Material

A high carbon CoCr alloy (hereafter HCCoCr) that complies with ASTM F75 standard was used as material. HCCoCr composition is shown in Table 6. "Double heat-treated" disks, i.e., solution treatment (ST) followed by hot isostatically pressing (HIP), of 38 mm in diameter and 4 mm thickness, were obtained from BIOMET Spain Orthopaedic (Valencia, Spain). The sample preparation consisted of grinding on SiC paper, followed by mechanical polishing with 3 μm diamond paste.

Table 6. Chemical composition (wt %) of High Carbon CoCr alloy (HCCoCr).

	C	Co	Cr	Mo	Ni	S	P	Al	W	Mn	Fe	Si	N	Ti	Cu
HC	0.22	62	29.4	6.4	0.1	0.004	0.001	0.01	0.03	0.7	0.16	0.7	0.16	-	-

3.2. Wear-Corrosion Tests under Electrochemical Control

Wear-corrosion experiments were carried out on a pin-on-disk tribometer, and 6-mm diameter alumina ball pins were used as HCCoCr disk counterpart. The HCCoCr disks were 38 mm in diameter and 4 mm thick. Both disks and pins were previously washed with double distilled water and cleaned in an ultrasonic ethanol bath for 10 min. The alumina pins were placed in a pin plastic holder and fixed on the load cell. A low normal load of 5 N was applied on the counterpart. The working electrode motion was provided by a rotating motor at a rotation rate of 120 rpm that produced, at the end of the alumina ball, a circular wear track (5 mm in diameter) on the HCCoCr disk surface.

The tribometer configuration consisted of an integrated electrochemical cell (3-electrode cell) including the HCCoCr disk as working electrode, a ring-shaped Pt wire counter electrode and a saturated Ag/AgCl reference electrode. All the potentials of the HCCoCr disks during the wear corrosion tests were measured versus the reference electrode. Wear-corrosion tests were performed in Phosphate Buffer Solution (PBS) containing the following composition: 0.2 g/L KCl, 0.2 g/L KH_2PO_4, 8 g/L NaCl, and 1.150 g/L Na_2HPO_4 (anhydrous) and this PBS solution was supplemented with 3 g/L hyaluronic acid, the approximate concentration reported for the synovial fluid of healthy joints [17].

The wear-corrosion behavior was studied simultaneously measuring the friction coefficient and electrochemical parameters. The wear-corrosion tests were performed as follows (Figure 8): (a) before wear (no sliding) by the measurement of the corrosion potential for 10 min and (b) under sliding (at 120 rpm and 5 N load) in two different ways: one where a simultaneous measurement of the corrosion potential and the coefficient of friction (COF) were performed for 40 min without applying polarization and the other, applying anodic potentiodynamic polarization and simultaneous measurement of current and coefficient of friction (COF) for 200 min. The anodic potentiodynamic polarization was applied from the corrosion potential to a polarization of 1 V at a scanning rate of 10 mV/min, and back curve was drawn until reaching the corrosion potential. The back curve was also measured to analyze the repassivation ability of the HCCoCr alloy. For comparative purposes, the anodic potentiodynamic polarization without wear in PBS and PBS-HA was also measured. All experiments were carried out in triplicate.

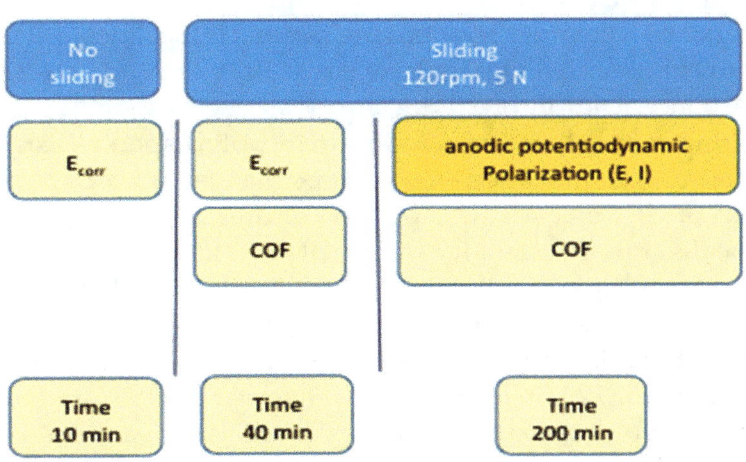

Figure 8. Schema of the experimental procedure of the wear-corrosion tests.

Surface characterization of the worn surface after wear-corrosion tests with polarization and without polarization was performed by profilometry and using a JEOL-6500F microscope equipped with a field Emission Gun (FEG) coupled to an Energy Dispersive X-ray (EDS) spectrometer. Secondary electron (SE) images were taken at 7.5 keV and EDS analysis was performed at 20 keV.

3.3. Isolation and Characterization of Particles

Debris from tribocorrosion tests performed in PBS, PBS containing 3 g/L hyaluronic acid (both without applying polarization), and in PBS supplemented with hyaluronic acid under anodic polarization was collected for the subsequent characterization. Metallic particles were isolated, purified, and characterized following the protocol developed by Billi et al. for metal particles [31]. This procedure allows exhaustive removal of organic and inorganic impurities from the metallic particles. To completely digest the hyaluronic acid, metal particles in PBS supplemented with 3 g/L HA were digested adapting the protocol developed by Kavanaugh et al. [32].

Wear-corrosion media (PBS and the digested hyaluronic acid solutions) containing metallic particles were rotated at 28 rpm in an orbital agitator for 24 h at room temperature to disperse the metal particles evenly before their isolation. The particles were then purified via density gradient centrifugation varying from 4446× *g* to 284,000× *g* (Beckman Optima L80 XP; Beckman Instruments, Fullerton, CA,USA) through multiple layers of denaturants and metal-selective high-density layers as was described [31,32]. This led to well-dispersed particles deposited onto a 5 mm × 5 mm featureless display silicon wafer (Ted Pella, Inc., Redding, CA, USA) coated with a monolayer of marine mussel glue (Cell-TakTM; BD Biosciences, San Jose, CA, USA). The silicon wafer was then coated with 10 Å iridium [31,32].

The morphology of metallic particles was studied with a field emission scanning electron microscope (FE-SEM) (Supra VP-40; Zeiss, Peabody, MA, USA) at a voltage of 15 kV and chemically analyzed by means of Energy-dispersive spectroscopy (EDS) analysis (Thermo Ultradry feature sizing system; Thermo Electron Scientific Instruments, Madison, WI, USA).

3.4. Macrophages Cell Cultures Assays

The biocompatibility of wear particles was tested in a mouse macrophage cell line (J774A.1) from DSMZ Human and Animal Cell Bank. Macrophages cell cultures were exposed to different concentrations of wear particles.

Wear particles obtained from the wear-corrosion tests were centrifuged and the particle pellet was weighted, UV sterilized for 15 min, and resuspended in sterile bidistillated water and maintained in aliquots at −20 °C until use. Wear particles, just before cell cultures assays, were thawed, resuspended by vigorously mixing with a vortex, and diluted at a concentration of 20 mg/mL in Dulbecco's Modified Eagle Medium (DMEM 41966; Gibco, BRL, Invitrogen, Thermofisher scientific, Paisley, UK) supplemented with 10% heat-inactivated fetal bovine serum (FBS; Gibco, BRL) and with a mixture of antibiotics (penicillin at 100 units/mL and streptomycin at 100 g/mL, Gibco, BRL), named as complete cell culture medium. A concentration of 20 mg/mL was used as stock solutions for the particles concentration tested in different cell assays. To assure a polydisperse distribution of the particles vigorous vortexing was applied in all experimental steps that required particles manipulation.

To evaluate the effect of HCCoCr particles on cell cultures, macrophages were seeded on 96-well culture plates at 75,000 cells/mL cell density in complete cell culture medium. A final volume of 100 µL of cell suspension in complete cell culture medium was added to each well of the 96-well plates. After 24 h in culture, cell media were removed and replaced by 100 µL of fresh complete cell culture medium containing the following concentrations of HCCoCr particles: 0, 0.5, 1 and 2 mg/mL. Cell cultures were maintained for 72 h in a cell culture chamber at 37 °C and 5% CO_2. Incubation time was selected based on the set-up of cell cultures assays for metallic particles studies carried out in the lab and is the most commonly used time point for cell viability studies [33]. Mitochondrial activity

(WST-1 assay) and plasma membrane damage (LDH assay) were used to evaluate the biocompatibility and cytotoxicity, respectively, as described below [29].

3.5. Mitochondrial Activity Measurement

Reduction of the WST-1 reagent (4-[3-4-iodophenyl)-2-(4-nitro-phenyl)-2H-5-tetrazolio]-1,3-benzene disulfonate (Roche Diagnostics GmbH, Mannheim, Germany)) was used to evaluate the effect of different concentrations of the HCCoCr wear particles on mitochondrial activity of macrophages cultures. The mitochondrial activity measurement is directly proportional to the number of metabolically active cells in culture. After 72 h in culture, 10 µL of the cell proliferation kit reagent WST-1 was added to each well containing 100 µL of fresh complete cell culture medium, and the mixture was incubated inside the cell culture incubator for 30 min. After incubation, 100 µL of each reaction mixture were transferred to a 96-well cell plate, and the absorbance of the samples was measured as differential absorbance, 415 nm minus 655 nm, in an iMark microplate absorbance reader (Bio-Rad, Hercules, CA, USA), using the absorbance given by complete cell culture medium as a blank. All experiments were carried out as independent triplicate.

3.6. Measurement of Lactate Dehydrogenase Activity

To measure and quantify the effect of HCCoCr wear particles on cell death and cell lysis, lactate dehydrogenase (LDH) activity was measured in the supernatants of cell cultures by an enzymatic assay using the Cytotoxicity Detection Kit^{plus} (Roche Diagnostics GmbH, Mannheim, Germany). Supernatants were collected from cell culture after being exposed for 72 h to different HCCoCr particles concentrations and were centrifuged for 5 min at 1024× *g*. The enzymatic assays were performed according to the LDH kit protocol provided by Roche Diagnostics (Mannheim, Germany). Complete cell culture medium was used as a control for absorbance baseline. LDH activity was measured based on differential absorbance, 490 nm minus 655 nm, in an iMark microplate absorbance reader (Bio-Rad, Hercules, CA, USA). LDH catalyzes the conversion of lactate to pyruvate, reducing NAD^+ to $NADH/H^+$, which is used by the catalyst to reduce a tetrazolium salt to a formazan salt, which is responsible for the change in absorbance at 490 nm. Quantification of LDH activity is used as an indicator of plasma membrane damage, as is a stable cytoplasmic enzyme present in all cells and rapidly release into the cell culture supernatant when the plasma membrane is damaged being a sign of cell death. The percentage of cytotoxicity is calculated taking as control a total cell lysate in the absence of any particles. The percentage cytotoxicity is calculated as described in the LDH kit protocol provided by Roche Diagnostics: Cytotoxicity (%) = [(exp. value − low control)/(high control − low control)] × 100; where experimental value (exp. value) corresponds to the absorbance of the treated sample in the study exposed to wear HCCoCr particles, low control is the absorbance from the untreated cell cultures with no particles that corresponds to spontaneous LDH released, and high control is the absorbance value obtained after total cell cultures lysis that corresponds to the maximum releasable LDH activity. The background absorbance corresponding to complete cell culture media was subtracted from the absorbance of all samples before cytotoxicity calculations. All experiments were carried out as independent triplicate.

3.7. Statistical Analysis of Data

3.7.1. Wear Particles Analysis Data

The experimental design used to determine the effect of two factors as the corrosive medium and the application of polarization on the dependent variable, that is, the chemical composition of the particles, was a 2^2 factorial design. In order to explain significant interaction, simple effects of one factor on the dependent variable at each single level of the other factor were computed. After this, simple effect pairwise comparisons were performed to detect levels of the second factor in which simple effects of the first factor on the dependent variable were significantly different.

Kruskal–Wallis [34] and Mann–Whitney [35] nonparametric tests were used to confirm the ANOVA results. A p-value < 0.05 was considered as significant. All the statistical analyses were performed with the Minitab® 17.1.0 software (Minitab Inc., State College, PA, USA) [36].

3.7.2. Biocompatibility Analysis Data

Mean differences on cytotoxicity effects between wear particles obtained in PBS (0.5 mg/mL) versus particles in PBS containing 3 g/L of hyaluronic acid (0.5 mg/mL) and between wear particles obtained in PBS containing 3 g/L HA (PBS-HA; 2 mg/mL) without versus with polarization application (PBS-HA+POL; 2 mg/mL) were studied with Student's t tests ($\alpha = 0.05$), respectively.

The effects of the particles, the concentration, and their interaction on the changes in mitochondrial respiratory activity of macrophages were analyzed with a two-way analysis of variance. A p value of ≤ 0.05 was considered significant. Mean pairwise comparisons were computed with a Tukey's test ($\alpha = 0.05$). Means with the same letter are not significantly different and means with different letters are significantly different.

All analyses were performed with the R software version 3.4.2 (R Core Team, Vienna, Austria, 2017) [37].

4. Conclusions

1. The wear particles collected after wear corrosion in PBS and PBS-HA were mainly composed of chromium oxide coming from the detachment of the passive film and phosphate adsorbed on the particle surface and/or adsorbed on the broken passive film.

2. Composition of the corrosive medium and polarization, applied to mimic the electrical interactions observed in living tissues, has an influence on the chemical composition of the particles. The wear particles detached after wear corrosion with polarization in PBS-HA have a chemical composition with a higher significant content of Cr and Co than those particles collected without polarization.

3. Biocompatibility in vitro assays here reported, measured by LDH release and mitochondrial respiratory activity, seem to indicate that particles from wear corrosion in PBS supplemented with 3 g/L of hyaluronic acid, an approximate concentration that is found in the synovial fluid of healthy joints, under anodic polarization produce in macrophages lower damage to the plasma membrane and are more biocompatible, most likely associated with particles chemical composition.

4. As more variables of the prosthesis environment are considered in in vitro assays to study cell-biomaterial interactions, as are the electric interactions, in order to have a closer view of the different processes that are taking place in vivo at the cell-biomaterial interface, a better knowledge of the biological consequences will be obtained.

5. Understanding these consequences of the electrical signals on the growth and development of cells and tissues should be applicable for the design of appropriate solutions and adequate treatments for orthopedic-bearing patients.

Author Contributions: Conceptualization, B.T.P.-M., M.L.E., M.C.G.-A., R.M.L.; Methodology, B.T.P.-M., M.E.L.F., I.D., A.K., F.B., M.L.E., M.C.G.-A., R.M.L.; Software, B.T.P.-M., M.L.E., M.C.G.-A., R.M.L., G.P., J.G.; Validation, B.T.P.-M., I.D., A.K., F.B., M.L.E., M.C.G.-A., R.M.L; Formal Analysis, B.T.P.-M., M.E.L.F., I.D., M.L.E., M.C.G.-A., R.M.L.; Investigation, B.T.P.-M., M.E.L.F., I.D., A.K., F.B., M.L.E., M.C.G.-A., R.M.L.; Resources, B.T.P.-M., M.L.E., M.C.G.-A., R.M.L.; Data Curation, B.T.P.-M., M.L.E., M.C.G.-A., R.M.L.; Writing-Original Draft Preparation, B.T.P.-M., M.L.E., M.C.G.-A., R.M.L.; Writing-Review & Editing, B.T.P.-M., M.L.E., M.C.G.-A., R.M.L.; Visualization, B.T.P.-M., M.L.E., M.C.G.-A., R.M.L.; Supervision, B.T.P.-M., M.L.E., M.C.G.-A., R.M.L.; Project Administration, B.T.P.-M., M.L.E., M.C.G.-A., R.M.L.; Funding Acquisition, B.T.P.-M., M.L.E., M.C.G.-A., R.M.L.

Acknowledgments: Authors wish to thank Guillermo Padilla PhD G.P. (Bioinformatics and Biostatics facility at Centro de Investigaciones Biológicas, CIB-CSIC) and J. Garrido J.G. (U. Autonoma Madrid, Dept. Psicol. Social & Metodol., Fac. Psicol.) for technical assistance in the statistical analysis of macrophages data and wear particles.

References

1. Fujiwara, N.; Kobayashi, K. *Macrophages in Inflammation in Current Drug Targets—Inflammation & Allergy*; Zaenker, K.S., Ed.; Bentham Science Publisher: Berlin, Germany, 2005; pp. 281–286. [CrossRef]
2. Poggio, C.E. Plasmacytoma of the mandible associated with a dental implant failure: A clinical report. *Clin. Oral Implant. Res.* **2007**, *18*, 540–543. [CrossRef] [PubMed]
3. McGuff, H.S.; Heim-Hall, J.; Holsinger, F.C.; Jones, A.A.; O'Dell, D.S.; Hafemeister, A.C. Maxillary osteosarcoma associated with a dental implant: Report of a case and review of the literature regarding implant-related sarcomas. *J. Am. Dent. Assoc.* **2008**, *139*, 1052–1059. [CrossRef] [PubMed]
4. Ferrier, J.; Ross, S.M.; Kanehisa, J.; Aubin, J.E. Osteoclasts and osteoblasts migrate in opposite directions in response to a constant electrical-field. *J. Cell. Physiol.* **1986**, *129*, 283–288. [CrossRef] [PubMed]
5. Levin, M.; Thorlin, T.; Robinson, K.R.; Nogi, T.; Mercola, M. Asymmetries in H+/K+-ATPase and cell membrane potentials comprise a very early step in left-right patterning. *Cell* **2002**, *111*, 77–89. [CrossRef]
6. Becker, R.O.; Spadaro, J.A.; Marino, A.A. Clinical experiences with low intensity direct-current stimulation of bone-growth. *Clin. Orthop. Relat. Res.* **1977**, *124*, 75–83. [CrossRef]
7. Levin, M. Large-scale biophysics: Ion flows and regeneration. *Trends Cell Biol.* **2007**, *17*, 261–270. [CrossRef] [PubMed]
8. Lokietek, W.; Pawluk, R.J.; Bassett, C.A. Muscle injury potentials source of voltage in undeformed rabbit tibia. *J. Bone Jt. Surg. Br.* **1974**, *56*, 361–369. [CrossRef]
9. McCaig, C.D.; Rajnicek, A.M.; Song, B.; Zhao, M. Controlling cell behavior electrically: Current views and future potential. *Physiol. Rev.* **2005**, *85*, 943–978. [CrossRef] [PubMed]
10. Gittens, R.A.; Olivares-Navarrete, R.; Tannenbaum, R.; Boyan, B.D.; Schwartz, Z. Electrical implications of corrosion for osseointegration of titanium implants. *J. Dent. Res.* **2011**, *90*, 1389–1397. [CrossRef] [PubMed]
11. Faes, T.J.; van der Meij, H.A.; de Munck, J.C.; Heethaar, R.M. The electric resistivity of human tissues (100 Hz–10 MHz): A meta-analysis of review studies. *Physiol. Meas.* **1999**, *20*, R1–R10. [CrossRef] [PubMed]
12. Borgens, R.B.; Jaffe, L.F.; Cohen, M.J. Large and persistent electrical currents enter the transected lamprey spinal-cord. *Proc. Natl. Acad. Sci. USA* **1980**, *77*, 1209–1213. [CrossRef] [PubMed]
13. Fukada, E.; Yasuda, I. On the piezoelectric effect of bone. *J. Phys. Soc. Jpn.* **1957**, *12*, 1158–1162. [CrossRef]
14. Guzelsu, N.; Demiray, H. Electro-mechanical properties and related models of bone tissues—Review. *Int. J. Eng. Sci.* **1979**, *17*, 813–851. [CrossRef]
15. Rubinacci, A.; Black, J.; Brighton, C.T.; Friedenberg, Z.B. Changes in bioelectric potentials on bone associated with direct-current stimulation of osteogenesis. *J. Orthop. Res.* **1988**, *6*, 335–345. [CrossRef] [PubMed]
16. Díaz, I.; Martínez-Lerma, J.F.; Montoya, R.; Llorente, I.; Escudero, M.L.; García-Alonso, M.C. Study of overall and local electrochemical responses of oxide films grown on CoCr alloy under biological environments. *Bioelectrochemistry* **2017**, *115*, 1–10. [CrossRef] [PubMed]
17. Hui, A.Y.; McCarty, W.J.; Masuda, K.; Firestein, G.S.; Sah, R.L. A systems biology approach to synovial joint lubrication in health, injury, and disease. *Wiley Interdiscip. Rev. Syst. Biol. Med.* **2012**, *4*, 15–37. [CrossRef] [PubMed]
18. Hodgson, A.W.E.; Kurz, S.; Virtanen, S.; Fervel, V.; Olsson, C.-O.A.; Mischler, S. Passive and transpassive behavior of CoCrMo in simulated biological solutions. *Electrochim. Acta* **2004**, *49*, 2167–2178. [CrossRef]
19. Bitar, D.; Parvizi, J. Biological response to prosthetic debris. *World J. Orthop.* **2015**, *6*, 172–189. [CrossRef] [PubMed]
20. Jacobs, J.J.; Roebuck, K.A.; Archibeck, M.; Hallab, N.J.; Glant, T.T. Osteolysis: Basic science. *Clin. Orthop. Relat. Res.* **2001**, *393*, 71–77. [CrossRef]
21. Dorr, L.D.; Bloebaum, R.; Emmanual, J.; Meldrum, R. Histologic, biochemical, and ion analysis of tissue and fluids retrieved during total hip-arthroplasty. *Clin. Orthop. Relat. Res.* **1990**, *261*, 82–95. [CrossRef]
22. Jacobs, J.J.; Urban, R.M.; Hallab, N.J.; Skipor, A.K.; Fischer, A.; Wimmer, M.A. Metal-on-metal bearing surfaces. *J. Am. Acad. Orthop. Surg.* **2009**, *17*, 69–76. [CrossRef] [PubMed]
23. Ponthiaux, P.; Wenger, F.; Drees, D.; Celis, J.P. Electrochemical techniques for studying tribocorrosion processes. *Wear* **2004**, *256*, 459–468. [CrossRef]

24. Yan, Y.; Yang, H.; Su, Y.; Qiao, L. Study of the tribocorrosion behaviors of albumin on a cobalt-based alloy using scanning Kelvin probe force microscopy and atomic force microscopy. *Electrochem. Commun.* **2016**, *64*, 61–64. [CrossRef]
25. Uesaka, S.; Miyazaki, K.; Ito, H. Age-related changes and sex differences in chondroitin sulfate isomers and hyaluronic acid in normal synovial fluid. *Mod. Rheumatol.* **2004**, *14*, 470–475. [CrossRef] [PubMed]
26. Igual-Muñoz, A.; Mischler, S. Effect of the environment on wear ranking and corrosion of biomedical CoCrMo alloys. *J. Mater. Sci. Mater. Med.* **2011**, *22*, 437–450. [CrossRef] [PubMed]
27. Lewis, A.C.; Kilburn, M.R.; Heard, P.J.; Scott, T.B.; Hallam, K.R.; Allen, G.C.; Learmonth, I.D. The Entrapment of Corrosion Products from CoCr Implant Alloys in the Deposits of Calcium Phosphate: A Comparison of Serum, Synovial Fluid, Albumin, EDTA, and Water. *J. Orthop. Res.* **2006**, *24*, 1587–1596. [CrossRef] [PubMed]
28. Man, K.; Jiang, L.-H.; Foster, R.; Yang, X.B. Immunological response to total hip arthroplasty. *J. Funct. Biomater.* **2017**, *8*, 33. [CrossRef] [PubMed]
29. Lozano, R.M.; Pérez-Maceda, B.T.; Carboneras, M.; Onofre-Bustamante, E.; García-Alonso, M.C.; Escudero, M.L. Response of MC3T3-E1 osteoblasts, L929 fibroblasts and J774 macrophages to fluoride surface-modified AZ31 magnesium alloy. *J. Biomed. Mater. Res. Part A* **2013**, *101*, 2753–2762. [CrossRef] [PubMed]
30. VanOs, R.; Lildhar, L.L.; Lehoux, E.A.; Beaulé, P.E.; Catelas, I. In vitro macrophage response to nanometer-size chromium oxide particles. *J. Biomed. Mater. Res. Part B* **2014**, *102B*, 149–159. [CrossRef] [PubMed]
31. Billi, F.; Benya, P.; Kavanaugh, A.; Adams, J.; McKellop, H.; Ebramzadeh, E. The John Charnley Award: An accurate and extremely sensitive method to separate, display, and characterize wear debris: Part 2: Metal and ceramic particles. *Clin. Orthop. Relat. Res.* **2012**, *470*, 339–350. [CrossRef] [PubMed]
32. Kavanaugh, A.E.; Benya, P.; Billi, F. A Method to Isolate and Characterize Wear Debris from Synovial Fluid and Tissues. In *Metal-On-Metal Total Hip Replacement Devices*; ASTM International: West Conshohocken, PA, USA, 2013. [CrossRef]
33. Wang, J.; Witte, F.; Xi, T.; Zheng, Y.; Yang, K.; Yang, Y.; Zhao, D.; Meng, J.; Li, Y.; Li, W.; et al. Recommendation for modifying current cytotoxicity testing standards for biodegradable magnesium-based materials. *Acta Biomater.* **2015**, *21*, 237–249. [CrossRef] [PubMed]
34. Kruskal, W.H.; Wallis, W.A. Use of Ranks in One-Criterion Variance Analysis. *J. Am. Stat. Assoc.* **1952**, *47*, 583–621. [CrossRef]
35. Mann, H.B.; Whitney, D.R. On a Test of Whether one of Two Random Variables is Stochastically Larger than the Other. *Ann. Math. Stat.* **1947**, *18*, 50–60. [CrossRef]
36. Minitab Inc. Minitab Statistical Software. (n.d.). Available online: www.minitab.com/en-us/ (accessed on 16 April 2018).
37. R Core Team. *R: A Language and Environment for Statistical Computing*; R Foundation for Statistical Computing: Vienna, Austria, 2017; Available online: https://www.R-project.org/ (accessed on 16 April 2018).

12

Finite Element Simulations of Hard-On-Soft Hip Joint Prosthesis Accounting for Dynamic Loads Calculated from a Musculoskeletal Model during Walking

Alessandro Ruggiero [1,*], Massimiliano Merola [2] and Saverio Affatato [2]

1 Department of Industrial Engineering, University of Salerno, Via Giovanni Paolo II, nr. 132, 84084 Fisciano, Italy

2 Medical Technology Laboratory, IRCCS—Rizzoli Orthopaedic Institute, Via di Barbiano, 1/10, 40136 Bologna, Italy; massimiliano.merola@ior.it (M.M.); affatato@tecno.ior.it (S.A.)

* Correspondence: ruggiero@unisa.it

Abstract: The hip joint replacement is one of the most successful orthopedic surgical procedures although it involves challenges to overcome. The patient group undergoing total hip arthroplasty now includes younger and more active patients who require a broad range of motion and a longer service lifetime for the replacement joint. It is well known that wear tests have a long duration and they are very expensive, thus studying the effects of geometry, loading, or alignment perturbations may be performed by Finite Element Analysis. The aim of the study was to evaluate total deformation and stress intensity on ultra-high molecular weight polyethylene liner coupled with hard material head during one step. Moving toward in-silico wear assessment of implants, in the presented simulations we used a musculoskeletal multibody model of a human body giving the loading and relative kinematic of the investigated tribo-system during the gait. The analysis compared two frictional conditions -dry and wet and two geometrical cases- with and without radial clearance. The loads and rotations followed the variability of the gait cycle as well as stress/strain acting in the UHWMPE cup. The obtained results allowed collection of the complete stress/strain description of the polyethylene cup during the gait and calculation of the maximum contact pressure on the lateral edge of the insert. The tensional state resulted in being more influenced by the geometrical conditions in terms of radial clearance than by the variation of the friction coefficients due to lubrication phenomena.

Keywords: total hip arthroplasty; musculoskeletal multibody model; dynamic loading; finite element analysis; radial clearance; dry and wet friction

---

1. Introduction

Total Hip Replacement (THR) is the most successful application of biomaterials in the short term in order to alleviate pain, restore joints, and increase functional mobility in diseased traumatized articulations [1–3]. A major limiting factor to the service life of THRs remains the wear of the polyethylene acetabular cup [4,5]. Preclinical endurance testing has become a standard procedure to predict the mechanical performance of new devices during their development. Wear tests are performed on different materials and designs used in prosthetic implants [1,6–8] to obtain quality assessment and acquire further knowledge about the tribological processes of joint prostheses. The objective of these investigations is to find out the wear rate and its dependence on the test conditions. In order to obtain realistic results, a wear test should reproduce the in vivo working conditions on the artificial implants [9].

It is well known that wear tests that are close to the in vivo conditions have a long duration and elevate costs [1,10,11]. The wear simulation is run for several million cycles, considering that one million cycles corresponds to one year in vivo [12–14]. The running-in period encompasses approximately the first half a million cycles; the steady-state wear is assessed by measuring the wear after the running-in period [15]. Wear is evaluated either gravimetrically, determining the weight loss of the components, or by measuring the volume of the material that has been removed, e.g., wear pit dimensions [9,16]. Lubricant absorption or creep of the loaded components, especially for polyethylene, is considered. Wear measurements are normally done at lubricant change stops, e.g., every 500,000 cycles.

Finite Element Analysis (FEA) has been widely used in many areas of biomechanics and medical engineering [17]. The numerical modelling tool of finite element analysis has been widely applied to study the behavior of articular cartilage, joints, and bone structures under compressive and tensile stresses. Structural applications include the design and development of joint prosthesis and fracture fixation devices. FEA enables to investigate parameters and boundary conditions, which are not accessible experimentally nor analytically. It has been applied to orthopedic devices to gain a deep understanding of the behavior of the bone-implant system and to support the design and pre-clinical testing of new devices. Thus, computational wear simulation can be a valuable complement to wear tests, e.g., in predictions of the lifetime of prostheses evaluating the effects of geometry, loading, or alignment perturbations.

As the first attempt to apply FEA to the orthopedic field dates back to 1972 [18], there have been four decades of developing and improving this methodology, along with the increase of computational power. Nevertheless, to make in silico wear simulation meaningful, better wear models are needed through advanced study design and corroboration with in vitro testing. The most intricate aspect of such models is the loading conditions acting on the implants, as their knowledge is still not fully reached. Few hip replacements have been subjected to direct load measures from Bergmann et al. [19–21], which limits the result validity to the subjects of the study. A more general load analysis can be obtained by muscular skeletal models, as it has been done by the authors [22], to study knee implants, or by van der Ploeg et al. [23], who used the multibody results as input for a FEA studying the micro-motions of a femoral stem.

In this work, a musculoskeletal multibody model was used in order to estimate the loads acting on the hip joint during walking. A finite elements analysis was then conducted using these loads and kinematic inputs. The study reports the results in terms of total deformation and stress intensity of an acetabular polyethylene liner coupled with a femoral head of a hard (ideally rigid) material.

2. Materials and Methods

2.1. Gait Cycles and Loads

In this study, the authors used a musculoskeletal modelling software to estimate loads acting on the hip joint during level walking. The simulation was performed with AnyBody Modelling System™ (AMS) [24]. To calculate the joint forces, knowledge of kinematic data and ground reaction forces that are used as input is required. These data are collected in gait analysis laboratories using special motion capture tools [25], which allows the measurement of a subject's gait through cameras that monitor markers on the subject's skin.

In inverse dynamics, the motion and the external loads on the body are known, and the aim is determining the internal forces. However, not enough equilibrium equations are available to find all the unknowns of the problem, therefore the calculation of the muscle forces is possible by the so-called redundancy problem. The solution of the muscle recruitment problem in the inverse dynamics approach is generally formulated as an optimization problem of the form:

$$\min G(f^{(M)}) \tag{1}$$

with

$$Cf = d \tag{2}$$

$$0 \leq f_i^{(M)} \leq N_i, i \in \{1, \ldots, n^{(M)}\}, \tag{3}$$

where G is the objective function (1), i.e., the assumed criterion of the recruitment strategy of the central nervous system, stated in terms of the muscle forces, and minimized with respect to all unknown forces in the problem, $f = \left(f^{(M)T} \; f^{(R)T} \right)^T$, (i.e., muscle forces and joint reactions). Equation (2) is the dynamic equilibrium equations, which enter as constraints into the optimization. C is the coefficient matrix for the unknown forces/moments in the system, d is a vector of the known applied loads and inertia forces. The non-negativity constraints on the muscle forces, Equation (3), states that muscle can only pull, not push and the upper bounds limit their capability, so N_1 is the strength of the muscle.

The most popular forms of the objective function G, calculated from the relative intensity and normalized for each muscle, are the polynomial criteria and the soft saturation criteria per Siemienski et al. [26]:

$$G(f^{(M)}) = \sum_{i=1}^{n^{(M)}} \left(\frac{f_i^{(M)}}{N_i} \right)^p \tag{4}$$

with $p = 2$, since it is established in the literature as predicting reasonable muscle activation patterns for the type of analyzed trial.

All segments of the biomechanical system are modelled as rigid bodies, neglecting effects such as the wobbly masses of soft tissues.

2.2. Finite Element Modelling

The finite elements model was realized through Ansys® Workbench commercial software (v.18.1, ANSYS Inc., Canonsburg, PA, USA). To minimize the computational complexity there were considered only the two major bearing components in a hip implant, namely the femoral head and the acetabular cup. The presence of the pelvic bone has been neglected, since its influence has a least effect on contact pressure [27]. The bodies of the FE model are shown in Figure 1, the mesh was realized through quadratic tetrahedral elements. Mesh convergence tests were performed, resulting in a total number of elements and nodes of 2012 and 3283, respectively, having 383 contact elements.

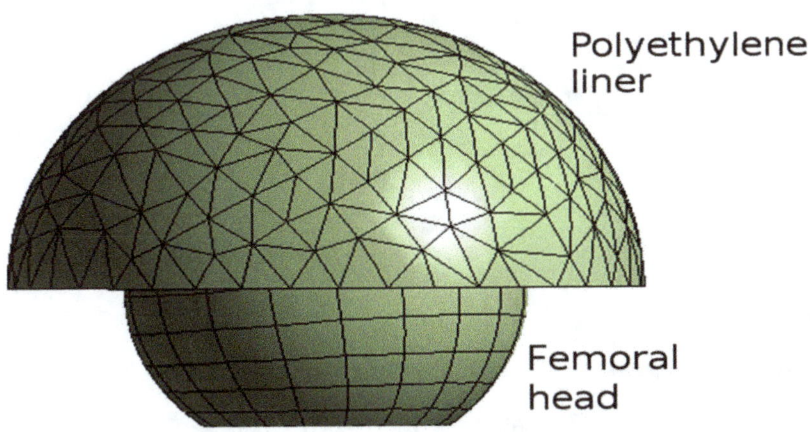

Figure 1. Mesh model of the femoral head and the polyethylene liner.

To solve the contact problem the Augmented Lagrange algorithm was used, considering an asymmetric behavior, which is recommended for the solution of frictional contacts. The femoral head was modelled as a rigid body, whereas for the polyethylene insert of the cup it was selected the Ultra-High-Molecular-Weight-Polyethylene (UHMWPE) GUR 1050 material, as it is one of the main polymer materials used for implant applications [28,29]; Table 1 summarizes its main parameters.

Table 1. UHMWPE GUR 1050 attributes.

Density ($kg{\cdot}m^{-3}$)	Young's Modulus (MPa)	Poisson's Ratio (-)	Bulk Modulus (MPa)	Shear Modulus (MPa)	Tensile Yield Strength (MPa)	Tensile Ultimate Strength (MPa)
930	690	0.43	1640	241	21	40

The material is assumed to be homogenous and isotropic. Even if roughness plays a key role on the tribological behavior of hip implants [30,31], the model surfaces are considered smooth, as in most of the models found in literature, for the ease of solution.

The study was conducted to understand the stress behaviour in dry conditions, as the presence of lubricant modifies the pressure distribution on the surfaces. However, as further knowledge, the influence of the friction coefficient was introudced, comparing a dry and a lubricated regime, namely, a DRY case, i.e., no lubrication, and a WET case, i.e., lubricated conditions. The mean values of the friction coefficient in lubricated conditions were extracted from experimental studies on the prosthesis tribological pairs [32,33]. Thus, a dry friction value of 0.13 and a mean wet friction value of 0.05 was selected.

The femoral head had a diameter of 28 mm, whereas the acetabular cup had a thickness of 5 mm. Moreover, two geometrical configurations of the coupled bodies were studied, and the simulations were executed considering the presence of the radial clearance (CC condition) and not considering it (NC condition). Radial clearance is the difference between the radius of the acetabular cup and the one of the femoral head (see Figure 2). Radial clearance, when considered, was 0.5 mm [34]; the results of the two configurations were then compared.

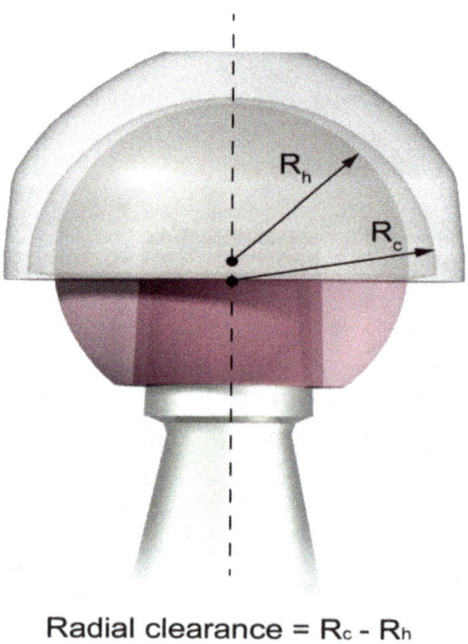

Figure 2. Radial clearance is the difference in radius of the acetabular cup and the femoral head. In this image the clearance is amplified for a better understanding.

The input data obtained by the multibody system were evaluated in a local coordinates system, which follows the movements of the femoral head. As the FE model requires a global coordinates system, a conversion was performed considering well-known geometric transformations [35]. Further force components and mesh orientations are defined with respect to a pelvic reference frame that coincides with the true anatomic superior, anterior, and lateral directions (see Figure 3). The tensional state and the total deformation were evaluated on the inner surface of the polyethylene liner.

3. Results

The forces and the rotations taking place along the three degrees of freedom were gained from the multibody analysis. The force components are the ones depicted in Figure 3. The three rotations around the axes are the *Flexion/Extension* (around z axes), *Abduction/Adduction* (around x axes) and *Inward/Outward* (around y axes).

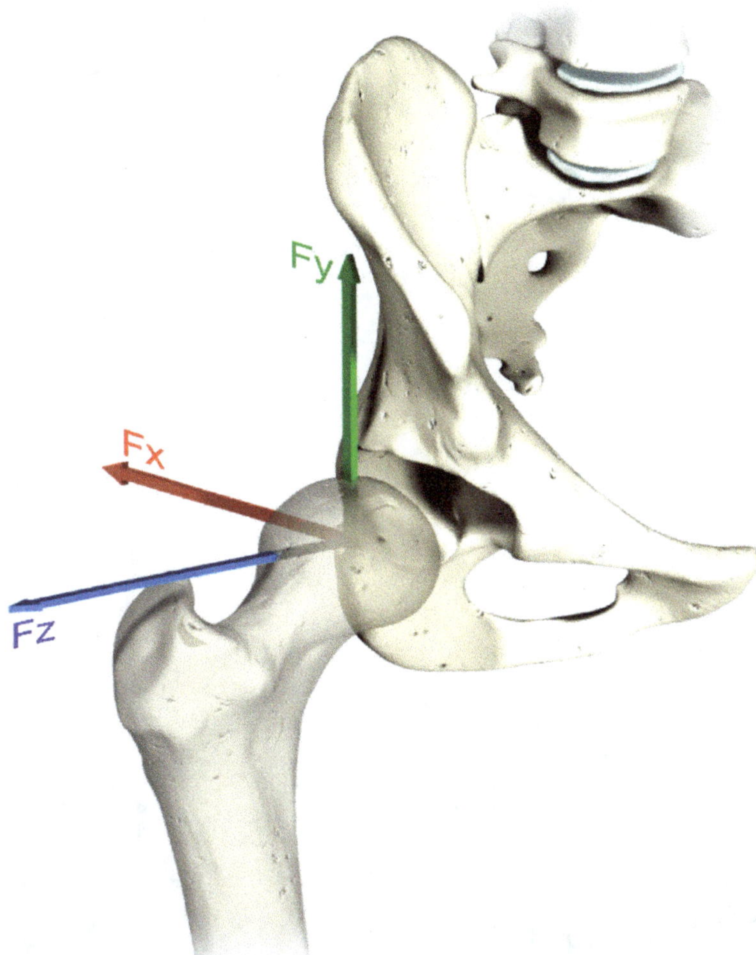

Figure 3. The three force vectors represented on a femoral head.

In Figure 4 the force components and the rotations derived from the model are shown. It is noticeable that the highest rotation is the *Flexion/Extension*, whereas the highest load is along the y axes. Forces and rotations so obtained were used as dynamic inputs for the finite element model.

In Figure 5 the pressure distribution on the internal surface of the cup in different instants of the cycle is shown, with regards to the dry NC condition as exemplificative case. Along with the different orientation of the femoral head it is possible to observe the pressure distribution on the polyethylene liner. Its highest values are found at 8% and 48% of the cycle (respectively Figure 5a,c). In the latter case the highest level of the *Anterior/Posterior* force was also found (see Figure 4), and the pressure is more concentrated in the edge zone of the insert. In the other two images, Figure 5b,d, at 26% and 93% of the cycle, the pressure reaches lower values and its mostly located in the central part of the inner hemisphere. The other geometrical and frictional cases are here omitted for brevity, but they presented a similar distribution of pressure, only leading different intensity of the tensional state.

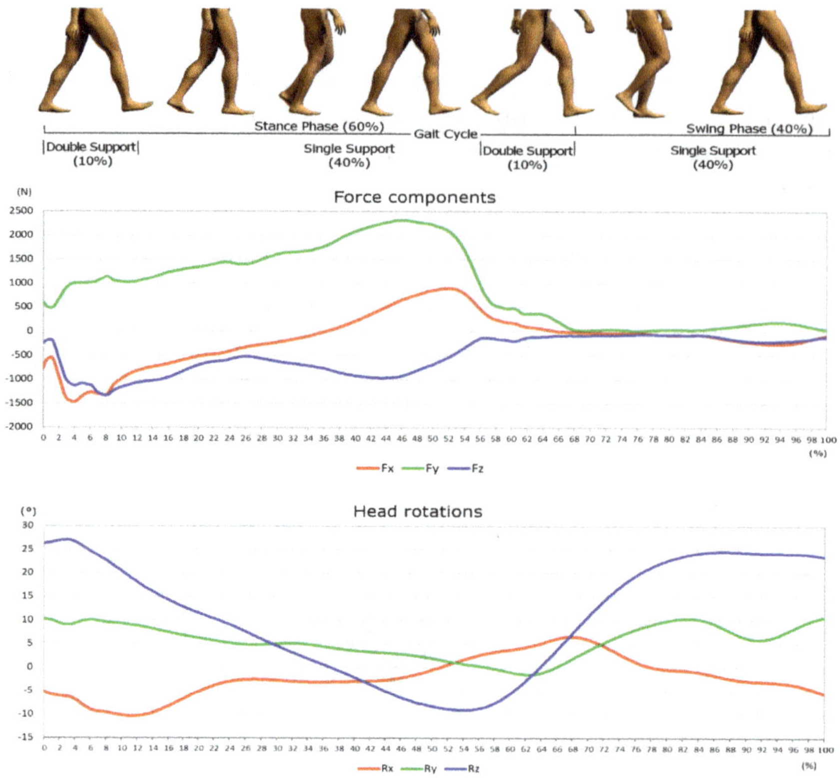

Figure 4. Forces components, in red Fx, in green Fy, in blue Fz. Head rotations, around *x* axes in red, *y* axes green and *z* axes blue.

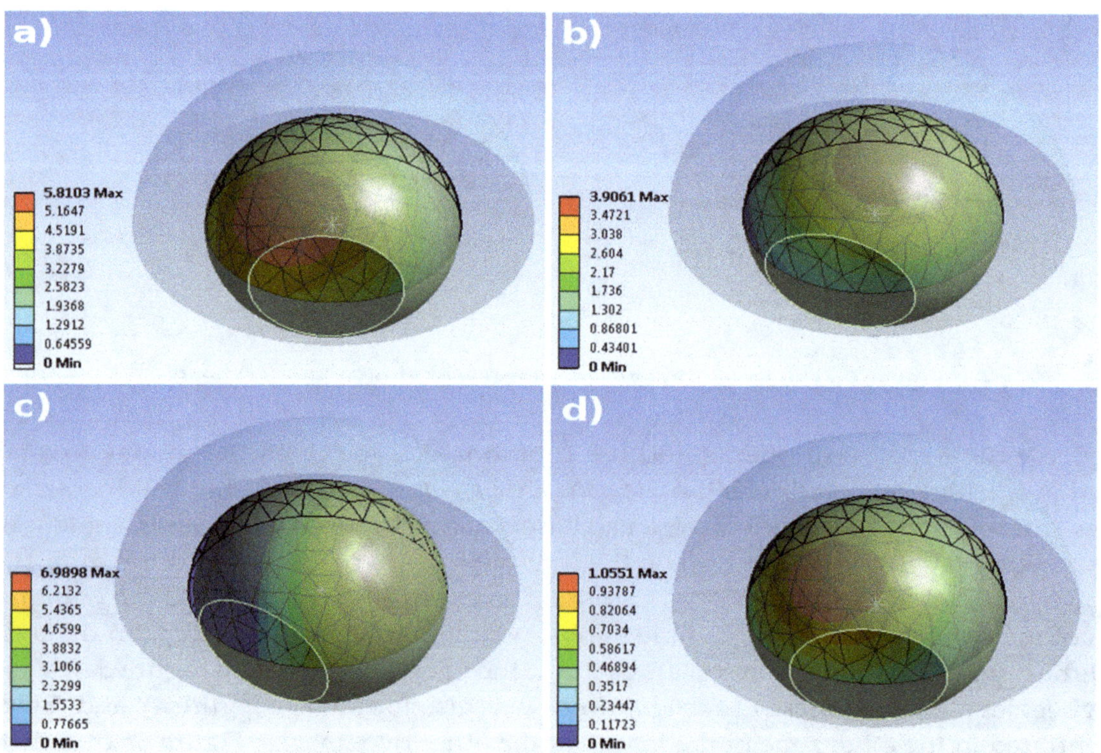

Figure 5. Pressure distribution on the internal surface of the acetabula cup. (**a**) NC case, dry condition; (**b**) NC case, wet condition; (**c**) CC case, dry condition; (**d**) CC case, wet condition.

Figures 6 and 7 present a summary of the maximum values of pressure and total deformation, comparing the two friction conditions and the two geometric configurations. In Figure 6a the maximum value of pressure is shown, for each part of the cycle. The maximum value throughout the walking cycle is equal to 7 MPa and it is found around 48% of the way through the cycle—agreeing with the dynamic analysis. A slight difference was found between the two friction cases, showing a higher peak value in the wet condition. In Figure 6c the maximum value of the total deformation is displayed; its highest value is again related to the wet case, reaching almost 0.6 mm. In Figure 6b,d the comparisons are shown, in terms of pressure and deformation, between the two friction cases considering the presence of the radial clearance (CC). In Figure 6b, the comparison highlights the almost complete lack of difference in the two friction conditions; the highest value reached is almost 10 MPa. However, in Figure 6d the curves have some differences, showing slightly higher values of total deformation in wet condition (maximum value of 1 mm and 0.9 mm for the wet and the dry case, respectively).

In Figure 7 the comparison of the two geometrical conditions is presented, with and without radial clearance (CC and NC, respectively). In Figure 7a, considering the boundary lubrication, the maximum pressure plot shows the large divergence in the two geometrical solutions. The highest values are almost 10 MPa and 6.7 MPa, for the CC and NC respectively. As well as the curves in Figure 7c, where the total deformation is shown, the highest values are found for the CC condition where it reaches almost 1 mm, whereas NC gives back at the most 0.6 mm. The curves in Figure 7b also brings out the divergences in the two geometrical configurations under dry friction, the pressure in CC being higher than the one found in NC; the values are almost the same as those already described in the wet condition. Figure 7d reports the maximum values of the total deformation, clearly showing the difference in the CC and NC conditions.

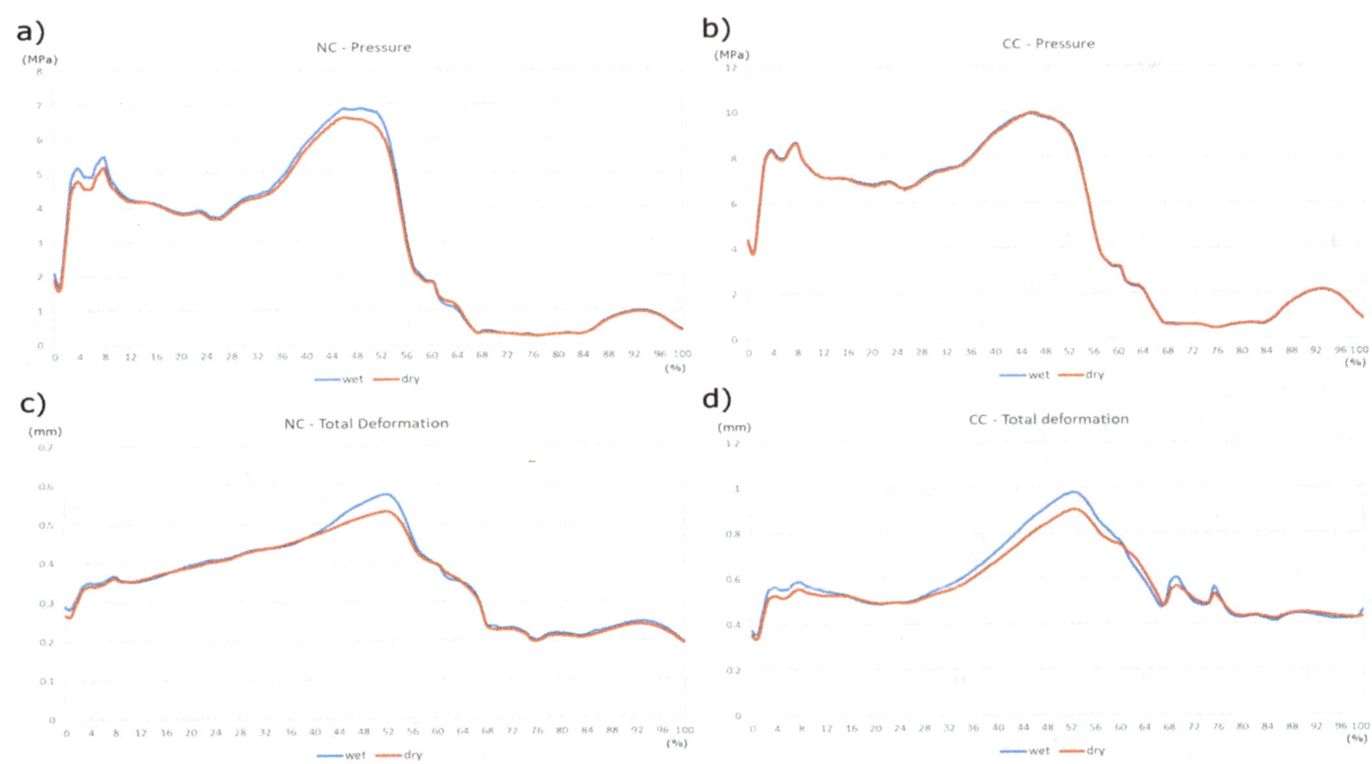

Figure 6. Comparison of result in the NC (**a**,**c**) and CC (**b**,**d**) cases, between the dry and wet conditions.

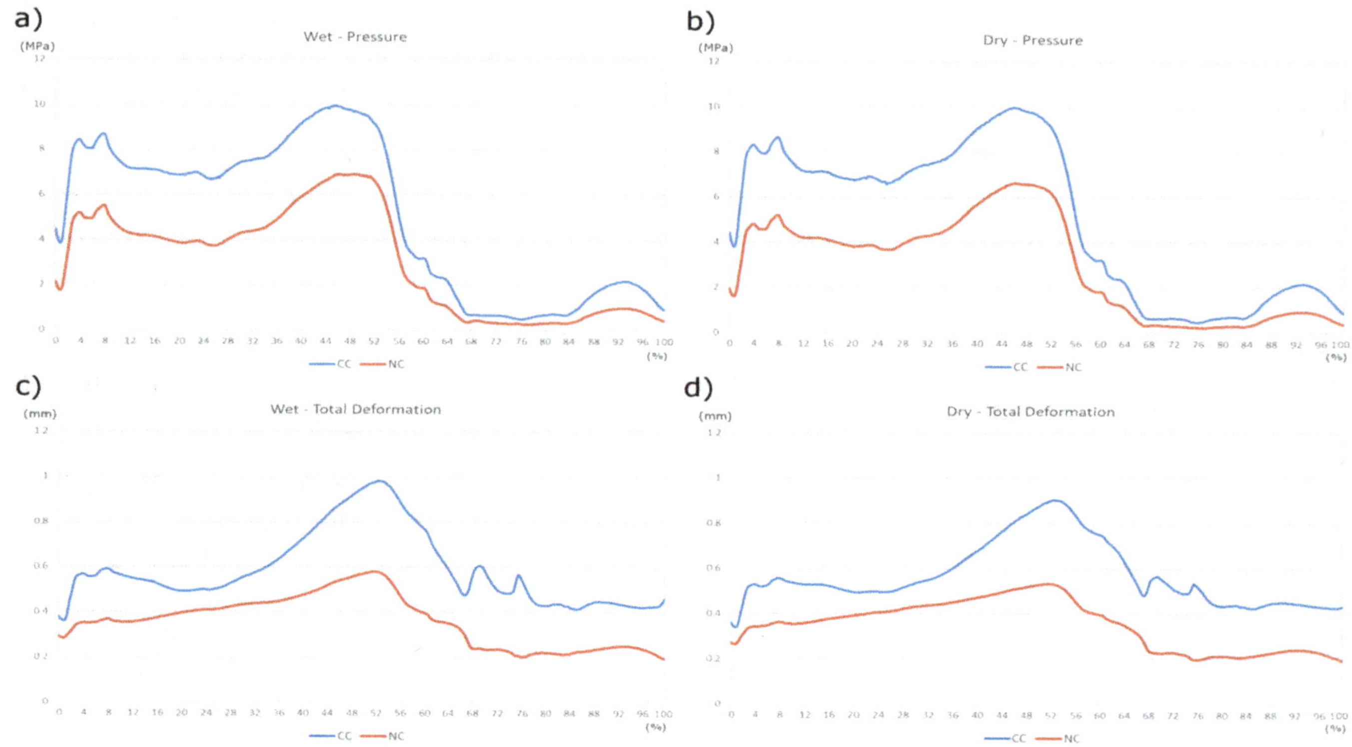

Figure 7. Comparison of result in the wet (**a**,**b**) and dry (**c**,**d**) condition, between the CC and NC cases.

4. Discussion

In this work, the forces and rotations acting on the hip joint during a complete gait cycle were first evaluated by solving the inverse dynamic problem. These data agree with the walking cycle variability [25], showing how the joint results more loaded during the stance phase than in the swing phase, when there is almost no contact between the foot and the ground. Furthermore, the highest loads is the axial (along the y axes) as expected and confirmed by a comparison with the standard ISO 14242-1:2012 [36]. Afterwards, these loads and rotation were used as dynamical input in the finite element model, obtaining the pressure distribution and the elastic deformation on each node of the surface during the whole gait cycle. The stress state of the internal surface of the UHMWPE liner reaches peaks of the order of 10 MPa, being in accordance with literature results [37–39]. Several authors [36,40,41] used simplified hip kinematic and gait load, such as one-dimensional vertical load or considered only the flexion/extension rotation [40], which does not represent actual physiological loading, plus these studies rely on ISO standards at the expense of a flexible design. In this regard, the original contribution of the study is the acquisition of stress and deformation distribution based on a multibody model. This offers the possibility to apply a wide variety of gaits and to consider the peculiarity of a specific class of patients, e.g., older or younger people. This could lead to the design of prosthesis which account the requirement of a patient, by simply characterize his activity through the multibody and finite elements model.

The comparison of the different working conditions allowed the conclusion that the presence of radial clearance strongly influences the tensional state of the coupled surfaces. Whereas, for a complete understanding of the lubrication influence on the tribology of hip implants the Reynolds equations must be involved [42], as varying the coefficient of friction does not allow the establishment of a sensible difference in results. In literature, the contact is usually assumed to be frictionless, justifying this hypothesis with negligible variation in contact pressure distribution. However, the presence of a frictional force has an influence to the location of the nominal contact point, as demonstrated by Mattei and Di Puccio in [35].

The reasons for the differences across the two geometrical conditions are ascribable to the different tensional state of the surfaces. In the geometry without radial clearance a conformal contact is realized, meaning that the contact is distributed along an area. On the other hand, when the radial clearance is considered, the contact become non-conformal, which implies that the contact is limited to a small area that increases its extension as the deformation rises. These differences in the area size led to the distinction of the pressure values, shown in the previous paragraph. As stated by Teoh et al. [37] the radial clearance plays a vital role in the wear process, finding that its extreme values (0.001 and 0.5 mm) led to the highest level of wear. In the study by Tudor et al. [43] the difference between the conditions of small loads with high clearances is highlighted, where the contact pressure tends to a Hertzian distribution, and high loads with small clearances, where the contact pressure tends to have a hyperbolic distribution. Furthermore, concerning the influence of the frictional force, in the study by Teoh et al. [37] they found that varying the friction coefficient between 0 and 0.3, only yielded a slightly variance of the wear rate.

5. Conclusions

This work is meant as a first step forward to the simplified hip kinematic and gait load. In this work we presented a dynamic load, derived by a multibody technique applied to a musculoskeletal model, considering the variability of the load direction during gait movement.

The main conclusions of the study are:

- multibody technique applied to a musculoskeletal model was proven to be a valid instrument to obtain a flexible design of implant, leading to the evaluation of load for a specific demanding task;
- load components and rotations match the variability between the stance and the swing phase of the leg during the gait;
- highest values of pressure on the inner surface of the polyethylene insert are found near its edge side;
- tensional state and elastic deformation are mainly influenced by the radial clearance rather than the friction coefficient.

The results of the present work offer the possibility to extend, in further studies, the range of kinematics and dynamics; an additional improvement could include lubrication to apply this set-up in a realistic scenario.

Acknowledgments: The authors would like to thank Simone Di Stasio (University of Salerno) for his help with the finite element model. This work was partially supported by the Italian Program of Donation for Research "5 per mille", year 2014, and by FARB 2016 obtained from University of Salerno.

Author Contributions: A.R. and S.A. conceived and designed the investigation; A.R. developed the dynamical analysis; M.M. performed the FEM model; M.M. and S.A. analyzed the data; A.R. and S.A. discussed the results; A.R., M.M. and S.A. wrote the paper.

Nomenclature

THR	Total Hip Replacement
AMS	AnyBody Modelling System
FEA	Finite Element Analysis
UHMWPE	Ultra-High-Molecular-Polyethylene
G	objective function
$f^{(M)}$	muscle forces
$f^{(R)}$	joint reaction
d	vector of applied loads and inertia forces
N_1	strength of the muscle

References

1. Affatato, S.; Freccero, N.; Taddei, P. The biomaterials challenge: A comparison of polyethylene wear using a hip joint simulator. *J. Mech. Behav. Biomed. Mater.* **2016**, *53*, 40–48. [CrossRef] [PubMed]
2. Learmonth, I.D.; Young, C.; Rorabeck, C. The operation of the century: Total hip replacement. *Lancet* **2007**, *370*, 1508–1519. [CrossRef]
3. Kurtz, S.; Ong, K.; Lau, E.; Mowat, F.; Halpern, M. Projections of Primary and Revision Hip and Knee Arthroplasty in the United States from 2005 to 2030. *J. Bone Jt. Surg.* **2007**, *89*, 780–785. [CrossRef]
4. Affatato, S.; Ruggiero, A.; Merola, M. Advanced biomaterials in hip joint arthroplasty. A review on polymer and ceramics composites as alternative bearings. *Compos. Part B Eng.* **2015**, *83*, 276–283. [CrossRef]
5. Rajaee, S.S.; Theriault, R.V.; Pevear, M.E.; Smith, E.L. National Trends in Primary Total Hip Arthroplasty in Extremely Young Patients: A Focus on Bearing Surface Usage From 2009 to 2012. *J. Arthroplast.* **2016**, *31*, 63–68. [CrossRef] [PubMed]
6. Affatato, S.; Bersaglia, G.; Emiliani, D.; Foltran, I.; Taddei, P.; Reggiani, M.; Ferrieri, P.; Toni, A. The performance of gamma- and EtO-sterilised UHMWPE acetabular cups tested under severe simulator conditions. Part 2: Wear particle characteristics with isolation protocols. *Biomaterials* **2003**, *24*, 4045–4055. [CrossRef]
7. Affatato, S.; Bersaglia, G.; Rocchi, M.; Taddei, P.; Fagnano, C.; Toni, A. Wear behaviour of cross-linked polyethylene assessed in vitro under severe conditions. *Biomaterials* **2005**, *26*, 3259–3267. [CrossRef] [PubMed]
8. Affatato, S.; Ruggiero, A.; Jaber, S.; Merola, M.; Bracco, P. Wear Behaviours and Oxidation Effects on Different UHMWPE Acetabular Cups Using a Hip Joint Simulator. *Materials* **2018**, *11*, 433. [CrossRef] [PubMed]
9. Grillini, L.; Affatato, S. How to measure wear following total hip arthroplasty. *Hip Int.* **2013**, *23*, 233–242. [CrossRef] [PubMed]
10. Affatato, S.; Zavalloni, M.; Spinelli, M.; Costa, L.; Bracco, P.; Viceconti, M. Long-term in-vitro wear performance of an innovative thermo-compressed cross-linked polyethylene. *Tribol. Int.* **2010**, *43*, 22–28. [CrossRef]
11. Affatato, S.; Testoni, M.; Cacciari, G.L.; Toni, A. Mixed oxides prosthetic ceramic ball heads. Part 2: Effect of the ZrO_2 fraction on the wear of ceramic on ceramic joints. *Biomaterials* **1999**, *20*, 971–975. [CrossRef]
12. Affatato, S.; Spinelli, M.; Zavalloni, M.; Mazzega-Fabbro, C.; Viceconti, M. Tribology and total hip joint replacement: Current concepts in mechanical simulation. *Med. Eng. Phys.* **2008**, *30*, 1305–1317. [CrossRef] [PubMed]
13. Dumbleton, J.H. *Tribology of Natural and Artificial Joints*; Elsevier: New York, NY, USA, 1981.
14. Petersen, D.; Link, R.; Wang, A.; Polineni, V.; Essner, A.; Sokol, M.; Sun, D.; Stark, C.; Dumbleton, J. The Significance of Nonlinear Motion in the Wear Screening of Orthopaedic Implant Materials. *J. Test. Eval.* **1997**, *25*, 239–245. [CrossRef]
15. Affatato, S.; Bersaglia, G.; Foltran, I.; Emiliani, D.; Traina, F.; Toni, A. The influence of implant position on the wear of alumina-on-alumina studied in a hip simulator. *Wear* **2004**, *256*, 400–405. [CrossRef]
16. Astarita, A.; Rubino, F.; Carlone, P.; Ruggiero, A.; Leone, C.; Genna, S.; Merola, M.; Squillace, A. On the Improvement of AA2024 Wear Properties through the Deposition of a Cold-Sprayed Titanium Coating. *Metals* **2016**, *6*, 185. [CrossRef]
17. Taylor, M.; Prendergast, P.J. Four decades of finite element analysis of orthopaedic devices: Where are we now and what are the opportunities? *J. Biomech.* **2015**, *48*, 767–778. [CrossRef] [PubMed]
18. Brekelmans, W.A.M.; Poort, H.W.; Slooff, T.J.J.H. A New Method to Analyse the Mechanical Behaviour of Skeletal Parts. *Acta Orthop. Scand.* **1972**, *43*, 301–317. [CrossRef] [PubMed]
19. Bergmann, G.; Graichen, F.; Rohlmann, A. Hip joint loading during walking and running, measured in two patients. *J. Biomech.* **1993**, *26*, 969–990. [CrossRef]
20. Bergmann, G.; Bergmann, G.; Deuretzabacher, G.; Deuretzabacher, G.; Heller, M.; Heller, M.; Graichen, F.; Graichen, F.; Rohlmann, A.; Rohlmann, A.; et al. Hip forces and gait patterns from rountine activities. *J. Biomech.* **2001**, *34*, 859–871. [CrossRef]
21. Bergmann, G.; Kniggendorf, H.; Graichen, F.; Rohlmann, A. Influence of shoes and heel strike on the loading of the hip joint. *J. Biomech.* **1995**, *28*, 817–827. [CrossRef]
22. Ruggiero, A.; Merola, M.; Affatato, S. On the biotribology of total knee replacement: A new roughness measurements protocol on in vivo condyles considering the dynamic loading from musculoskeletal multibody model. *Meas. J. Int. Meas. Confed.* **2017**, *112*. [CrossRef]
23. Van der Ploeg, B.; Tarala, M.; Homminga, J.; Janssen, D.; Buma, P.; Verdonschot, N. Toward a more realistic prediction of peri-prosthetic micromotions. *J. Orthop. Res.* **2012**, *30*, 1147–1154. [CrossRef] [PubMed]

24. Damsgaard, M.; Rasmussen, J.; Christensen, S.T.; Surma, E.; de Zee, M. Analysis of musculoskeletal systems in the AnyBody Modeling System. *Simul. Model. Pract. Theory* **2006**, *14*, 1100–1111. [CrossRef]
25. Vaughan, C.; Davis, B.L.; O'Connor, J.C. The man data set from "Dynamics of Human Gait". *Hum. Kinet. Publ.* 1992. Available online: https://isbweb.org/data (accessed on 6 April 2018).
26. Siemienski, A. Soft saturation—An idea for load sharing between muscles. Application to the study of human locomotion. In *Biolocomotion: A Century of Research Using Moving Pictures*; Cappozzo, A., Marchetti, M., Tosi, V., Eds.; Promograph: Rome, Italy, 1992; pp. 293–303.
27. Barreto, S.; Folgado, J.; Fernandes, P.R.; Monteiro, J. The Influence of the Pelvic Bone on the Computational Results of the Acetabular Component of a Total Hip Prosthesis. *J. Biomech. Eng.* **2010**, *132*, 54503. [CrossRef] [PubMed]
28. Kurtz, S.M.; Villarraga, M.L.; Herr, M.P.; Bergström, J.S.; Rimnac, C.M.; Edidin, A.A. Thermomechanical behavior of virgin and highly crosslinked ultra-high molecular weight polyethylene used in total joint replacements. *Biomaterials* **2002**, *23*, 3681–3697. [CrossRef]
29. Laurian, T.; Tudor, A. Some Aspects Regarding the Influence of the Clearance on the Pressure Distribution in Total Hip Joint Prostheses. In Proceedings of the National Tribology Conference RotTrib03, Galati, Romania, 24–26 September 2003.
30. Merola, M.; Ruggiero, A.; de Mattia, J.S.; Affatato, S. On the tribological behavior of retrieved hip femoral heads affected by metallic debris. A comparative investigation by stylus and optical profilometer for a new roughness measurement protocol. *Measurement* **2016**, *90*, 365–371. [CrossRef]
31. Affatato, S.; Ruggiero, A.; Merola, M.; Logozzo, S. Does metal transfer differ on retrieved Biolox® Delta composites femoral heads? Surface investigation on three Biolox® generations from a biotribological point of view. *Compos. Part B Eng.* **2017**, *113*, 164–173. [CrossRef]
32. Ruggiero, A.; D'Amato, R.; Gómez, E. Experimental analysis of tribological behavior of UHMWPE against AISI420C and against TiAl6V4 alloy under dry and lubricated conditions. *Tribol. Int.* **2015**, *92*, 154–161. [CrossRef]
33. Ruggiero, A.; D'Amato, R.; Gómez, E.; Merola, M. Experimental comparison on tribological pairs UHMWPE/TIAL6V4 alloy, UHMWPE/AISI316L austenitic stainless and UHMWPE/AL_2O_3 ceramic, under dry and lubricated conditions. *Tribol. Int.* **2016**, *96*, 349–360. [CrossRef]
34. Shen, F.-W.; Lu, Z.; McKellop, H.A. Wear versus Thickness and Other Features of 5-Mrad Crosslinked UHMWPE Acetabular Liners. *Clin. Orthop. Relat. Res.* **2011**, *469*, 395–404. [CrossRef] [PubMed]
35. Mattei, L.; di Puccio, F. Wear Simulation of Metal-on-Metal Hip Replacements with Frictional Contact. *J. Tribol.* **2013**, *135*, 21402. [CrossRef]
36. Matsoukas, G.; Willing, R.; Kim, I.Y. Total Hip Wear Assessment: A Comparison Between Computational and In Vitro Wear Assessment Techniques Using ISO 14242 Loading and Kinematics. *J. Biomech. Eng.* **2009**, *131*, 41011. [CrossRef] [PubMed]
37. Teoh, S.H.; Chan, W.H.; Thampuran, R. An elasto-plastic finite element model for polyethylene wear in total hip arthroplasty. *J. Biomech.* **2002**, *35*, 323–330. [CrossRef]
38. Maxian, T.A.; Brown, T.D.; Pedersen, D.R.; Callaghan, J.J. A sliding-distance-coupled finite element formulation for polyethylene wear in total hip arthroplasty. *J. Biomech.* **1996**, *29*, 687–692. [CrossRef]
39. Gao, Y.; Jin, Z.; Wang, L.; Wang, M. Finite element analysis of sliding distance and contact mechanics of hip implant under dynamic walking conditions. *Proc. Inst. Mech. Eng. Part H J. Eng. Med.* **2015**, *229*, 469–474. [CrossRef] [PubMed]
40. Bevill, S.L.; Bevill, G.R.; Penmetsa, J.R.; Petrella, A.J.; Rullkoetter, P.J. Finite element simulation of early creep and wear in total hip arthroplasty. *J. Biomech.* **2005**, *38*, 2365–2374. [CrossRef] [PubMed]
41. Maxian, T.A.; Brown, T.D.; Pedersen, D.R.; Callaghan, J.J. Adaptiive finite element modeling of long-term polyethylene wear in total hip arthroplasty. *J. Orthop. Res.* **1996**, *14*, 668–675. [CrossRef] [PubMed]
42. Di Puccio, F.; Mattei, L. Biotribology of artificial hip joints. *World J. Orthop.* **2015**, *6*, 77. [CrossRef] [PubMed]
43. Tudor, A.; Laurian, T.; Popescu, V.M. The effect of clearance and wear on the contact pressure of metal on polyethylene hip prostheses. *Tribol. Int.* **2013**, *63*, 158–168. [CrossRef]

13

Comparison of Titanium and Bioresorbable Plates in "A" Shape Plate Properties—Finite Element Analysis

Rafał Zieliński [1,*], Marcin Kozakiewicz [1] and Jacek Świniarski [2]

1 Department of Maxillofacial Surgery, Medical University of Lodz, 1st Haller Plac, 90-647 Lodz, Poland; qed@op.pl
2 Department of Strength of Materials and Structures, Technical University of Lodz, Stefanowskiego 1/15, 90-924 Lodz, Poland; jacek.swiniarski@p.lodz.pl
* Correspondence: bkost@op.pl

Abstract: (1) Background: The main disadvantage of rigid fracture fixation is remain material after healing period. Implementation of resorbable plates prevents issues resulting from left plates. The aim of this study is to compare the usage of bioresorbable and titanium "A" shape condyle plate in condylar fractures. (2) Methods: Thickness of 1.0 mm, height of 31 mm, and width of 19 mm polylactic acid (PLLA) and titanium "A" shape plate with 2.0 mm-wide connecting bar and 9 holes were tested with finite element analysis in high right condylar neck fracture. (3) Results: On bone surface the highest stress is on the anterior bridge around first hole (approx. 100 MPa). The highest stress on screws is located in the first screw around plate in the anterior bridge and is greater in titanium (150 MPa) than PLLA (114 MPa). (4) Conclusion: Pressure on bone in PLLA osteosynthesis is two times higher than in titanium fixation. On small areas where pressure on bone is too high it causes local bone degradation around the fracture and may delay the healing process or make it impossible. Fixation by PLLA is such flexible that bone edges slide and twist what may lead to degradation of callus.

Keywords: mandible condylar fractures; surgical treatment; titanium; PLLA; finite element analysis

---

1. Introduction

Open reduction internal fixation is the method of choice in mandibular condyle fractures [1–3]. Although it demands the surgical skills because of the risk of facial palsy. Titanium alloys are still gold standard in terms of osteosynthesis fixation systems, however, bioresorbable plates and screws are also used in condyle fractures. The main disadvantage of metal plates is when the necessity of removal of osteosynthesis material appears (especially extraoral scars or facial nerve palsy) [4]. Loosening of metal plates or screws which might not be visible on radiographs also demand removal [5–7]. According to the literature there are a few reasons where removing of metal plates should be performed: metallosis, corrosion, thermal dysaesthesia, difficulties with future radiological diagnosis, malpositioning, and the migration of osteosynthesis material, particularly in craniofacial surgery [8,9].

Insertion of resorbable screws demand tapping because of the mechanical properties of the material. In long screws there is high risk of fracture of the neck of the screw. Cutting of the threads take much time and any other additional manipulation is linked with the possibility of displacement of condylar fragments. In the "bone welding" method, screws are not inserted such as self-tapping screws but resorbable pins are placed by ultrasound activation [10–13]. The pin is put into the drilled hole and link with osseointegrate with spongy bone.

There are various ways how to perform rigid internal fracture fixation in the condylar area (base, middle, high neck, and head) and it significantly changed in the last decade. To our knowledge, there are no published reports concerning what fixation system and which material provide functionally stable fixation in fractures of the condylar neck of the mandible.

The aim of the study is to compare by means of finite element analysis (FEA) one of the bioresorbable type of "A" shape condyle plate and screws made of polylactic acid (PLLA) versus titanium grade 5 alloy (Ti6Al4V).

2. Materials and Methods

2.1. The Plate

Recently developed resorbable plate (ChM company, Lewickie, Poland, www.chm.eu) has been tested. Manufacturer applied their own new PLLA polymer. Figure 1 shows the design of A-shape condylar plate (ACP) made of resorbable material. The height and the width of the PLLA plate are 31 mm and 19 mm, respectively, whereas the thickness is 1.0 mm. The first bridge of ACP is parallel to posterior border of the mandibular ramus (compression area) and the second is parallel to the sigmoid notch (traction area). The width of the bridge is 2.5 mm. Bridges of ACP are strictly designed according to known compression and traction lines in the mandibular ramus (Figure 2) [14]. There are three linearly located holes on inferior tails of the bridges. Superiorly, the bridges converge and has triangular 3 hole group. Two tails are connected by means of 2.0 mm wide bar. The connecting bar has been designed according to compression line of condylar neck [15].

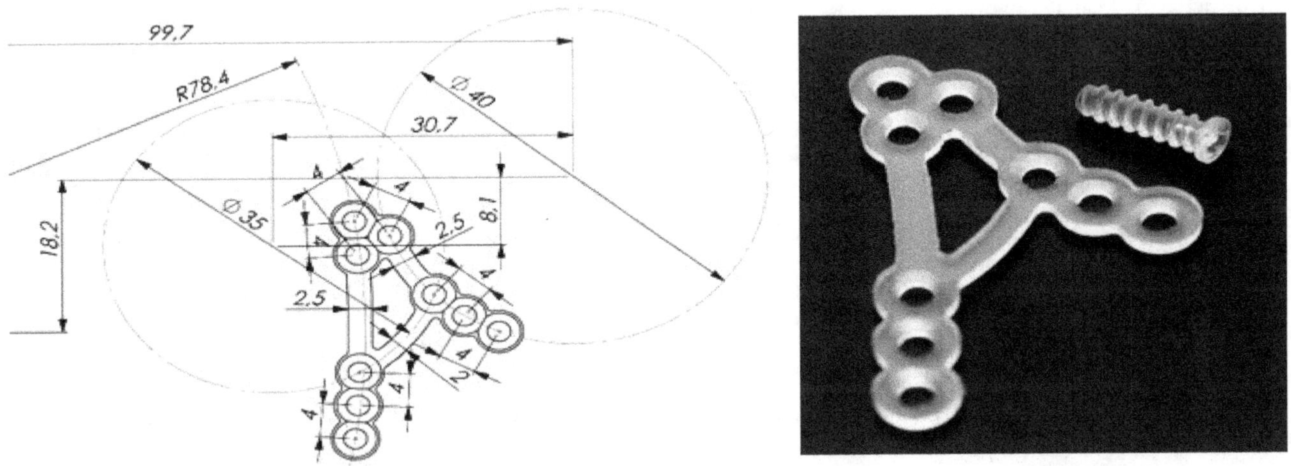

Figure 1. Right side shows the photo of resorbable polylactic acid (PLLA) A-shape right plate and screw whereas on the left side sketch with the dimensions. The height and the width of "A" shape plate are 31 mm and 19 mm respectively whereas the thickness is 1.0 mm. The width of the bridge is 2.5 mm. There are three linearly located holes on inferior tails of the bridges. Superiorly, the bridges converge and has triangular 3-hole group. Two tails are connected by means of 2.0 mm wide bar.

2.2. Material Properties

Mechanical properties have been implemented to calculations are following: Young modulus for Ti-6Al-4V Grade 5 is 140 GPa, Poisson coefficient was 0.3, Yield stress Re = 880 MPa, ultimate tensile stress Rm = 960 MPa, plasticity modulus Ep = 1.4 GPa. For polymer material PLLA: Young modulus 3.5 GPa, Poisson coefficient was 0.35 [16], durability of stretch from 195 MPA to 240 MPa. For mandible material following data were adopted: Young modulus 14 GPa, Poisson coefficient 0.28. Bone is the material that is not described by Hooke's law and it does not have neither linearly elastic characteristic nor plasticity modulus.

Static tensile (Instron 5989 with extensometer, Zwick/Roell, Ulm, Germany) test according to ISO 6892-1 [16] was performed in order to verify the properties of Ti-6Al-4V grade 5. The test results are shown in the graph above (Figure 2). Properties of bone and PLLA have been set on the basis of the literature [17].

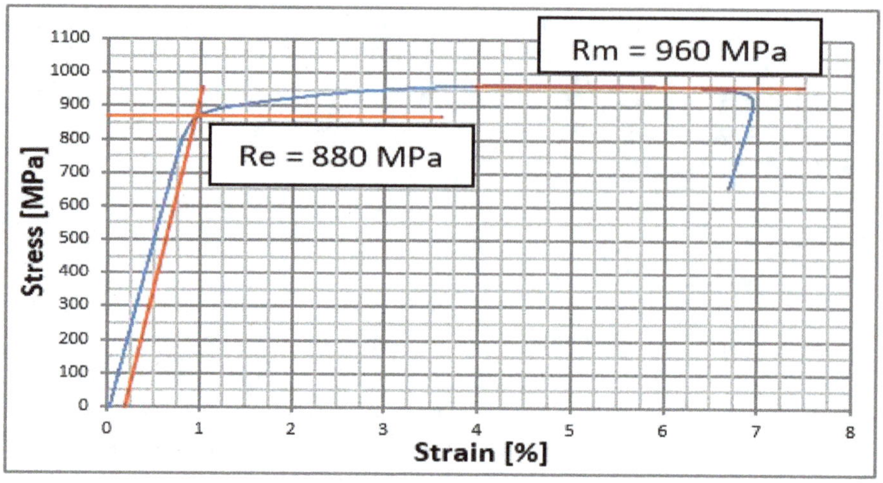

Figure 2. Stress strain curve for the Ti-6Al-4V Grade 5 titanium alloy.

2.3. Finite Element Analysis

Finite element models are helpful for simulating endurance of 3D complex models [18–20].

In the study FEM (Finite Element Method) was used for the comparison between bone end movements just after the open rigid internal fixation by titanium and PLLA plates.

During stretching bone is nonlinearly elastic and after achieving endurance on stretching or squeezing it breaks. In real life bone is not isotropic material but orthotropic, with precise mechanical properties that are different in each layer and maximal load forces in bone depends on direction of loading. Mathematical methods especially for orthotropy are linearly-elastic till the moment of bone destruction. There are several restrictions that in significant way influence on FEM results. Drawing conclusions are made on the basis of the FEM researcher and modelling of biomechanical structure and degree of its simplicity was the basis for the researchers' team. Discussion about FEM results presented as comparison between titanium osteosynthesis and PLLA for the same one.

Authors of this study know advantages and disadvantages of finite element method and restrictions of this method. The software for preparing FEM and simulation was Ansys version 18.2 (Ansys Inc., Canonsburg, PA, USA, www.ansys.com). The proper name of used element is SOLID187 individual name for ANSYS. Users of other software might not know this name whereas tetrahedron tet10 is used for other systems. Mathematical model FEM was solved with material and construction unlinearity using significant displacements. Total size of the quest was DOF (degree of freedom) = 4350480.

2.4. Models

In the Figure 3 mandible 3D model was shown with fixation bone ends in high fracture of condylar neck. Osteosynthesis was designed according to physiology and loaded by forces (purple colour shows forces from muscles) direction and value described by Ramos [21].

In real fractures ragged contours are observed, whereas mathematical model of friction refers to flat surfaces that irregularities are not designed and surface is described as coefficient of friction. In the study to simulate surface degradation by fracture not physical, a (extremely high) coefficient of friction of $\mu = 0.8$ was adopted. The highest coefficient of friction that is gained in machine construction is $\mu = 0.65$, found in brake blocks in aircraft.

The plates were fixed with mandible on basis of continuous displacement. There is initial state of strain between screws and bone because of screw fixation. Contact situation can decrease the stiffness of the connection screw–bone in order to save some time on calculations authors have decided to eliminate the threads on the screw and perform continuous displacements between simplified model of the screw and bone.

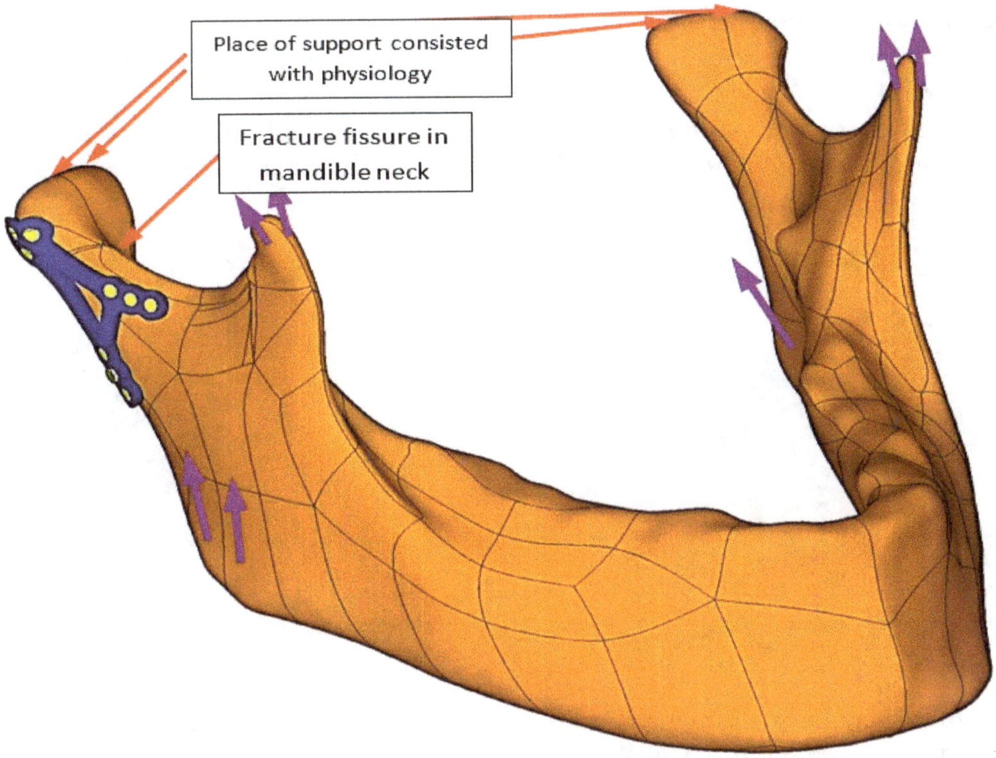

Figure 3. 3D model with plate fixation of high neck condylar fracture (red indicators). Fixation has its physiological support points and it was loaded by muscles forces (purple indicators). In the Figure 3 purple indicators have been described in the literature [20].

3. Results

Authors compared the state of bone ends in contact, pressure in contact, displacement in contact, dimension of fissure in contact and comparison maximal equivalent stress distribution in mandible and in osseofixation system.

In the Figure 4a in titanium fixation half of contact area is marked in yellow color. It means that in such a fixation contact is open. Open contact is the reason of so called mechanical silence which might block healing of fracture. However, it is possible that in such conditions collagen mesh may appear and vessels from the region may grow. As a result callus becomes calcified.

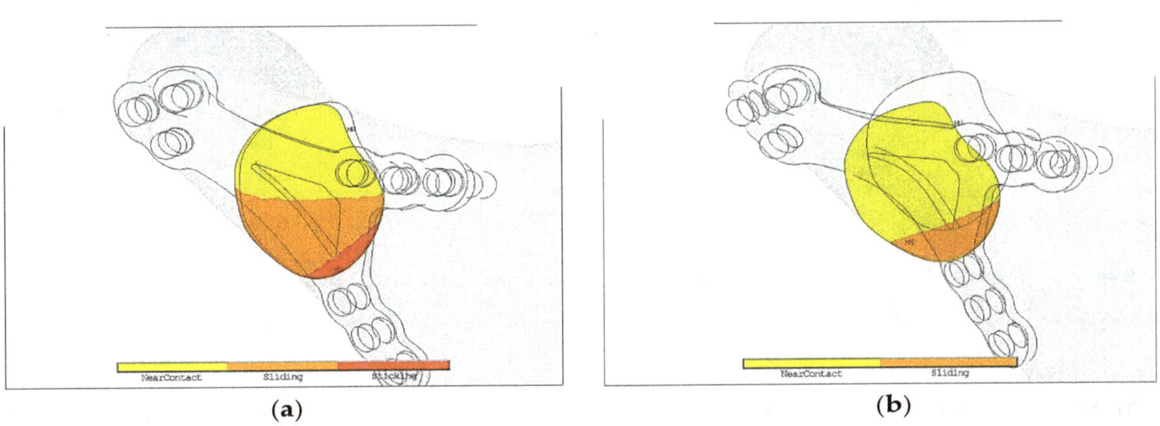

Figure 4. Contact status just after following plate fixation in the maximal loading according to the literature [16]: (**a**) Ti-6Al-4V plate fixation—insignificant displacement at the expense of high contact surface of bone ends during loading thanks to which appearance of minimal twisting of bone ends appeared, (**b**) PLLA plate fixation—significant displacement of bone ends thanks to which high twist appeared.

Orange color shows bone in contact but it is slip so there is possibility of displacement. Cutting forces cause displacement of bone ends and also destroy the gentle collagen mesh preventing calcification, that would never calcified. As a result bone does not heal properly.

Red color describes condition where both parts of bones do not displace to each other. As Figure 5b proves in PLLA fixation is much worse environment that obstruct the healing process in comparison to titanium alloy plate.

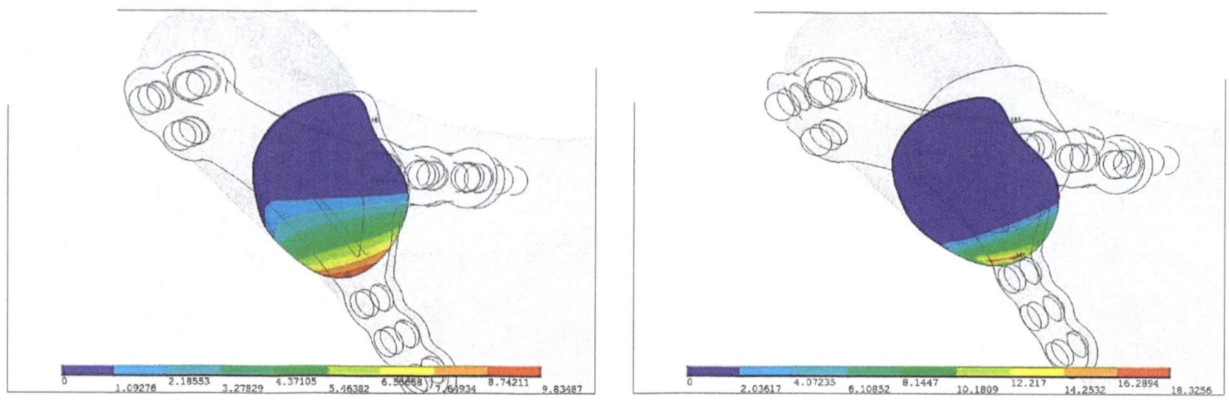

(a) (b)

Figure 5. Displacements of pressure in mandibular bone ends just after plate fixation in the maximal loading according to the literature [16]: (**a**) Ti-6Al-4V plate fixation, $p_{max} = 9.8$ MPa, (**b**) PLLA plate fixation, $p_{max} = 18.3$ MPa.

As Figure 5a shows surface pressure in contact $p_{max} = 9.8$ MPa are almost twice lower than in PLLA $p_{max} = 18.3$ MPa but the area of contact is significantly higher in plate made in Ti-6Al-4V than in PLLA, shown on Figure 5b. Greater area of surface pressure makes healing process faster and as a result it proves osseofixation stiffness.

In Figure 6 displacements of bone ends in fracture plane are shown. Blue area shows the fissure and relative displacements in plane is indeterminable. Displacement on contact surface in Ti-6Al-4V plate is $u_{max} = 0.01$ mm and is 10 times lower than PLLA plate $u_{max} = 0.1$ mm.

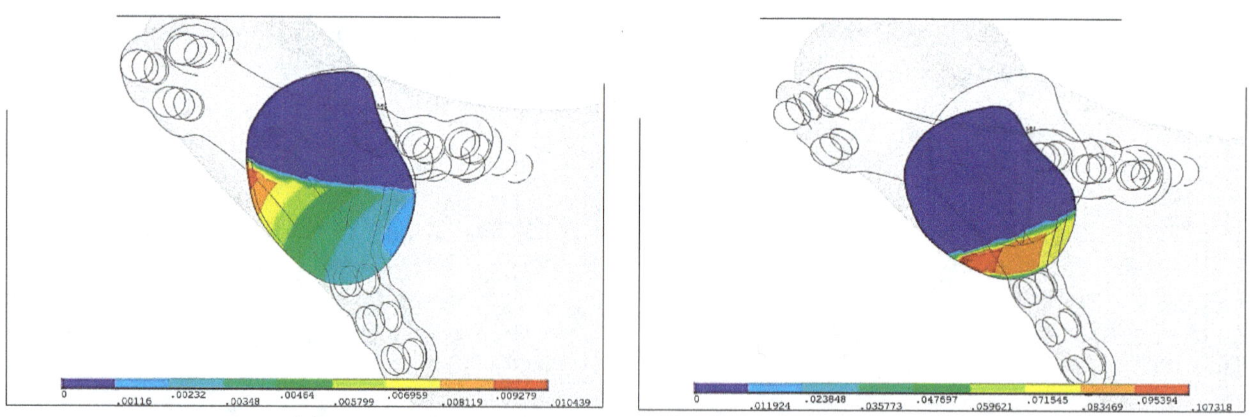

(a) (b)

Figure 6. Displacements of bone ends just after plate fixation in the maximal loading according to the literature [16]: (**a**) Ti-6Al-4V plate fixation, $u_{max} = 0.01$ mm, (**b**) PLLA plate fixation, $u_{max} = 0.1$ mm.

In Figure 7 size of fissures in plate fixation were compared. Red color means that surface is in contact. Colors from orange to blue means fissure is getting wider. In Ti-6Al-4V plate the widest fissure is $g_{max} = 0.0057$ mm whereas in PLLA plate fixation it is $g_{max} = 0.024$ mm.

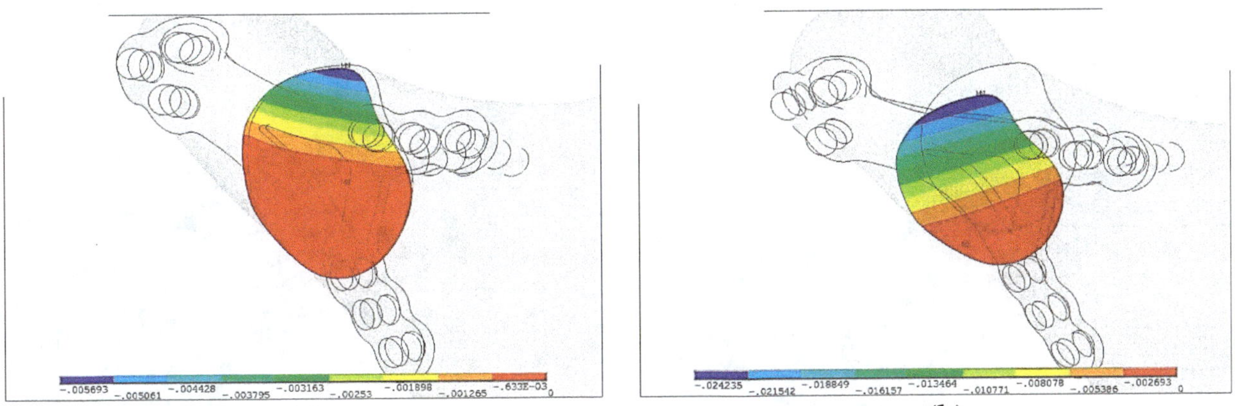

(a) (b)

Figure 7. The size of the fissure between bone ends just after plate fixation in the maximal loading according to the literature [16]: (**a**) Ti-6Al-4V plate fixation, g_{max} = 0.0057 mm, (**b**) PLLA plate fixation, g_{max} = 0.024 mm.

Color from blue to red means increasing stresses from 0 to maximum marked on red. In the Figure 8, reduced stresses distribution according to von Mises on PLLA plate with fixing screws made in Ti-6Al-4V and PLLA were the following: $\sigma_{red\ max}$ = 234 MPa and $\sigma_{red\ max}$ = 76 MPa respectively. Reduced stresses are 4 times lower in PLLA screws than in Ti-6Al-4V grade 5 plate. The fact of paramount importance is that Young modulus for Ti-6Al-4V grade 5 is forty times higher than PLLA. Plate made in more flexible material (PLLA) is prone to higher deformation than Ti-6Al-4V. Titanium alloy grade 5 allow for higher loading forces and make the osseofixation much rigid. Thus titanium alloy material make the healing process easier because of the immobilization of the bone ends. In any of discussed situation, yield stress was not exceeded.

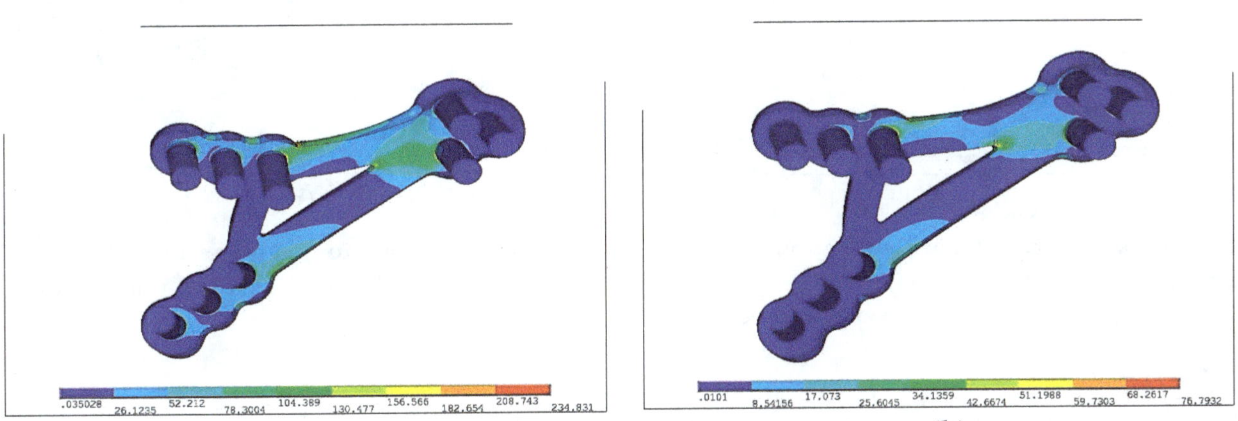

(a) (b)

Figure 8. Equivalent stress distribution on plates according to von Mises hypothesis following plate fixation in the maximal loading according to the literature [16]: (**a**) Ti-6Al-4V plate fixation, $\sigma_{red\ max}$ = 234 MPa, (**b**) PLLA plate fixation, $\sigma_{red\ max}$ = 76 MPa; Colors from blue to red means stresses from 0 to maximum.

In the Figure 9, reduced stresses distribution according to von Mises on Ti-6Al-4V and PLLA plate were $\sigma_{red\ max}$ = 87 MPa and PLLA—$\sigma_{red\ max}$ = 91 MPa, respectively. In both cases stresses are comparable. In order to precise the difference of stresses on bone after fixation, strain has been reduced to 30 MPa.

Grey color on Figure 10 shows strain above the scale. Comparing 10(a) and 10(b) figures Ti-6Al-4V plate and screws indicates the center of strains is around last screws in lower part of mandible. In PLLA plate the highest stress is around the hole that is located near the fracture. This location is at risk during surgical fixation because of secondary fractures during plate fixation that restricts possibility of PLLA usage.

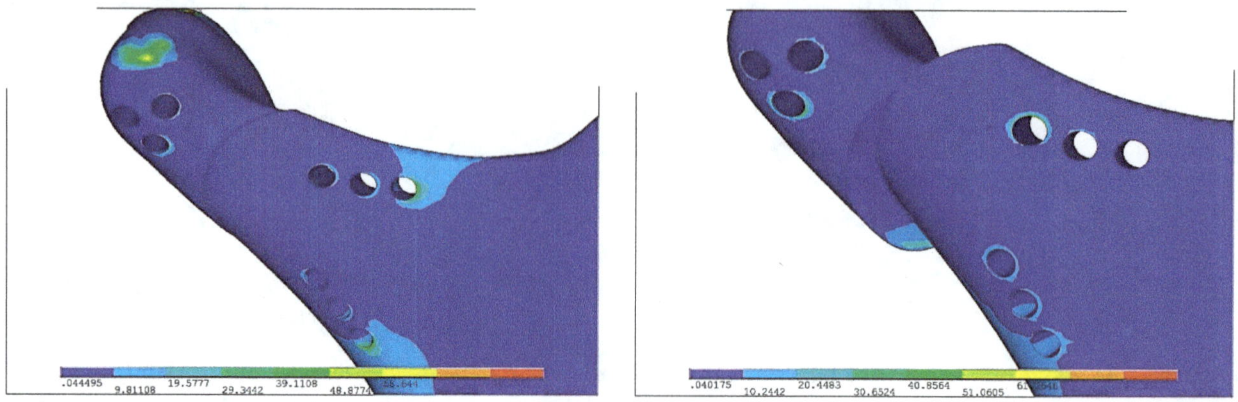

(a) (b)

Figure 9. Equivalent stress distribution in mandibular condyle according to von Mises hypothesis just after plate fixation in the maximal loading according to the literature [16]: (**a**) Ti-6Al-4V plate fixation, $\sigma_{red\ max}$ = 87MPa, (**b**) PLLa plate fixation, $\sigma_{red\ max}$ = 91MPa; Colors from blue to red means increasing stresses from 0 to maximum.

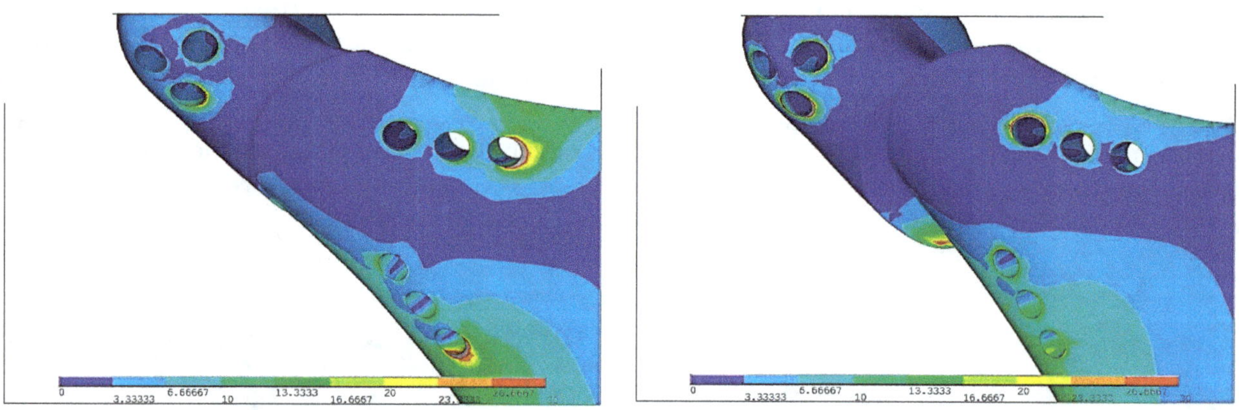

(a) (b)

Figure 10. Reduced stress distribution in mandibular condyle according to von Mises hypothesis just after plate fixation in the maximal loading according to the literature [16]: (**a**) Ti-6Al-4V plate fixation, (**b**) PLLA plate fixation; Stresses have been reduced to $\sigma_{red\ max}$ = 30 MPa.

4. Discussion

Bioresorbability is the most desire feature and titanium alloy does not have it. After fixation bone ends osseointegrate in the proper way when the material is useless. Bioresorbable fixation decomposes and the patient's state will be the same as before the surgical procedure "restitution ad integrum". Titanium alloys that are commonly used in osteosynthesis are deprived of such a feature. Implantation of titanium fixation stays with a patient till the end of the life unless it was screwed out by the surgeon. In some cases especially when a patient grows implantation of plate and screws demand removal immediately after bone healing. It required second surgery made in postsurgical scar and facial nerve branch re-preparation (Figure 1). That may lead to permanent facial nerve palsy, thus bioresorbable materials have found its application in maxillofacial surgery.

Surgeons often during the operation in the most cases tighten in the screws without dynamometer key. It might be assumed that every single screw might be screwed with different torque and as a result stress on every screw is different. This matter has been omitted in order to simplify the procedure as well. Authors have focused on modelling of the contact of the bone ends just after the fracture and comparison of fixation materials taking into consideration only contact between bone ends. On the basis of computed tomography 3D model of edentulous mandible has been designed. Loading on the model is described as loading area transformed to the notches. Supports in temporomandibular joint have been defined as superior notch and linked on the real contact surface by Rigid Body Element (RBE). Such modelling ensures free rotation around joint. On the surface where earlier geometrically teeth have been extracted, degree of freedom are linked with the process of biting (in the direction perpendicular to the surface where teeth have been extracted).

Just after fixation, a patient who fulfils diet precautions and low forces on chewing is able to function almost normally. However, if a surgeon wants to achieve total biodegradability of fixation, then PLLA is the material of choice. The most important factor regarding durability is to perform stresses less than yield stress in order to prevent from irreversible deformation of screws and plates. That is why maxillofacial surgeon asks patients not to overload jaws regarding biting tough food especially after the surgery. Process of making new bone takes about 2 weeks and after this time new bone starts to load forces [22]. By using PLLA materials time of compulsory low forces chewing lengthens from a few days to a few months.

Plates made in PLLA or PLGA are biodegradable in comparison to Ti-6Al-4V. In terms of pressure in fracture, displacement, strain condition Ti-6Al-4V is superior to polymer/composite materials apart from biodegradability. PLLA osteosynthesis indicates that in comparison to titanium alloy fixation contact surface plate with slightly sliding between bones and plates is only 30%. Moreover, displacement between bones has occurred. In the Figure 3 it is easy to notice that in titanium fixation, so called mechanical silence occurs on half of the area after fracture whereas in case of PLLA plate only 20% of the area is in mechanical silence thus bone healing is not possible. Comparing PLLA to titanium alloy small area of concentration of the forces were observed. That is why pressure on bone in PLLA osteosynthesis is twice higher than in titanium fixation. On small areas where pressure on bone is too high it may cause local bone degradation around the fracture (i.e., bone atrophy by compression) and it might be the reason of delay in the healing process or make it impossible. The same conclusion might be assumed by observing cutting forces in the fracture shown in the Figure 4. The higher forces the higher displacement in fracture plane. In significant displacement of bone fragments in fracture fissure, collagen fibres tear and inhibit the healing process (Figure 5). Using PLLA plate has another negative feature if it comes to displacement in fracture plane. Osteosynthesis by means of PLLA is such flexible that strong biting might cause opening of fracture fissure resulting in sliding and twisting that lead to degradation of callus. Using PLLA plates require additional immobilization such as intermaxillary traction or liquid diet. Fixation cannot be overloaded otherwise bone healing process was inhibited.

Author Contributions: Conceptualization, M.K. and J.Ś.; methodology, J.Ś.; software, J.Ś.; validation, J.Ś., M.K. and R.Z.; formal analysis, M.K.; investigation, R.Z.; resources, J.Ś.; data curation, J.Ś.; writing—original draft preparation, R.Z.; writing—review and editing, R.Z., J.Ś., M.K.; visualization, J.Ś., R.Z., M.K.; supervision, J.Ś., M.K.; project administration, M.K., J.Ś.; funding acquisition, M.K.

Acknowledgments: ChM (www.chm.eu) for support the study.

References

1. Eckelt, U.; Schneider, M. Open versus closed reduction of condylar process fractures—A prospective randomized multicenter study with regard to fracture localisation. *Int. J. Oral Maxillofac. Surg.* **2009**, *38*, 478. [CrossRef]
2. Eckelt, U.; Schneider, M.; Erasmus, F.; Gerlach, K.L.; Kuhlisch, E.; Loukota, R.; Rasse, M.; Schubert, J.; Terheyden, H. Open versus closed treatment of fractures of the mandibular condylar process—A prospective randomized multi-center study. *J. Craniomaxillofac. Surg.* **2006**, *34*, 306–314. [CrossRef]

3. Hlawitschka, M.; Loukota, R.; Eckelt, U. Functional and radiological results of open and closed treatment of intracapsular (diacapitular) condylar fractures of the mandible. *Int. J. Oral Maxillofac. Surg.* **2005**, *34*, 597–604. [CrossRef] [PubMed]
4. Eckelt, U.; Hlawitschka, M. Clinical and radiological evaluation following surgical treatment of condylar neck fractures with lag screws. *J. Craniomaxillofac. Surg.* **1999**, *27*, 235–242. [CrossRef]
5. Schneider, M.; Lauer, G.; Eckelt, U. Surgical treatment of fractures of the mandibular condyle: A comparison of long-term results following different approaches—Functional, axiographical, and radiological findings. *J. Craniomaxillofac. Surg.* **2007**, *35*, 151–160. [CrossRef] [PubMed]
6. Klotch, D.W.; Lundy, L.B. Condylar neck fractures of the mandible. *Otolaryngol. Clin. N. Am.* **1991**, *24*, 181–194.
7. Choi, B.H.; Yoo, J.H. Open reduction of condylar neck fractures with exposure of the facial nerve. *Oral Surg. Oral Med. Oral Pathol. Oral Radiol. Endod.* **1999**, *88*, 292–296. [CrossRef]
8. Lizuka, T.; Lindqvist, C. Rigid internal fixation of mandibular fractures. An analysis of 270 fractures treated using the AO/ASIF method. *Int. J. Oral Maxillofac. Surg.* **1992**, *21*, 65–69.
9. Kim, Y.K.; Yeo, H.H.; Lim, S.C. Tissue response to titanium plates: A transmitted electron microscopic study. *J. Oral Maxillofac. Surg.* **1997**, *55*, 322–326. [CrossRef]
10. Pilling, E.; Mai, R.; Theissig, F.; Stadlinger, B.; Loukota, R.; Eckelt, U. An experimental in vivo analysis of the resorption to ultrasound activated pins (Sonic weld) and standard biodegradable screws (ResorbX) in sheep. *Br. J. Oral Maxillofac. Surg.* **2007**, *45*, 447–450. [CrossRef] [PubMed]
11. Eckelt, U.; Nitsche, M.; Muller, A.; Pilling, E.; Pinzer, T.; Roesner, D. Ultrasound aided pin fixation of biodegradable osteosynthetic materials in cranioplasty for infants with craniosynostosis. *J. Craniomaxillofac. Surg.* **2007**, *35*, 218–221. [CrossRef]
12. Meissner, H.; Pilling, E.; Richter, G.; Koch, R.; Eckelt, U.; Reitemeier, B. Experimental investigations for mechanical joint strength following ultrasonically welded pin osteosynthesis. *J. Mater. Sci. Mater. Med.* **2008**, *19*, 2255–2259. [CrossRef] [PubMed]
13. Pilling, E.; Meissner, H.; Jung, R.; Koch, R.; Loukota, R.; Mai, R.; Reitemeier, B.; Richter, G.; Stadlinger, B.; Stelnicki, E.; et al. An experimental study of the biomechanical stability of ultrasound-activated pinned (SonicWeld Rx + Resorb-X) and screwed fixed (Resorb-X) resorbable materials for osteosynthesis in the treatment of simulated craniosynostosis in sheep. *Br. J. Oral Maxillofac. Surg.* **2007**, *45*, 451–456. [CrossRef]
14. Meyer, C.; Kahn, J.L.; Boutemi, P.; Wilk, A. Photoelastic analysis of bone deformation in the region of the mandibular condyle during mastication. *J. Cranio-Maxillofac. Surg.* **2002**, *30*, 160–169. [CrossRef]
15. Kozakiewicz, M.; Swiniarski, J. "A" shape plate for open rigid internal fixation of mandible condyle neck fracture. *J. Cranio-Maxillofac. Surg.* **2014**, *42*, 730–737. [CrossRef]
16. *Metallic Materials—Tensile Testing—Part 1: Method of Test at Room Temperature*; ISO 6892-1; International Organization for Standardization: Geneva, Switzerland, 2016.
17. Maurer, P.; Holweg, S.; Knoll, W.D.; Schubert, J. Study by finite element method of the mechanical stress of selected biodegradable osteosynthesis screws in sagittal ramus osteotomy. *Br. J. Oral Maxillofac. Surg.* **2002**, *40*, 76–83. [CrossRef] [PubMed]
18. Hart, T.R.; Hennebel, V.; Thongpreda, N.; Van Buskirk, W.C.; Anderson, R.C. Modelling the biomechanics of the n audible: A three-dimensional finite element study. *J. Biomech.* **1992**, *25*, 261–286. [CrossRef]
19. Field, C.; Ichim, I.; Swain, M.V.; Chan, E.; Darendeliler, M.A.; Li, W.; Li, Q. Mechanical responses to orthodontic loading: A 3-dimensional finite element multi-tooth model. *Am. J. Orthod. Dentofacial. Orthop.* **2009**, *135*, 174–181. [CrossRef] [PubMed]
20. Ichim, I.; Kieser, J.A.; Swain, M.V. Functional significance of strain distribution in the human mandible under masticatory load: Numerical predictions. *Arch. Oral Biol.* **2007**, *52*, 465–473. [CrossRef] [PubMed]
21. Ramos, A.; Completo, A.; Relvas, C.; Mesnard, M.; Simoes, J.A. Straight, Semi-anatomic and anatomic TMJ implants: The influence of condylar geometry and bone fixation screws. *J. CranMaxillofac. Surg.* **2011**, *39*, 343–350. [CrossRef]
22. Marsell, R.; Einhorn, T. The biology of fracture healing. *Injury* **2011**, *42*, 551–555. [CrossRef] [PubMed]

14

Materials for Hip Prostheses

Massimiliano Merola and Saverio Affatato *

Laboratorio di Tecnologia Medica, IRCCS—Istituto Ortopedico Rizzoli, Via di Barbiano, 1/10 40136 Bologna, Italy; merola@tecno.ior.it

* Correspondence: affatato@tecno.ior.it

Abstract: Replacement surgery of hip joint consists of the substitution of the joint with an implant able to recreate the articulation functionality. This article aims to review the current state of the art of the biomaterials used for hip implants. Hip implants can be realized with different combination of materials, such as metals, ceramics and polymers. In this review, we analyze, from international literature, the specific characteristics required for biomaterials used in hip joint arthroplasty, i.e., being biocompatible, resisting heavy stress, opposing low frictional forces to sliding and having a low wear rate. A commentary on the evolution and actual existing hip prostheses is proposed. We analyzed the scientific literature, collecting information on the material behavior and the human-body response to it. Particular attention has been given to the tribological behavior of the biomaterials, as friction and wear have been key aspects to improve as hip implants evolve. After more than 50 years of evolution, in term of designs and materials, the actual wear rate of the most common implants is low, allowing us to sensibly reduce the risk related to the widespread debris distribution in the human body.

Keywords: biomaterials; ceramic; friction; hip; implants; polyethylene; prosthesis; simulator; wear

---

1. Introduction

The hip is one of the most important joints that support our body, having the task of joining the femurs with the pelvis. The smooth and spherical head of the femur fits perfectly into the natural seat of the acetabulum, which is a cup-shaped cavity; the whole joint is wrapped in very resistant ligaments that make the joint stable. The hip joint is subjected to high daily stresses, having to bear the weight of the upper part of the body. Thus, especially with advancing age, these stresses can jeopardize its functioning.

Osteoarthritis of the hip is one of the most widespread alterations of the hip: it is a condition that causes intense pain due to a stiffening of the joint itself. The surface of the femoral head, due to arthritis, can undergo some alterations, becoming porous and causing damage to the entire joint complex. Osteoarthritis of the hip, as a degenerative pathology, involves irreversible damage due to which in many cases it is necessary to resort to the substitution of the compromised joint with an artificial one. A hip prosthesis is an artificial joint designed to perform the same functions as the natural one and which is surgically implanted. The surgical operation is referred to as Total Hip Arthroplasty (THA).

This paper aims to exhaustively review the state of the art of the biomaterials used as hip joint medical devices. More in depth, our review focuses on advantages, disadvantages and future perspectives regarding the use of biomaterials: polymers, metals, ceramics, and composites. This perspective may provide a clearer insight into how biomaterials research sets up the basis for the design of innovative devices for improved solutions to orthopaedic clinical problems.

1.1. History

Since its first application, the development of design and materials of hip prosthesis continuously progressed. Its development is one of the most challenging issues of the century in the field of implant technology [1]. Several materials were used for this scope: glass, polymers, metal alloys, ceramics, composites, etc., trying to combine biocompatibility and fatigue resistance, stiffness, toughness, withstanding static and dynamic loads, and high resistance to mechanical and chemical wear [2,3]. All these biomaterials were developed with the aim to improve the patient's quality life, avoiding repeated surgery. First attempts at hip surgery date back to 1750, in England, willing to heal arthritis cases [4]. In 1840, the first idea of healing the hip was to replace it with a prosthesis [5]. This procedure was limited to resurfacing or replacing the acetabular part of the femoral head. To do so a wooden block was installed between the damaged terminal parts of the hip articulation. Due to wear particles released into the body, this procedure ended up being disastrous. Biological elements were therefore applied to solve the compatibility issue: skin, muscle tissue, pig bladder and gold foil [6]. Only several decades later were used different artificial materials, such as rubber, zinc, glass, wax and silver plates [4]. In 1880, Prof. Themistocles Glück implanted, for the first time, an ivory ball and socket prosthesis fixed to the bone by screws [7]. Later on, finding that human body could not accept large quantities of external material, he experimented with a mixture of plaster of Paris in combination with powder pumice and resin.

Different materials were also introduced: in 1919, Delbet used rubber to replace a femoral head, whereas Hey-Groves used ivory nail in 1922 to simulate the articular surface of the femoral head [5]. In 1925, Marius Smith-Petersen introduced the first glass and bakelite femoral cup, defining the mold arthroplasty technique, that consisted of a hollow hemisphere adapted over the femoral head [8]. In 1938, Philip Wiles performed the first THA, employing a custom-made implant in stainless steel that was fixed to the bone tissue with screws and bolts. In 1950, Austin Moore introduced hemiarthroplasty, a new kind of hip implant, consisting of the replacement of the femoral head and part of the femoral neck using a long-stemmed element. The stem fitted into the femur cavity without cement, substituting around 31 cm of the proximal part of the bone, whereas the ball was placed on the hip acetabulum. This procedure was satisfactory, even though loosening of the implant was still a problem [5]. In Figure 1 are some of the mentioned hip prostheses designs.

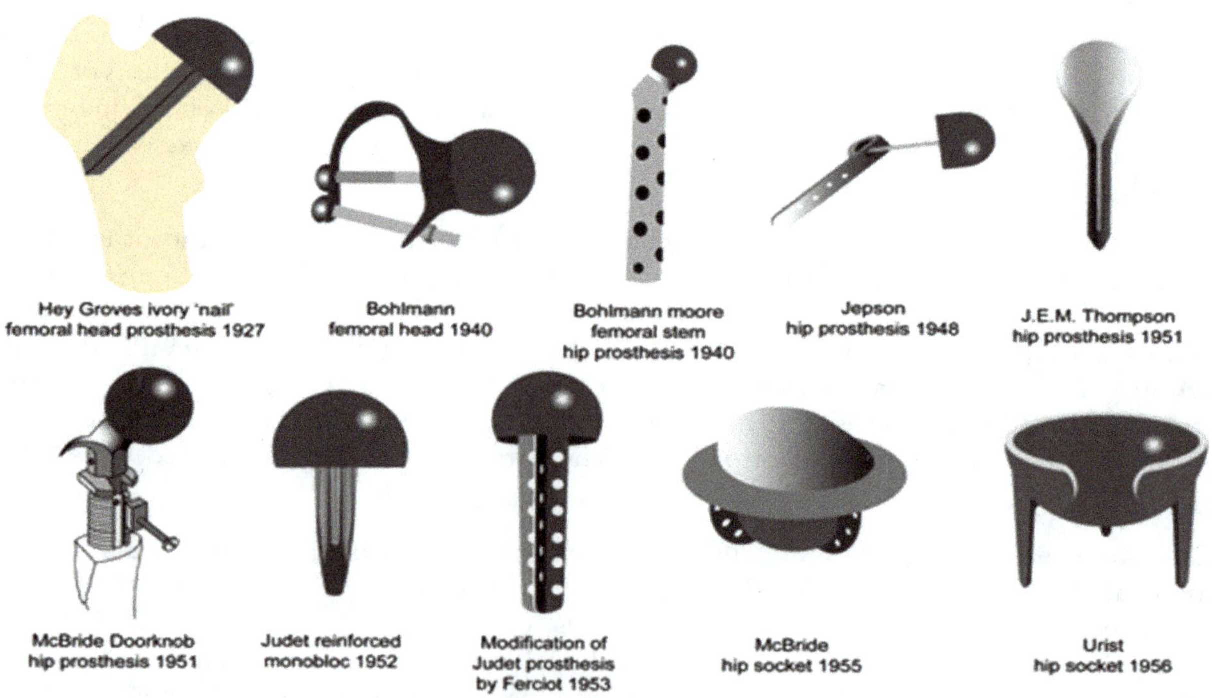

Figure 1. Evolution of the prostheses design.

In 1960, the orthopedic surgeon, San Baw, started performing hip replacements, and in twenty years of work, over 300 ivory hip replacements, with an 88% rate of success [9]. The recognized pioneer of THA, as currently known, is believed to be Sir John Charnley. During the 60's, he defined the concept of Low Friction Arthroplasty (LFA). His first prosthesis was made of a stainless-steel stem, fixed with acrylic cement, and a 22.2-mm diameter head coupled with a polytetrafluoroethylene (PTFE) cup, as shown in Figure 2. PTFE was unsuitable for prosthetic bearing, as it caused wear and tear that leaded to inflammatory reactions. To solve these issues, Sir Charnley adopted other polymer materials, such as high-density polyethylene (HDPE), and ultra-high molecular weight polyethylene (UHMWPE). He also used cement fixation for the acetabular cup [10]. With this combination, the wear effects were reduced, due to the smaller contacting surface and the hard-on-soft coupling. Sir Charnely made many variations to the original design of his LFA, which led to thousands of successful operations.

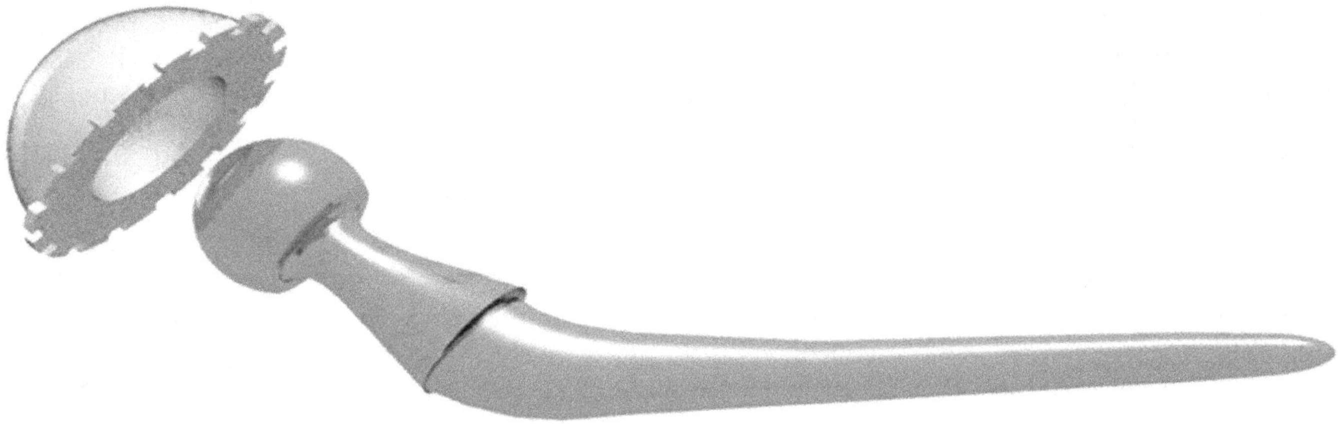

Figure 2. Charnley's first LFA.

1.2. Current Materials

Four main types of bearings are studied and applied in THA: metal-on-polyethylene (MoP), metal-on-metal (MoM), ceramic-on-ceramic (CoC), and ceramic-on-polyethylene (CoP). Recently, hybrid combinations were introduced such as ceramic heads and metallic inserts (CoM) [11,12]. Many factors influence the choice between these types of bearing, such as the implant cost, age and activity level of the patient, complications during surgery, etc. MoM articulations were introduced first in 1950, by McKee and Farrar, leading to unsatisfactory results as two out of three implants were removed after 1 year due to loosening and the third removed for fracture [13–15]. After many improvements of the bearings, they were reintroduced in 1960, when the wear rate ranged from 1 to 5 mm^3 per year (which was roughly 20 times lower than that registered for metal on polyethylene) [16,17]. MoM articulations were used for both total hip replacements and hip resurfacing (HR), which have the advantage of preserving the femoral head and neck, resulting in a less invasive operation and a lower dislocation rate. When, during the 2000s, the issues of metal debris came to light, the MoM replacements were almost stopped completely. In the early middle 2000s, these implants were used in more than one out of five cases in the UK and up to one-third in the US. Today, they are used in less than 1% of the total surgical operations [18]. MoM articulations have been used again in the last two decades, thanks to the appearance of new surface finishing techniques [6] that improve their wear resistance. On the other hand, MoM bearings aim to ensure high wear resistance, good manufacturability and low friction torque. However, even if lower wear volume is associated with such implants, very small particles are produced [19]. The amount of metal ions present in the serum and their potential toxic effects both locally and systemically are a cause for concern [19]. Moreover, polishing wear, promoted by wear debris, produced by the abrasive action of carbides, has been shown in retrieved Co-Cr alloy hip implants [19].

Up to the middle of the 1990s, the most widespread hip implant was MoP couples that worked well in older and less active patients [20]. Two relevant problems were still a concern: aseptic loosening as result of inadequate initial fixation caused by particle-induced osteolysis around the implant and hip dislocation.

In the 80's, when aseptic loosening and osteolysis arose as main issues in metal-on-polymers hip implants, the firsts CoC couples were launched, starting with alumina and zirconia [21–23]. Zirconia ceramics have been introduced for orthopedic implants as a secondary ceramic material along with alumina for several years. Major advantages of ceramics for THA are their hardness, scratch resistance, and the inert nature of debris [24]. These characteristics promote the use of CoC bearings, and the inert nature of the wear debris result in them being the best choice for young patients. On the other hand, their use is expensive, and implants require an excellent surgical insertion to preclude chipping of contact surfaces.

The introduction of an innovative hybrid hard-on-hard bearing ceramic head and metallic insert claimed to reduce ion release and wear particle production and possibly the breakage of the ceramic insert rim [25–27]. In in vitro studies on CoM hip implants [12,28], smaller particles and lower wear have been found.

Nowadays hip joint prostheses are made with metals, ceramics and plastic materials. Most used are titanium alloys, stainless steel, special high-strength alloys, alumina, zirconia, zirconia toughened alumina (ZTA), and UHMWPE. Usually, stems and necks are composed of metals, whereas femoral heads can be both metal and ceramic, and the acetabulum can be made of metals, ceramics or polymers. There are several combinations that can be realized by using these materials with the aim of coupling with the fewest concerns and the highest long-term success odds.

Hereafter, we present an overall evaluation of biomaterials (polymers, metals, ceramics) for THA.

2. Polymers

Polymer materials were the first choice for low friction hip replacements, as proven by Charnely. Highly stable polymeric systems such as PTFE, UHMWPE or polyetheretherketone (PEEK) have been investigated due to their excellent mechanical properties and their high wear resistance. Nevertheless, when implanted, acetabular cups made of polyethylene generate debris that is attacked by the body's immune system [29]. This leads to bone loss, also known as osteolysis; furthermore, since the debris accumulates in the area close to the implant, the bone loss leads to loosening of the implant stem. This results in the needs of a revision, namely, another surgery. Revision for loosening is four times higher than the next leading reason (dislocation at 13.6%) and is more severe in young patients [30].

2.1. PTFE

PTFE has a high thermal stability; it is hydrophobic, stable in most types of chemical environments, and generally considered to be inert in the body [31]. It was used by Charnley in his firsts THA, but exhibited two main drawbacks, which were found only after implantation in 300 patients [32]. The material had a very high wear rate, equal to 0.5 mm per month [33], and PTFE produced voluminous masses of amorphous material due to the vast number of foreign-body giant cells [34]. Furthermore, this debris elicited an intense foreign-body reaction that Charnley verified by injecting two specimens of finely divided PTFE into his own thigh [35].

Charnley tried to use a composite material based on PTFE reinforced with glass fibers (known as Fluorosint), finding poor performance in vivo, despite its fine behavior in vitro. The composite, after one year of implantation, developed a pasty surface that could be easily worn away. Plus, the filler acted abrasively and lapped the metal counter-face. Moreover, this composite material showed a higher rate of infection (20%) and loosening (57%) than the other materials employed [36].

2.2. UHMWPE

Charnley introduced UHMWPE in 1962, urged by the failure of PTFE as a bearing material and sustained by the promising behavior in laboratory tests [37]. The polymer is characterized by its excellent wear resistance, low friction and high impact strength. It is created by the polymerization of ethylene, and it is one of the simplest polymers. Its chemical formula is $(–C_2H_4–)_n$, where n is the degree of polymerization, being the number of repeating units along the chain. The average degree of n is a minimum of 36,000 [38], having a molecular weight of at least 1 million g/mole as defined by the standard [39].

During the 1980s and early 1990s, aseptic loosening and osteolysis emerged as major problems in the orthopedic field, and these problems were perceived to limit the lifespan of joint replacements [40]. To limit the wear particle concentration and improve the overall mechanical characteristics, efforts have been made to improve the overall characteristics of UHMWPE for hip implants. In the 90s, scientists were able to correlate changes in the physical properties of the UHMWPE with the in vivo degradation of mechanical behaviors. UHMWPE was typically sterilized by gamma irradiation, with a mean dose of 25 to 40 kGy. This process resulted in the formation of free radicals, which are the precursors of oxidation-induced embrittlement. Only in the past decade did the radiation crosslinking achieve common diffusion. This process of crosslinking combined with thermal treatment has emerged to increase wear and oxidation resistance of the polymer, and a large number of laboratory and clinical studies indicated positive outcomes [41–44]. Crosslinked polyethylene is commonly abbreviated as PEX or XLPE. Currently, there are different treatments, including irradiation and melting, irradiation and annealing, sequential irradiation with annealing, irradiation followed by mechanical deformation, and irradiation and stabilization with vitamin E [45]. Crosslinking also affects the mechanical properties of UHMWPE, corresponding usually to a decrease in the toughness, ultimate mechanical properties, stiffness, and hardness of the polymer [46]. These factors could negatively influence the device performance in vivo [47]. Free radicals may form during the manufacturing process, allowing for oxidative changes in the XLPE. As a consequence, the wear resistance of the polymer is expected to decline, the opposite behaviour constitutes a sort of paradox. Muratoglu et al. [46] studied the wear behavior of UHMWPE, finding drastic changes as a consequence of crosslinking; these authors found that this process reduces the ability of molecules to orient and reorient, inhibiting this mechanism responsible for wear. It also appeared that the level of crosslinking, found in the study, overwhelmed the effects of reduced mechanical and physical properties in controlling the wear behaviour of UHMWPE. For the best outcome, XLPE should be cross-linked at a correct level of radiation, and then re-melted to remove the free radicals [48]. The exceeding free radicals that did not react to form cross-links through irradiation must be eliminated to prevent the formation of oxidized species and their recombination. The removal can be realized through two different methods: annealing or remelting; highly cross-linked polyethylene (HXLPE) has demonstrated superior wear resistance compared to gamma-sterilized materials [46]. By annealing below the peak melting point of the polymer, some of the crystalline regions are melted and the free radical concentration is reduced, but it is still measurable. On the other hand, through post-irradiation remelting, residual free radicals are reduced to undetectable levels, as measured by state-of-the-art electron spin resonance instrument. By this process, crystallinity is reduced after the melting step due to the hindrance by the new crosslinks, so the mechanical strength and fatigue resistance of the polymer decrease [49]. Several clinical studies have been realized on the in vivo oxidation of remelted or annealed XLPEs, even if our knowledge is restricted to what might happen during the first decade of implantation [50].

Muratoglu et al. [51] analyzed retrieved XLPE acetabular liners, finding minimal oxidation, but they discovered that the oxidation increases during shelf storage in air, producing severe damage. They assumed that two mechanisms could alter the oxidative stability of UHMWPE, the in vivo cyclic loading and the absorption of lipids. Lipids are able to react with oxygen and thus extract hydrogen atoms from the polyethylene chains, provoking the initiation of free radicals.

Rinitz et al. [52] investigated short- and middle-term retrievals made of remelted and annealed HXLPEs to determine whether oxidation can lead to mechanical property changes through oxidative chain scissions.

Their studies proved crosslink density decreases, corresponding to augmented oxidation for some highly cross-linked, thermally stabilized materials. Other clinical studies highlighted fast in vivo oxidation rates of post-irradiation thermally treated retrievals [53].

Successful outcomes are reached by HXLPE liners associated with a delta ceramic femoral head, as found by Kim et al. [54], finding an annual penetration rate of the femoral head of around 0.022 mm/year. Hamai et al. compared the clinical wear rates of annealed and remelted HXLPE liners by means of radiographs on 36 matched pairs of hip explants. They found significantly greater creep in the remelted than the annealed, but no significant differences between the steady state wear rates. The retrospective study of Takada et al. [55] compared the wear behavior between the second-generation annealed and first-generation remelted HXLPEs. Involving 123 primary THA, their study confirmed excellent wear resistance of both types of HXLPE, but found that second-generation annealed HXLPE had a better wear resistance than first-generation remelted HXLPE in a short-term follow-up. Also, D'antonio et al. [56] reported the wear rate of second-generation annealed HXLPE, which compared to a conventional polyethylene, represented a reduction of 72–86% (depending on other studies results). They further found a reduction of 58%, when comparing the linear wear of the second- and first-generation annealing HXLPE.

Crystallinity of the polymer is a function of the irradiation dose and of the thermal treatment [57]. Irradiation leads to smaller chains with augmented mobility, whereas the change in crystallinity after the thermal procedure depends on the temperature reached. If the treatment is realized below the melting point of 137 °C, the chain mobility rises, yielding higher crystallinity [58,59]. If the procedure is performed at higher temperature, the crystallization of the polymer, during the cool-down to ambient temperature, occurs in the presence of cross-linking, which decreases the crystallinity of the polymer and improve the wear resistance with small changes in toughness [58].

Basically, the mechanisms by which UHMWPE improves its chains occurs via plastic deformation of the polymer, with molecular alignment in the direction of motion that results in the formation of fine, drawn-out fibrils oriented parallel to each other [60]. As a result of this arrangement, the UHMWPE wear surface may strengthen along the direction of sliding, while it weakens in the transverse direction. In light of this, there is a will to realize reinforced polymers with high strength such as self-reinforced UHMWPE [61]. This composite is basically a non-oriented matrix of UHMWPE where reinforcement particles of the same material have been dispersed, resulting in a polymer with excellent biocompatibility, increased mechanical properties and the chance to be sterilized and cross-linked such as the traditional UHMWPE [61].

In Figure 3 are presented typical PE prostheses designs.

In the recent years, a different approach was developed to stabilize polyethylene. Blending vitamin E with polymers was firstly meant as a hygienically safe stabilization, Tocopherol compounds were proposed as a stabilizer for polyolefin in the 1980s [62]. In 1994, Brach del Prever et al. [63] introduced UHMWPE blended with vitamin E for a prosthetic implant. In 2007, the first vitamin E-diffused, irradiated UHMWPE hip implant was clinically introduced in the United States (Biomet Inc., Warsaw, IN, USA) [64]. The blending led to the interruption of the oxidation cycle by decreasing the reactivity of the radical species, giving origin to a third generation of polyethylenes [64–66]. If vitamin E-stabilized, irradiated UHMWPE undergoes accelerated aging at high temperatures and/or in the presence of pure oxygen, it will be oxidatively more stable than gamma-sterilized or high-dose irradiated UHMWPE [67,68]. In vitro studies supported the hypothesis that vitamin E-blending would enhance the oxidative stability of XLPEs. There are also some drawbacks in the procedure: increasing the concentration of vitamin E in the blend is not viable, the obstacle of cross-linking in the presence of vitamin E prescribes the use of a lower concentration [69]. Therefore, a balance is needed to obtain elevate cross-linking density and high oxidative stability.

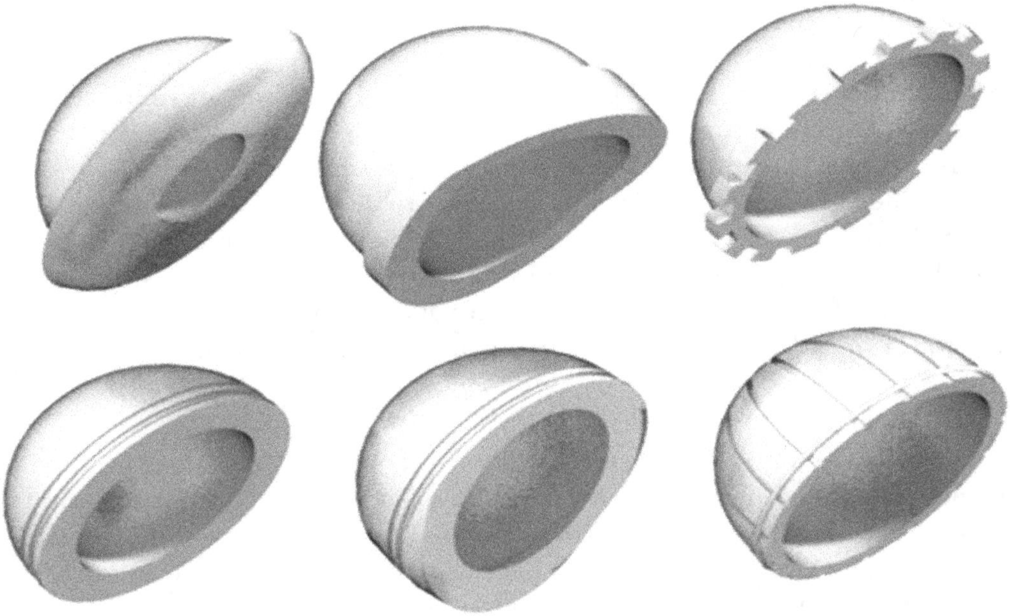

Figure 3. Some of the designs that are achieved with polyethylene for the acetabular cup.

2.3. PEEK

Polyether-ether-ketone (PEEK) is a well-known biocompatible polymer used in orthopedic applications [70]. It has been considered as an alternative joint arthroplasty bearing material due to its favorable mechanical properties and the biocompatibility of its wear debris [71]. PEEK had been used as biomaterials, in particular in the spine, since the 1980s [72,73], due to its structure that confers outstanding chemical resistance, inertness, and thermal stability for in vivo conditions. In 1998, Wang and coworkers [74] tested acetabular cups made of PEEK on a hip simulator for 10 million cycles. They observed a reduction in the wear rate of almost two orders of magnitude in comparison to a conventional UHMWPE/metal or UHMWPE/ceramic couple. However, despite the good promises deriving from in vitro, low contact stress situations, when in high contact stress environments, there are questions about the suitability of this material as acetabular cups or knee tibial components [75,76]. No clinical data of its use are available.

3. Metals

Metallic materials have wide applications in the medical and bioengineering fields and are widespread as orthopedic implants components. The most common traditional metals used for THA are stainless steels, titanium alloys (Ti6Al4V) and—mainly—cobalt-chromium-molybdenum alloys. The latter have good corrosion resistance compared to other metals, and high toughness, high wear resistance and higher hardness (HV = 350) than other metals and polymers.

3.1. Cobalt Chromium Molybdenum Alloys

MoM articulation is typically produced from cobalt-chromium-molybdenum (CoCrMo) alloys. CoCrMo alloys are composed of 58.9–69.5% Co, 27.0–30% Cr, 5.0–7.0% Mo, and small amount of other elements (Mn, Si, Ni, Fe and C). These metallic alloys can be divided in 2 categories: high-carbon alloys (carbon content >0.20%) and low-carbon alloys (carbon content <0.08%) [77,78]. In addition, metallic alloys can be manufactured using 2 different techniques such as casting and forging; the grain size of the forged alloy is typically less than 10 μm, whereas the grain size of the cast material ranges from 30 to 1000 μm [79]. Intensive studies were done on the metallurgy for CoCrMo alloys with carbon; nevertheless, there is no complete phase diagram. This is mainly due to the complex phases existing in the system. Various carbide species, such as $M_{23}C_6$, and M_6C can take place based on the heat treatment [80]. The differences in the microstructure of the carbides, their chemical composition, and nano-hardness are related to wear performances.

Cobalt and chromium are both present in the environment and in food. They are necessary to human beings as trace elements in the body but are toxic when highly concentrated. Patients with Co-Cr metal-on-metal pairings are exposed to wear with release of cobalt and chromium into the synovial fluid. These are capable of migrating to the blood before being expelled through the urine [81,82]. There is poor knowledge on the effects of circulating Co and Cr; they may affect mainly biological and cellular functions with potential effects on the immune system, mutagenesis, and carcinogenesis. In patients with metal-on-metal hip implant, elevated levels of circulating Co and Cr ions may be generated, and there is a positive linear correlation with a lymphocytic reactivity [83,84].

3.2. Other Metal Alloys

Metallic materials have high module of elasticity, which limits stress distribution from implant to bone. Therefore, new metallic components have been developed with lower elastic modulus and higher corrosion and wear resistance. There is continuous research for new metallic alloys for application in hip prostheses to obtain a better biocompatibility along with superior mechanical properties. Still, it is mandatory to find a compromise between the many optimal characteristics desired for an implant material. Co-Cr-Mo alloys have low chemical inertness but high wear resistance, whereas stainless steel alloys have low strength and ductility. Zirconium (Zr) and tantalum (Ta) are refractory metals—due to their great chemical stability and elevate melting point—and are very resistant to corrosion, due to the stability of the oxide layer. As vanadium is a relatively toxic metal, some attempts were made to replace it in the widespread Ti-6Al-4V alloys. To improve biocompatibility and mechanical resistance, this Ti-6Al-4V alloys was replaced with iron (Fe) or niobium (Nb), realizing the improved alloys Ti-5Al-2.5Fe and Ti-6Al-7Nb. These alloys with respect to the traditional Ti-6Al-4V have greater dynamic hardness and lower elastic module, allowing a better implant/bone stress distribution. A new class of titanium alloys introduced into the orthopedic field uses molybdenum in concentration greater than 10%. Its presence stabilizes the β-phase at room temperature; these are referred to as β-Ti alloys. Having 20% less elastic modulus, they behave closer to real bones and have better shaping possibilities. Femoral stems made of a β titanium alloy have been used as part of modular hip replacements since the early 2000's but were recalled in 2011 by the US Food & Drug Administration (FDA) due to elevated levels of wear debris. Yang and Hutchinson [85] found that the dry wear behaviour of a β titanium alloy (TMZF (Ti-12Mo-6Zr-2Fe (wt.%)) is very similar to that of Ti64, whereas their behaviour is completely different in simulated body fluid, where the wear of TMZF is significantly accelerated. Another recently introduced metal material is the oxidized zirconium (Oxinium, by Smith & Nephew), with a metal core and abrasion-resistant ceramic surface. The niobium alloy of zirconium has proven to decrease the UHMWPE wear rate and particle production considerably [86]. In Figure 4 it is possible to see the design of metal implants with different material renderings.

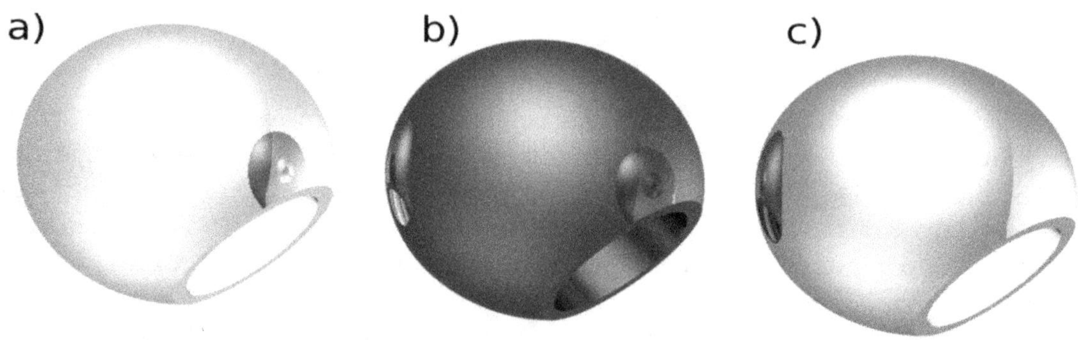

Figure 4. Metal femoral heads: (**a**) stainless-steel; (**b**) Oxinium; (**c**) CoCrMo.

The revision rate of large head metal-on-metal and resurfacing hips is significantly higher than that of conventional total hip replacements. The revision of these bearings has been linked to high wear as a consequence of edge loading, which happens when the head-cup contact patch extends over the cup rim [87]. Underwood et al. [88] highlighted that using hip implants with low clearance, having more conformal contact and so a larger contact patch, increases the risk of edge loading and therefore intense wear.

4. Ceramics

The word ceramics derives from Greek, *keramos*, meaning potter or pottery. Ceramics were defined by Kingery [89] as "the art and science of making and using solid articles, which have, as their essential component, and are composed in large part of, inorganic nonmetallic materials". It is likely to say that a ceramic is whatever material is neither a metal, a semiconductor or a polymer. Ceramics are used to build engineering components when wear resistance, hardness, strength and heat resistance are required. Ceramics were also defined as "the materials of the future", as they are derived from sand that is about 25% of the earth's crust as compared to 1% for all metals [90]. In the lasts decades, ceramic materials have exhibited great appealing and diffusion thanks to their chemical and physical characteristics, attracting the interest of biomedical scientists and companies [91]. Ceramic materials were introduced in the THA more than twenty years ago to overcome the major issue of polyethylene wear [92].

4.1. Alumina

Alumina was introduced in THA implants in 1971, when Boutin realized alumina-on-alumina hip coupling, leading to good clinical results [93,94]. Alumina ceramic has been one of the main ceramics to be used in THA, relying on its good tribological properties, meaning a favorable frictional behavior and a high wear resistance [95]. On the other hand, it has weaker mechanical resistance than other materials. It showed good performances in compression, but weak resistance to tensile stresses [96]. Alumina ceramics have been used in clinical applications for their tribological properties due to their hardness [97]. Among the ceramics, alumina is probably the most commonly used material.

The alumina used for hip replacements was different from the first generation of the material used for industrial applications. In particular, the first generation of alumina showed poor microstructure with low density, scarce purity, and large grain size. This generation of alumina was unsuited for biomedical use. The continuous efforts performed in this field allowed researchers to purify and improve this process, leading to an alumina for medical use, commercially known as Biolox® [21,92]. The ISO 6474 standard, introduced in 1980, aimed to improve the quality of alumina for THA and to decrease the fracture occurrence. Alumina performance is related to different aspects, such as the density, the purity and the grain size. The last one, in particular, influences the wear rate, as it decreases with smaller grain size [92]. In the 90's alumina hip implants were improved with the arrival of Biolox® forte on the market, which could rely on innovations in the production process to furnish much better mechanical characteristics [21,92]. It was realized using improved raw material, with smaller gain size, low level of impurities and sintered in air. Biolox® forte has a density of 3.98 g/cm^3 and grain size of 3.2 m, whereas for Biolox®, these values are 3.96 g/cm^3 and 4.2 m [98].

Recently, concerns have been raised because of some clinical reports on the presence of audible noise in some ceramic-on-ceramic THA patients [99]. The so-called "clicks" or "grinds" have been described after THA, regardless of whether metal-on-polyethylene, metal-on-metal, or ceramic-on-ceramic bearings were used [100]. The "squeak" appears to be limited, however, to hard-bearing couples. It is probably related to implant design or cup orientation and the exact etiology of squeaking is the object of debates; there is neither a specific definition for post-surgery squeaking nor a universal categorization for the sound [101].

4.2. Zirconia

Zirconia has high toughness and good mechanical properties; among all the monolithic ceramics, it has outstanding crack resistance [102]; these are the main reasons that made zirconia a very widespread alternative to alumina for THA. Firsts attempts were focused on magnesia partially stabilized zirconia (MgPSZ), that did not satisfy the wear resistance requirements [103]. Therefore, further developments were focused on yttria stabilizing oxide (Y-TZP), a ceramic that is completely formed by submicron-sized grains, representing the current standard for clinical application [104]. A picture of such a ceramic femoral head is shown in Figure 5.

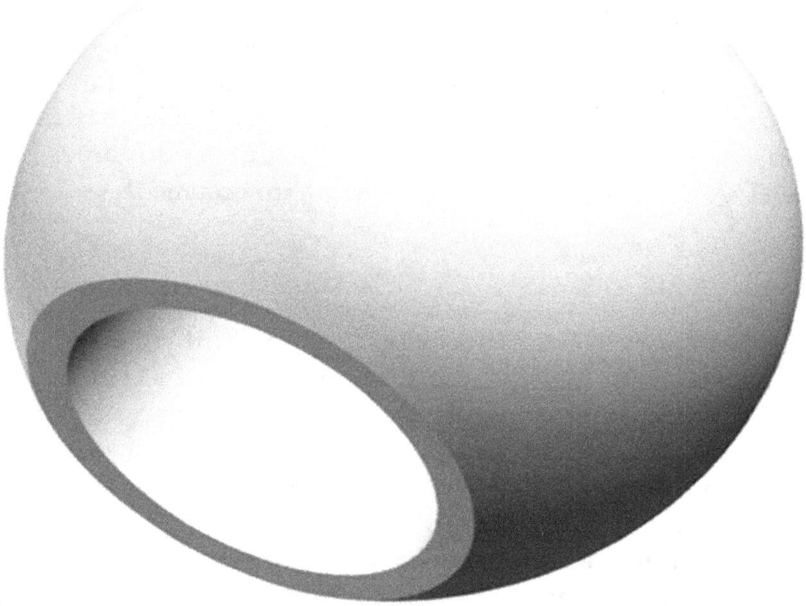

Figure 5. Zirconia femoral head.

Y-TZP is composed of tetragonal grains sized less than 0.5 μm, the faction of which retained at room temperature depends on the size, the distribution and the concentration of the yttria stabilizing oxide [96]. Such microstructural parameters define the mechanical properties of the Y-TZP. The tetragonal grains can transform into monoclinic grains, producing 3–4% volume expansion [105], which is the reason behind the toughness of the ceramic and its ability to dissipate the fracture energy. When a pressure acts on grains, e.g. a crack advancing in the material, they shift to the monoclinic phase, dissipating the crack energy in two ways: the T-M transformation and the volume expansion [106]. There are also metastable tetragonal phase particles, of which formation depends on grain size, stabilizing oxide concentration and matrix constraint. Above 100°C, the metastable particles in a wet environment can spontaneously transform into monoclinic particles [107]. As the transformation progresses, a decrease in material density and in strength and toughness of the ceramic can be observed. The structure of Y-TZP at room temperature is realized by submicron sized grains that grow during the sintering; it is therefore necessary to start from submicron size powders (e.g., 0.02 μm) and to introduce some sintering aid to limit the phenomenon [9].

With respect to metals, Y-TZP shows superior wettability properties that allows for fluid film formation between the articulating surfaces of an implant. Even if in clinical practice the Y-TZP femoral heads were only coupled with UHMWPE cups, tests performed on Y-TZP vs. alumina returned positive results [108]. From the wide investigation campaign on the wear performance of UHMWPE vs. zirconia, there is a general agreement on the fact that the wear is not higher than

UHMWPE vs. alumina [109–111]. Discrepancies in results derive mostly from the differences in the bulk materials used in laboratories, in their finishes, testing procedures etc. There is great concern in the orthopedic community regarding the future of Zirconia as prosthesis. The market has decreased more than 90% between 2001 and 2002 (corresponding with the recall and abandon of Prozyr®, by Saint Gobain) [112]. More than 600000 femoral heads used in Y-TZP have been implanted worldwide, mostly in EU and US. The debate on the Y-TZP future is due to its pros and cons; it exhibits the best mechanical properties (resistance to crack propagation) but is prone to aging in the presence of water.

Zirconia manufacturers tried to shrink this problem, claiming that it was limited under in vivo conditions until 2001 when around 400 femoral heads failed in a short period. This event was related to accelerated ageing affecting two batches of Prozyr® [112]. Even if the reason was identified to be processed controlled, this event led to catastrophic impact on the use of the Y-TZP, pushing some surgeons to go back to other solutions. The ageing problem and the Prozyr® event are still an issue, and further efforts are required to gain confidence from the orthopedic society. In this way, the future seems to be based on the combination of zirconia and alumina to obtain advanced composites.

4.3. Zirconia Toughened Alumina

In the second half of the 1970s, a new class of ceramic-based composite materials developed. This new composite material was realized by introducing up to 25% wt. of zirconia into an alumina matrix; this composite material is known as zirconia toughened alumina (ZTA). The addition of a fraction of zirconia to alumina results in a composite material of increased toughness [109,110,113]. In the 2000s, the first ZTA material introduced in a clinic was a composite known under the trade name of Biolox® Delta [114]. A picture of such a ceramic femoral head is shown in Figure 6.

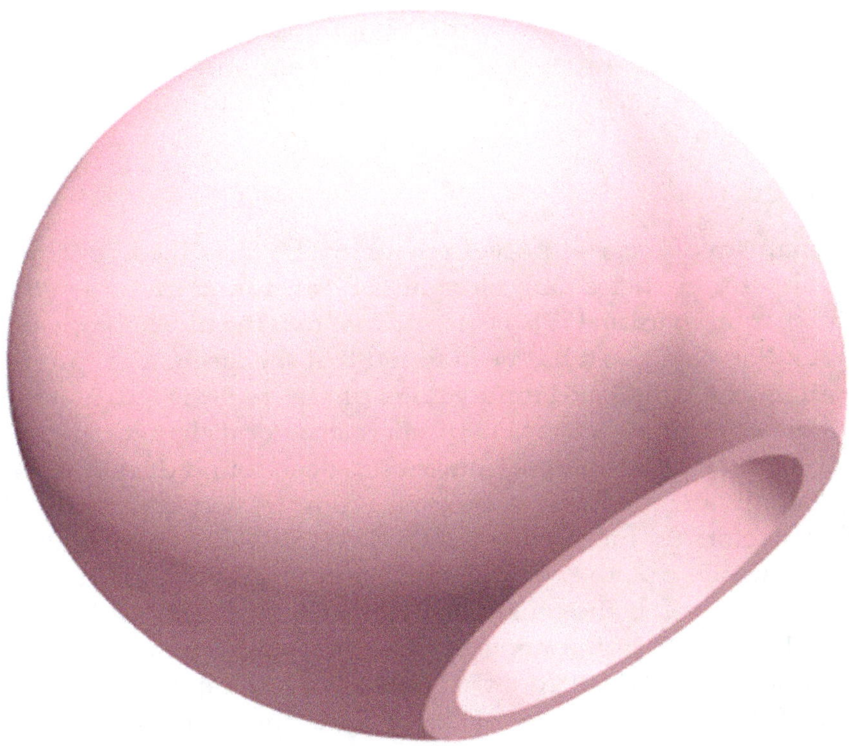

Figure 6. Biolox® Delta femoral head.

This material provides elevate resistance to the onset of cracking and to crack propagation [115,116]. This ZTA composite combines the best characteristics of both alumina and zirconia: the strength and toughness of alumina and the excellent wear resistance, chemical and hydrothermal stability of the alumina. This combination is realized through the uniform distribution of nano-sized particles of yttria-stabilized tetragonal zirconia (Y-TZP) in the alumina matrix. A small percentage of chromium oxide (Cr_2O_3) is added to counterbalance the hardness reduction caused by the zirconia presence. Strontium oxide (SrO) is added to the material, during the sintering process, to form strontium aluminate ($SrAl_{12-x}Cr_xO_{19}$) platelets [117]. These flat and elongated crystals dissipate cracks energy and limit their advance, as it would require extra energy for the crack to overtake the crystal. The final composite is a mixture of roughly 75% alumina, 25% zirconia, and less than 1% chromium oxide and strontium oxide [96]. Deville et al. [118] found that Alumina Y-TZP composites exhibit significant ageing, but this process was far slower than usually observed in Y-TZP ceramics, which is ascribable to the presence of the alumina. On the other side, the presence of zirconia aggregates was recognized as the main cause of ageing sensitivity [119]. Realizing an optimal dispersion at acid pH can avoid the formation of zirconia aggregates, but as soon as the percolation threshold level (16 vol.%) is exceeded, ageing cannot be avoided.

These composites achieve a fracture toughness (K_{IC}) up to 12 $MPa \cdot m^{1/2}$ and a bending strength up to 700 MPa. Due to the different elastic moduli of the two components, cracks will tend to move across the less stiff zirconia particles, inducing their T-M phase transformation that dissipates the crack energy.

5. Wear Behavior

Among the bearing surfaces involved in total hip arthroplasty, the biomaterials are submitted to sliding friction, producing particle debris, which, in turn, initiate an inflammatory reaction ultimately leading to osteolysis [120]. Wear is defined as a cumulative surface damage phenomenon in which material is removed from a body in the form of small particles, primarily by mechanical processes [121]. The wear mechanism is the transfer of energy with removal or displacement of material and in that follows an explanation of the mechanisms of wear observed with different biomaterials.

Pertinent literature was obtained from the Scopus database. The key words "hip joint replacement," "hip prostheses," "in vitro wear," "in vivo wear," and "THA" were searched in various combinations, and results were narrowed based on relevance to this review. Only articles from peer-reviewed journals were included.

5.1. Wear of Polyethylene

The primary mechanism of wear of polyethylene in THA is adhesive/abrasive, leading to the formation of sub-micron sized particles [33]. Elongated fibrils found in retrieved acetabular elements are precursors for this wear mechanism [58]. There is proof that the morphology of UHMWPE changes due to mechanical input. For example, it has been found that the mechanical properties of the polymer are dependent on both its crystalline and amorphous phases wear is led, at a micro-scale, by cyclic plastic deformation of the articulating surface [38]. Microstructural changes are correlated with plastic deformation in UHMWPE, in that lamellar alignment has been found during tests of cyclic tension, as well as decreased crystallinity in monotonic tension and compression specimens taken past yield [122].

There are different factors that influence the UHMWPE wear; some of them are related to the material itself, other are mostly due to the whole implant design. In the first category, is the nature or quality of the powder, as well as the tensile-rupture energy, the manufacturing process and the sterilization procedure. UHMWPE components can be obtained from ram-extruded bars; this process leads to internal inconsistencies or "dead zones". The dead zones can lower the molecular weight and increase the wear rate of the final component [123]. Furthermore, the so-obtained elements tend to have micro-shred on their surface that can cause the third-body wear process. If the component is realized through heat stamping, as the melted outer layer cools, crystallization begins. The differential cooling leads to internal stresses resulting in a final element with anisotropic strength properties, vulnerable to oxidation degradation.

In the adhesion/abrasion wear mechanism, the surface conditions of the femoral head component, in particular its roughness and hardness, are key aspects. The hardness of the head material should be higher than that of the acrylic bone cement. If so, in a cemented arthroplasty, there will be less likely for third-body wear at bearing surfaces. To minimize the UHMWPE wear rate, the counter-body should be very hard and have a low contact angle (less than 70°); further, the head should be as smooth as possible and inert to oxidation.

5.2. Wear of Metals

The dynamic loading these implants undergo, together with the corrosiveness of physiological fluids can enhance the degradation processes. The combined effect of wear and corrosion does not consist of a simple sum of the two but more as a synergy realized between them called tribo-corrosion. Tribo-corrosion is defined as an "irreversible transformation of material in tribological contact caused by simultaneous physicochemical and mechanical surface interactions" [124]. In the last decades, a scaring occurrence of inflammatory reactions has been seen in patients with large head MoM THA, often with signs of tribo-corrosion at the head-neck interface. Tribo-corrosion arises not only at MoM bearing surfaces, but also at metal/metal modular junctions where micro-motions between the two components are possible.

More frequently, the wear of metal bearings can be distinguished in three main processes and their combinations: abrasive wear, due to either two or three bodies, adhesive wear and fatigue wear. However, other types of wear such as corrosive can occur. The corrosion resistance of metals relies on the passive layer formed on their surface in contact with a corrosive environment. Metals react with an oxygen-rich biological environment, realizing a thin protective oxidative coating – generally 2–5 nm thick – that limits corrosion. The oxidative layer forms immediately when exposed to in vivo conditions, but it does not last forever. Regarding the passive metals, wear can break the oxide layer on the surface, accelerating the dissolution of the base metal. The coatings can be scratched or rubbed off when surface contact happens. Even though the oxide layer spontaneously reforms, in restoring the protection of the surface, there is a rise in corrosion currents during the process, which causes the degradation of the material along with the release of metallic ions [125]. Once the film is worn out, the implant can release metal ions and particulates. The presence of these elements realizes third body wear that intensely increases wear rates. This damaging process applied on the coating, and metal ions released, and reformation of new coatings is known as *oxidative wear* [122]. The propensity of the layer to breakdown derives from the difference between the resting and breakdown potential. Regarding the CoCr alloys, the difference is high but corrosion can still happen under certain conditions. However, localized corrosion is not so common in CoCr alloys, which typically fail by trans-passive dissolution [125].

Galvanic corrosion can arise when different metals are in contact with each other, but also when the contact is between the same metal being partly under corrosion and partly under tribo-corrosion conditions. This type of galvanic contact is typical of modular implants, as in the neck-head contact.

Wear particles occurring in MoP implants are within the size range required for phagocytosis by macrophages, which is considered to be a cause of aseptic loosening [126]. On the other hand, particles generated by MoM implants belong to the nanometer scale, which reduces macrophage reaction. Nevertheless, the distribution of these particles within the body can have different biological effects and could be responsible for cytotoxicity, hypersensitivity and eventually carcinogenesis.

Investigations on retrieved 1st and 2nd generation MoM hip prostheses have shown linear penetrations of roughly 5 mm/year, which corresponds to a wear volume of approximately 1 mm^3/year, two orders of magnitude lower than conventional polyethylene acetabular cups. The wear of hard-on-hard articulations such as MoM hip prostheses has two separate stages. Elevated bedding in the wear period occurs during the first million cycles or first year in vivo. Afterwards, a lower steady-state wear period occurs as the bearing surfaces have been subjected to the self-polishing action of the metal wear particles, which may act as a solid-phase lubricant. In vitro investigations, realized by hip simulators, generally show steady-state wear rates to be lower than those reported in vivo. The wear of tested MoM hip prostheses, 1 mm^3/million cycles, is much lower than the more widespread polyethylene-on-metal bearings, 30-100 mm^3/million cycles [19].

Each type of Co-Cr alloy has different characteristics that influence the wear rates of an implant. These properties comprise carbon percentage, manufacturing procedure and surface finishing. High carbon alloys have an initial wear of 0.21 mm^3/million cycles for the cast implants and 0.24 mm^3/million cycles for the wrought implants, whereas, alloys with a low carbon concentration have a significantly greater wear rate of 0.76 mm^3/million cycles. The high percent carbon alloys show superior wear resistance as compared to the low percent carbon alloys with the assumption that there was no additional variation in other parameters.

In the human hip joint, wear can be designated as reciprocating sliding wear, because the contact area is smaller than the stroke of the wear path. Furthermore, the wear paths of the back and forth section of the cycle do not lie on the same geometrical lines, which lead to sliding wear. Even though, in sliding as well as in reciprocating sliding wear, all the other wear process—adhesion, abrasion, surface fatigue and tribochemical reactions—may be present at the same time [127].

5.3. *Wear of Ceramics*

Ceramic-on-ceramic implants have a life expectancy longer than implants with other combinations because of their very low wear rate. This clinical result led to the success of the ceramic implants: since 1990, alumina components were implanted more than 3.5 million times, whereas zirconia elements were used more than 600k times [128]. Nevertheless, ceramic is a brittle material and fractures can happen under adverse circumstances. Fracture probability is low (0.004–0.35% for alumina heads) but does occur [129]. The main causes of head fractures are local stress concentrations that are ascribed to taper interface contamination or damage or to loosening of the head on the taper [130,131].

Affatato et al. [113] tested different ceramic configurations, i.e., pure alumina vs. alumina composite. The wear rate was lower for the pure alumina than for the alumina composites. Still, no statistically significant differences were observed between the wear behaviours of these materials at a 95% level of confidence. In different work, Affatato and co-workers [11] carried out wear tests to compare the tribo-behaviour of different sizes of ceramic components. Two different batches of alumina Biolox® Forte (28 mm vs. 36 mm) were tested on a hip simulator under bovine calf serum for five million cycles. They found that the 36 mm Biolox® forte size showed less weight loss than the 28 mm Biolox® Forte size.

Nevelos et al. [132] studied the behavior of CoC bearings realized with hot isostatically pressed alumina and compared with the standard alumina ones. They found a reduction of the wear rate for the hot-pressed prosthesis when working under standard conditions. Different behavior was observed under Gelofusione® (4% w/v solution of succinylated gelatin) and water lubricants, where the non-hot-pressed ceramic showed a lower wear rate. Even so, the results were significantly affected by uncertainties as testified by the large error bars. It is worth noting that the wear rates reported by the authors, under standard testing conditions, were an order of magnitude lower than the majority of reported clinical wear rates for in vivo ceramic prostheses [133,134].

A summary of the in vitro tests realized on the different combinations of materials is presented in Tables 1 and 2, for soft and hard bearings, respectively.

Table 1. Soft bearings' wear rates found in vitro through simulators.

Soft Bearings	Paired Materials *	Overall Wear Rate (mm^3/Mc)	Ref.
MoP	CoCr—XLPE	6.71 ± 1.03	[135]
	Biolox®Delta—XLPE	2.0 ± 0.3 **	[136]
CoP	CoCrMo—XLPE	4.09 ± 0.64	[137]
	Alumina—XLPE	3.35 ± 0.29	[138]
	Alumina—PE	34	[139]
	ZTA—PE	80	[140]

* all the abbreviations are reported at the end of the manuscript. ** only in this case the unit of measure is mg/Mc.

Table 2. Hard bearings wear rates found *in vitro* through simulators.

Hard Bearings	Paired Materials *	Overall Wear Rate (mm^3/Mc)	Ref.
CoM	CoMplete	0.129 ± 0.096	[141]
	Biolox®Delta - CoCrMo	0.02 ± 0.01	[142]
	Biolox®Delta-CoCrMo	0.87	[28]
CoC	Biolox®Forte-Biolox®Forte	0.052	[28]
	Alumina-Alumina	0.03	[143]
	ATZ-ATZ	0.024	[143]
	ATZ-ATZ	0.06 ± 0.004	[144]
	ZTA-ZTA	0.14 ± 0.10	[144]
	ATZ-ZTA	0.18	[145]
	ATZ-Alumina	0.20	[145]
	Alumina-Alumina	0.74 ± 1.73	[144]
	Biolox®Delta-Biolox®Delta	0.10	[146]
MoM	CoCrMo-CoCrMo	0.60 ± 0.18	[142]
	CoCrMo-CoCrMo	0.11 ± 0.055	[147]

* all the abbreviations are reported at the end of the manuscript.

6. Discussion

Since its first application, THA has evolved in both terms of material and design. After a first experimental phase, that went along many failures, the UHMWPE was established as the most widespread material to be used as acetabular component. The arrival of CoCrMo destabilized its supremacy for a while but the combination of the two resulted in great pairing. Ceramics are the most recent materials introduced in the orthopaedic field, having the best tribological behavior, they rapidly achieved great success. During the 1970s and 1980s, the great majority of hip prostheses in clinical use incorporated a polyethylene acetabular liner bearing against a femoral ball of metal or ceramic. The willing to resolve the issues of hip implants pushed many researchers to study the various combinations of materials and to introduce some variation of their characteristics. These alternatives included highly cross-linked, thermally stabilized polyethylenes against metal, composite ceramics. The latter composites realized with ceramic matrix are the most successful ones.

The biomaterials used in the orthopedic field play a vital role, and their validation through in vitro tests is of paramount importance. The main objective in the field of biomaterials for hip implants is the reduction of failure incidences. We believe that knowledge of wear rate is an important aspect in the pre-clinical validation of prostheses. Wear tests are executed on materials and designs used in prosthetic hip implants to control their final quality and obtain auxiliary knowledge on the tribological processes. Researchers should not forget that other issues still impact the life expectancy of the prostheses, such as the sensitivity of the cup position and edge loading in ceramic bearings. Therefore, several steps forward are required to improve the overall performance of the implants, such as the ability to sustain high demand activities—for young patients—and preserve the bone from retro-acetabular loss.

New implant concepts, such as hip resurfacing and shorter cementless hip stems, are today mostly used in Europe and may also influence the future of hip arthroplasty. Considering that the number of patients who undergo total joint arthroplasty, and consequently revision, is increasing due to an aging population, patients remain the principal players in this process. There is also an increase in the economic health expense, so it is necessary to reduce the number of revisions to reduce these costs. Knowledge of the behavior of individual prostheses in certain clinical conditions may help in this matter. Nowadays there are many prosthetic models on the market and few scientific evidence of good methodological quality to support the use of most of them. Under these conditions, it is difficult to monitor the use of prosthetic devices and ensure the traceability of the patients in the case of adverse events.

Many countries are adopting a registry for post-marketing surveillance in order to collect data on joint prosthetic performance. Registries can be compiled at the international, national or regional level but also locally, such as in hospitals [148]. Through the registers, it is possible to evaluate the effectiveness of an implant, its lifetime and performance for the treatment of specific cases. Registries are an important tool for research; they allow the identification of patients with a certain condition or outcome for prospective observational studies of large size. In this way, the registry can educate the surgeon to select the best type of prosthesis and surgical technique. Consequently, the healthcare resource will be properly used.

7. Conclusions and Future Prospects

The future of total hip replacement should be perceived as a divergent tendency for developed and developing countries. Advances in technology, improved materials and better understanding of natural tissue reactions will certainly result in breakthroughs of implant selection. Due the ageing of the population, the number of joint replacement surgery has increased in the last years [149]. Consequently, also the number of revision surgeries is growing, as the life expectancy of patients is longer than that of prostheses [150,151].

Current trends in prosthesis design emphasise the use of biocompatible materials that are strong enough to withstand the more active lifestyles of many patients, whilst generating minimal wear debris. As the main issue affecting the long term durability of prosthesis is wear and the propagation of wear particles, vast research is currently being undertaken to improve such biomaterials to give an "infinitive prosthesis life". Analysis of component wear is therefore essential for future progress; retrieval analysis of a well-functioning bearing prosthesis could help in improved the biomaterials. Controversy regarding the safety of metal-on-metal bearing surfaces still remains, particularly in relation to metal ion release and potential hypersensitivity reactions [152–154]. Ceramic-ceramic implants have been demonstrated to provide the lowest wear rates in comparison to other material options possible for ceramic-on-ceramic THA [9,98,155]. Trends in material development are also strongly influenced by the desire to improve hip function and stability through the use of increased head diameters [97]. Today, there is a large number of prosthetic models on the market and limited scientific evidence of good methodological quality to support their usage; the expected costs of treatment in a decade perspective amount to a fraction of what they turned out to be. Worldwide, countries should develop strategies to tackle the problem of increasing demand for medical services in a more simplified and inexpensive way, as they may not even be capable of absorbing the technology in the absence of infrastructure, lack of training and know-how. Prevention, i.e., appropriate dietary and lifestyle modifications, may be important to reduce hip implants. In addition, as mentioned above, countries should adopt registries for post-marketing surveillance. Such registries should collect all data on joint prostheses performance in order to evaluate the effectiveness of an implant, its lifetime and performance for the treatment of specific cases. In this way, the registry can educate the surgeon on the best type of prosthesis and surgical technique or to improve preoperative planning [3]. Consequently, the healthcare resource will be properly used. In conclusion, based on the increase in hip implants in young and older patients, the development of new biomaterials correlated with the lower wear-rate, and the systematic collection of limited essential information on the surgery and the definition of a single endpoint, the failure of the system and its replacement, allow us to monitor the device over time after its market introduction. This may help the surgeons to improve the quality life of the patient in the near future.

Acknowledgments: The authors would like to thank Luigi Lena (IRCCS – Istituto Ortopedico Rizzoli, Bologna-Italy) for his help with the original pictures.

Abbreviations

Alumina toughened	ATZ
Ceramic-on-ceramic	CoC
Ceramic-on-metal from	CoMplete
Cross-linked	XLPE
Metal-on-metal	MoM
Metal-on-polyethylene	MoP
Polytetrafluoroethylene	PTFE
Polyetheretherketone	PEEK
Total hip arthroplasty	THA
Ultra-high molecular weight polyethylene	UHMWPE
Zirconia toughened alumina	ZTA

References

1. Learmonth, I.D.; Young, C.; Rorabeck, C. The operation of the century: total hip replacement. *Lancet* **2007**, *370*, 1508–1519. [CrossRef]
2. Aherwar, A.; Singh, A.K.; Patnaik, A. Current and future biocompatibility aspects of biomaterials for hip prosthesis. *AIMS Bioeng.* **2015**, *3*, 23–43. [CrossRef]
3. Affatato, S. *Perspectives in Total Hip Arthroplasty: Advances in Biomaterials and Their Tribological Interactions*; Affatato, S., Ed.; Elsevier Science: Amsterdam, The Netherlands, 2014; ISBN 1782420398.
4. Gomez, P.; Morcuende, J.A. Early attempts at hip arthroplasty-1700s to 1950s. *Iowa Orthop J.* **2005**, *25*, 25–29. [PubMed]
5. Pramanik, S.; Agarwal, A.K.; Rai, K.N. Chronology of Total Hip Joint Replacement and Materials Development. *Trends Biomater. Artif. Organs* **2005**, *19*, 15–26.
6. Knight, S.R.; Aujla, R.; Biswas, S.P. Total Hip Arthroplasty - over 100 years of operative history. *Orthop. Rev. (Pavia)* **2011**, *3*. [CrossRef] [PubMed]
7. Muster, D. Themistocles Gluck, Berlin 1890: A pioneer of multidisciplinary applied research into biomaterials for endoprostheses. *Bull. Hist. Dent.* **1990**, *38*, 3–6. [PubMed]
8. Hernigou, P. Smith-Petersen and early development of hip arthroplasty. *Int. Orthop.* **2014**, *38*, 193–198. [CrossRef] [PubMed]
9. Zivic, F.; Affatato, S.; Trajanovic, M.; Schnabelrauch, M.; Grujovic, N. *Biomaterials in Clinical Practice: Advances in Clinical Research and Medical Devices*; Springer: Berlin, Germany, 2018; ISBN 3319680250.
10. McKee, G.K. Total hip replacement - past, present and future. *Biomaterials* **1982**, *3*, 130–135. [CrossRef]
11. Affatato, S.; Spinelli, M.; Squarzoni, S.; Traina, F.; Toni, A. Mixing and matching in ceramic-on-metal hip arthroplasty: an in-vitro hip simulator study. *J. Biomech.* **2009**, *42*, 2439–2446. [CrossRef]
12. Fisher, J.; Firkins, P.J.; Tipper, J.L.; Ingham, E.; Stone, M.H.; Farrar, R. In-vitro wear performance of contemporary alumina: Alumina bearing couple under anatomically-relevant hip joint simulation. In *Reliability and Long Term Results of Ceramics in Orthopedics*; Toni, A., Willmann, G., Eds.; Thieme Verlag: Stuttgart, Germany, 2001; pp. 1291–1298.
13. Triclot, P. Metal-on-metal: History, state of the art (2010). *Int. Orthop.* **2011**, *2*, 201–206. [CrossRef]
14. Kumar, N.; Arora, G.N.C.; Datta, B. Bearing surfaces in hip replacement - Evolution and likely future. *Med. J. Armed Forces India* **2014**, *70*, 371–376. [CrossRef] [PubMed]
15. Molli, R.G.; Lombardi, A.V.; Berend, K.R.; Adams, J.B.; Sneller, M.A. Metal-on-metal vs Metal-on-improved polyethylene bearings in total hip arthroplasty. *J. Arthroplast.* **2011**, *6*, 8–13. [CrossRef] [PubMed]
16. Topolovec, M.; Cör, A.; Milošev, I. Metal-on-metal vs. metal-on-polyethylene total hip arthroplasty tribological evaluation of retrieved components and periprosthetic tissue. *J. Mech. Behav. Biomed. Mater.* **2014**, *34*, 243–252. [CrossRef] [PubMed]
17. Huang, D.C.T.; Tatman, P.; Mehle, S.; Gioe, T.J. Cumulative revision rate is higher in metal-on-metal THA than metal-on-polyethylene THA: Analysis of survival in a community registry. *Clin. Orthop. Relat. Res.* **2013**, *471*, 1920–1925. [CrossRef] [PubMed]

18. National Joint Registry for England, Wales and Northern Ireland. *11th Annual Report 2014*. 2014. Available online: http://www.njrcentre.org.uk/njrcentre/News-and-Events/NJR-11th-Annual-Report (accessed on 1 February 2019).
19. Fisher, J.; Hu, X.Q.; Stewart, T.D.; Williams, S.; Tipper, J.L.; Ingham, E.; Stone, M.H.; Davies, C.; Hatto, P.; Bolton, J.; Riley, M.; Hardaker, C.; Isaac, G.H.; Berry, G. Wear of surface engineered metal-on-metal hip prostheses. *J. Mater. Sci. Mater. Med.* **2004**, *15*, 225–235. [CrossRef] [PubMed]
20. Hu, D.; Tie, K.; Yang, X.; Tan, Y.; Alaidaros, M.; Chen, L. Comparison of ceramic-on-ceramic to metal-on-polyethylene bearing surfaces in total hip arthroplasty: a meta-analysis of randomized controlled trials. *J. Orthop. Surg. Res.* **2015**, *10*, 22. [CrossRef] [PubMed]
21. Bader, R.; Willmann, G. Ceramic cups for hip endoprostheses. 6: Cup design, inclination and antetorsion angle modify range of motion and impingement. *Biomed. Tech.* **1999**, *44*, 212–219.
22. Henssge, E.J.; Bos, I.; Willman, G. Al2O3 against Al2O3 combination in hip endoprostheses. Histological investigations with semiquantitative grading of revision and autopsy cases and abrasion measures. *J. Mater. Sci. Mater. Med.* **1994**, *5*, 657–661. [CrossRef]
23. Macchi, F.; Willman, G. Allumina Biolox forte: evoluzione, stato dell'arte e affidabilità. *Lo Scalpello* **2001**, *15*, 99–106.
24. Morrison, J.C.; Ward, D.; Bierbaum, B.E.; Nairus, J.; Kuesis, D. Ceramic-on-ceramic bearings in total hip arthroplasty. *Clin. Orthop. Relat. Res.* **2002**, *405*, 158–163. [CrossRef]
25. Barnes, C.L.; DeBoer, D.; Corpe, R.S.; Nambu, S.; Carroll, M.; Timmerman, I. Wear performance of large-diameter differential-hardness hip bearings. *J. Arthroplast.* **2008**, *23*, 56–60. [CrossRef]
26. Sauvé, P.; Mountney, J.; Khan, T.; De Beer, J.; Higgins, B.; Grover, M. Metal ion levels after metal-on-metal Ring total hip replacement: a 30-year follow-up study. *J. Bone Jt. Surg. Br.* **2007**, *89*, 586–590. [CrossRef] [PubMed]
27. Toni, A.; Traina, F.; Stea, S.; Sudanese, A.; Visentin, M.; Bordini, B.; Squarzoni, S. Early diagnosis of ceramic liner fracture. Guidelines based on a twelve-year clinical experience. *J. Bone Jt. Surg. Am.* **2006**, *88* (Suppl. 4), 55–63. [CrossRef]
28. Affatato, S.; Spinelli, M.; Zavalloni, M.; Traina, F.; Carmignato, S.; Toni, A. Ceramic-on-metal for total hip replacement: mixing and matching can lead to high wear. *Artif. Organs* **2010**, *34*, 319–323. [CrossRef] [PubMed]
29. Orishimo, K.F.; Claus, A.M.; Sychterz, C.J.; Engh, C.A. Relationship between polyethylene wear and osteolysis in hips with a second-generation porous-coated cementless cup after seven years of follow-up. *J. Bone Joint Surg. Am.* **2003**, *85-A*, 1095–1099. [CrossRef] [PubMed]
30. Bozic, K.J.; Kurtz, S.M.; Lau, E.; Ong, K.; Vail, T.P.; Berry, D.J. The Epidemiology of Revision Total Hip Arthroplasty in the United States. *J. Bone Jt. Surgery-American Vol.* **2009**, *91*, 128–133. [CrossRef] [PubMed]
31. Ramakrishna, S. *Biomaterials: A Nano Approach*; CRC Press: Boca Raton, FL, USA, 2010.
32. Stauffer, R.N. Ten-year follow-up study of total hip replacement. *J. Bone Jt. Surg. Am.* **1982**, *64*, 983–990. [CrossRef]
33. Sinha, R.K. *Hip Replacement: Current Trends and Controversies*; Marcel Dekker: New York City, NY, USA, 2002.
34. Maguire, J.K.; Coscia, M.F.; Lynch, M.H. Foreign Body Reaction to Polymeric Debris Following Total Hip Arthroplasty. *Clin. Orthop. Relat. Res.* **1987**, *216*, 213–223. [CrossRef]
35. Charnley, J. Tissue reaction to the polytetrafluoroethylene. *Lancet* **1963**, *II*, 1379. [CrossRef]
36. Schreiber, A.; Huggler, A.H.; Dietschi, C.; Jacob, H. Complications After Joint Replacement — Longterm Follow-Up, Clinical Findings, and Biomechanical Research. In *Engineering in Medicine*; Springer: Berlin, Heidelberg, 1976; pp. 187–202.
37. Wroblewski, B.M.; Fleming, P.A.; Siney, P.D. *Charnley Low-Frictional Torque Arthroplasty of the Hip*; Springer: Berlin, Germany, 1999; Volume 81.
38. Sobieraj, M.C.; Rimnac, C.M. Ultra high molecular weight polyethylene: mechanics, morphology, and clinical behavior. *J. Mech. Behav. Biomed. Mater.* **2009**, *2*, 433–443. [CrossRef]
39. *ISO 11542-1:2001-Plastics—Ultra-High-Molecular-Weight Polyethylene (PE-UHMW) Moulding and Extrusion Materials—Part 1: Designation System and Basis for Specifications*; International Organization for Standardization: Geneva, Switzerland, 2001.
40. Harris, W.H. Wear and periprosthetic osteolysis: the problem. *Clin. Orthop. Rel. Res.* **2001**, *393*, 66–70. [CrossRef]

41. Wroblewski, B.M.; Siney, P.D.; Dowson, D.; Collins, S.N. Prospective clinical and joint simulator studies of a new total hip arthroplasty using alumina ceramic heads and cross-linked polyethylene cups. *J. Bone Jt. Surg. Br.* **1996**, *78*, 280–285. [CrossRef] [PubMed]
42. McKellop, H.; Shen, F.; Lu, B.; Campbell, P.; Salovey, R. Development of an extremely wear-resistant ultra high molecular weight polythylene for total hip replacements. *J. Orthop. Res.* **1999**, *17*, 157–167. [CrossRef] [PubMed]
43. Gul, R.M. *Improved UHMWPE for Use in Total Joint Replacement*; Dept. of Materials Science and Engineering, Massachusetts Institute of Technology: Cambridge, MA, USA, 1997.
44. Shen, F.-W.; McKellop, H.A.; Salovey, R. Irradiation of chemically crosslinked ultrahigh molecular weight polyethylene. *J. Polym. Sci. Part B Polym. Phys.* **1996**, *34*, 1063–1077. [CrossRef]
45. Muratoglu, O.K.; Bragdon, C.R. Highly Cross-Linked and Melted UHMWPE. In *UHMWPE Biomaterials Handbook: Ultra High Molecular Weight Polyethylene in Total Joint Replacement and Medical Devices*; Kurtz, S.M., Ed.; William Andrew: Norwich, NY, USA, 2015; ISBN 0323354351.
46. Muratoglu, O.K.; Bragdon, C.R.; O'Connor, D.O.; Jasty, M.; Harris, W.H.; Gul, R.; McGarry, F. Unified wear model for highly crosslinked ultra-high molecular weight polyethylenes (UHMWPE). *Biomaterials* **1999**, *20*, 1463–1470. [CrossRef]
47. Harris, W.H.; Muratoglu, O.K. A Review of Current Cross-linked Polyethylenes Used in Total Joint Arthroplasty. *Clin. Orthop. Relat. Res.* **2005**, *430*, 46–52. [CrossRef]
48. Burnett, S.J.; Abos, D. Total hip arthroplasty: Techniques and results. *BB Med. J.* **2010**, *52*, 455–464.
49. Oral, E.; Ghali, B.W.; Muratoglu, O.K. The elimination of free radicals in irradiated UHMWPEs with and without vitamin e stabilization by annealing under pressure. *J. Biomed. Mater. Res. Part B Appl. Biomater.* **2011**, *97 B*, 167–174. [CrossRef]
50. Puppulin, L.; Miura, Y.; Casagrande, E.; Hasegawa, M.; Marunaka, Y.; Tone, S.; Sudo, A.; Pezzotti, G. Validation of a protocol based on Raman and infrared spectroscopies to nondestructively estimate the oxidative degradation of UHMWPE used in total joint arthroplasty. *Acta Biomater.* **2016**, *38*, 168–178. [CrossRef]
51. Muratoglu, O.K.; Wannomae, K.K.; Rowell, S.L.; Micheli, B.R.; Malchau, H. Ex Vivo Stability Loss of Irradiated and Melted Ultra-High Molecular Weight Polyethylene. *JBJS* **2010**, *92*, 2809–2816. [CrossRef]
52. Reinitz, S.D.; Currier, B.H.; Levine, R.A.; Van Citters, D.W. Crosslink density, oxidation and chain scission in retrieved, highly cross-linked UHMWPE tibial bearings. *Biomaterials* **2014**, *35*, 4436–4440. [CrossRef] [PubMed]
53. Currier, B.H.; Currier, J.H.; Mayor, M.B.; Lyford, K.A.; Van Citters, D.W.; Collier, J.P. In Vivo Oxidation of γ-Barrier–Sterilized Ultra–High-Molecular-Weight Polyethylene Bearings. *J. Arthroplast.* **2007**, *22*, 721–731. [CrossRef] [PubMed]
54. Kim, Y.-H.; Park, J.-W.; Kim, J.-S. Alumina Delta-on-Highly Crosslinked-Remelted Polyethylene Bearing in Cementless Total Hip Arthroplasty in Patients Younger than 50 Years. *J. Arthroplast.* **2016**, *31*, 2800–2804. [CrossRef] [PubMed]
55. Takada, R.; Jinno, T.; Koga, D.; Miyatake, K.; Muneta, T.; Okawa, A. Comparison of wear rate and osteolysis between second-generation annealed and first-generation remelted highly cross-linked polyethylene in total hip arthroplasty. A case control study at a minimum of five years. *Orthop. Traumatol. Surg. Res.* **2017**, *103*, 537–541. [CrossRef] [PubMed]
56. D'Antonio, J.A.; Capello, W.N.; Ramakrishnan, R. Second-generation annealed highly cross-linked polyethylene exhibits low wear. *Clin. Orthop. Relat. Res.* **2012**, *470*, 1696–1704. [CrossRef] [PubMed]
57. Bhateja, S.K. Radiation-induced crystallinity changes in linear polyethylene: Influence of aging. *J. Appl. Polym. Sci.* **1983**, *28*, 861–872. [CrossRef]
58. Muratoglu, O.K.; Bragdon, C.R.; O'Connor, D.O.; Skehan, H.; Delany, J.; Jasty, M.; Harris, W.H. The Effect Of Temperature On Radiation Crosslinking Of Uhmwpe For Use In Total Hip Arthroplasty. In *46th Annual Meeting*; Orthopaedic Research Society: Orlando, FL, USA, 2000.
59. Oral, E.; Beckos, C.G.; Muratoglu, O.K. Free Radical Elimination In Irradiated Uhmwpe Through Crystal Mobility In Phase Transition To The Hexagonal Phase. *Polymer (Guildf)* **2008**, *49*, 4733–4739. [CrossRef]
60. Bracco, P.; Bellare, A.; Bistolfi, A.; Affatato, S. Ultra-High Molecular Weight Polyethylene: Influence of the Chemical, Physical and Mechanical Properties. *Materials (Basel)* **2017**, *10*, 791. [CrossRef]

61. Deng, M.; Shalaby, S.W. Properties of self-reinforced ultra-high-molecular-weight polyethylene composites. *Biomaterials* **1997**, *18*, 645–655. [CrossRef]
62. Dolezel, B.; Adamirova, L. Method of hygienically safe stabilization of polyolefines against thermoxidative and photooxidative degradation. *Czechoslovakian Social. Repub.* **1982**, *221*, 403.
63. Brach del Prever, E.M.; Camino, G.; Costa, L.; Crova, M.; Dallera, A.; Gallianro, P. Impianto Protesico Contenente un Componente di Materiale Plastico. Italian Patent 1271590, May 1994.
64. Bracco, P.; Oral, E. Vitamin E-stabilized UHMWPE for Total Joint Implants: A Review. *Clin. Orthop. Relat. Res.* **2011**, *469*, 2286–2293. [CrossRef] [PubMed]
65. Affatato, S.; De Mattia, J.S.; Bracco, P.; Pavoni, E.; Taddei, P. Wear performance of neat and vitamin E blended highly cross-linked PE under severe conditions: The combined effect of accelerated ageing and third body particles during wear test. *J. Mech. Behav. Biomed. Mater.* **2016**, *64*, 240–252. [CrossRef] [PubMed]
66. Kurtz, S.; Bracco, P.; Costa, L. Vitamin-e-Blended UHMWPE Biomaterials. In *UHMWPE Biomaterials Handbook*; Elsevier: Amsterdam, The Netherlands, 2009; pp. 237–247, ISBN 9780123747211.
67. Oral, E.; Rowell, S.L.; Muratoglu, O.K. The effect of α-tocopherol on the oxidation and free radical decay in irradiated UHMWPE. *Biomaterials* **2006**, *27*, 5580–5587. [CrossRef] [PubMed]
68. Oral, E.; Wannomae, K.K.; Hawkins, N.; Harris, W.H.W.H.; Muratoglu, O.K.O.K. α-Tocopherol-doped irradiated UHMWPE for high fatigue resistance and low wear. *Biomaterials* **2004**, *25*, 5515–5522. [CrossRef] [PubMed]
69. Kurtz, S.M.; Bracco, P.; Costa, L.; Oral, E.; Muratoglu, O.K. Vitamin E-Blended UHMWPE Biomaterilas. In *UHMWPE Biomaterials Handbook: Ultra High Molecular Weight Polyethylene in Total Joint Replacement and Medical Devices*; Kurtz, S.M., Ed.; Elsevier: Norwich, NY, USA, 2015; p. 840, ISBN 0323354351.
70. Anguiano-Sanchez, J.; Martinez-Romero, O.; Siller, H.R.; Diaz-Elizondo, J.A.; Flores-Villalba, E.; Rodriguez, C.A. Influence of PEEK Coating on Hip Implant Stress Shielding: A Finite Element Analysis. *Comput. Math. Methods Med.* **2016**, *2016*, 6183679. [CrossRef]
71. Cowie, R.M.; Briscoe, A.; Fisher, J.; Jennings, L.M. PEEK-OPTIMA ™ as an alternative to cobalt chrome in the femoral component of total knee replacement: A preliminary study. *Proc. Inst. Mech. Eng. Part H J. Eng. Med.* **2016**, *230*, 1008–1015. [CrossRef]
72. Kurtz, S.; Devine, J.N. PEEK biomaterials in trauma, orthopedic, and spinal implants. *Biomaterials* **2007**, *28*, 4845–4869. [CrossRef]
73. Kurtz, S. *PEEK Biomaterials Handbook*; Elsevier: Amsterdam, The Netherlands, 2012; ISBN 9781437744637.
74. Wang, A.; Lin, R.; Polineni, V.K.; Essner, A.; Stark, C.; Dumbleton, J.H. Carbon fiber reinforced polyether ether ketone composite as a bearing surface for total hip replacement. *Tribol. Int.* **1998**, *31*, 661–667. [CrossRef]
75. Grupp, T.M.; Utzschneider, S.; Schröder, C.; Schwiesau, J.; Fritz, B.; Maas, A.; Blömer, W.; Jansson, V. Biotribology of alternative bearing materials for unicompartmental knee arthroplasty. *Acta Biomater.* **2010**, *6*, 3601–3610. [CrossRef]
76. Brockett, C.L.; Carbone, S.; Abdelgaied, A.; Fisher, J.; Jennings, L.M. Influence of contact pressure, cross-shear and counterface material on the wear of PEEK and CFR-PEEK for orthopaedic applications. *J. Mech. Behav. Biomed. Mater.* **2016**, *63*, 10–16. [CrossRef] [PubMed]
77. Affatato, S.; Traina, F.; Ruggeri, O.; Toni, A. Wear of metal-on-metal hip bearings: Metallurgical considerations after hip simulator studies. *Int. J. Artif. Organs* **2011**, *34*, 1155–1164. [CrossRef]
78. Ihaddadene, R.; Affatato, S.; Zavalloni, M.; Bouzid, S.; Viceconti, M. Carbon composition effects on wear behaviour and wear mechanisms of metal-on-metal hip prosthesis. *Comput. Methods Biomech. Biomed. Engin.* **2011**, *14*, 33–34. [CrossRef]
79. Davis, J.R. *ASM Specialty Handbook: Nickel, Cobalt, and Their Alloys*; ASM International: Almere, The Netherlands, 2000; ISBN 978-0-87170-685-0.
80. Clemow, A.J.T.; Daniell, B.L. Solution treatment behavior of Co-Cr-Mo alloy. *J. Biomed. Mater. Res.* **1979**, *13*, 265–279. [CrossRef]
81. Delaunay, C.; Petit, I.; Learmonth, I.D.; Oger, P.; Vendittoli, P.A. Metal-on-metal bearings total hip arthroplasty: The cobalt and chromium ions release concern. *Orthop. Traumatol. Surg. Res.* **2010**, *96*, 894–904. [CrossRef]
82. Brodner, W.; Bitzan, P.; Meisinger, V.; Kaider, A.; Gottsauner-Wolf, F.; Kotz, R. Elevated serum cobalt with metal-on-metal articulating surfaces. *J. Bone Jt. Surg. Br.* **1997**, *79*, 316–321. [CrossRef] [PubMed]

83. Hallab, N.J.; Anderson, S.; Stafford, T.; Glant, T.; Jacobs, J.J. Lymphocyte responses in patients with total hip arthroplasty. *J. Orthop. Res.* **2005**, *23*, 384–391. [CrossRef] [PubMed]
84. Jacobs, J.J.; Hallab, N.J.; Skipor, A.K.; Urban, R.M. Metal degradation products: a cause for concern in metal-metal bearings? *Clin. Orthop. Relat. Res.* **2003**, *417*, 139–147. [CrossRef]
85. Yang, X.; Hutchinson, C.R. Corrosion-wear of β-Ti alloy TMZF (Ti-12Mo-6Zr-2Fe) in simulated body fluid. *Acta Biomater.* **2016**, *42*, 429–439. [CrossRef]
86. Good, V.; Ries, M.; Barrack, R.L.; Widding, K.; Hunter, G.; Heuer, D. Reduced Wear With Oxidized Zirconium Femoral Heads. *J. Bone Jt. Surgery-american Vol.* **2003**, *85*, 105–110. [CrossRef]
87. Langton, D.J.; Jameson, S.S.; Joyce, T.J.; Hallab, N.J.; Natu, S.; Nargol, A.V.F. Early failure of metal-on-metal bearings in hip resurfacing and large-diameter total hip replacement. *J. Bone Jt. Surg. Br.* **2010**, *92-B*, 38–46. [CrossRef]
88. Underwood, R.J.; Zografos, A.; Sayles, R.S.; Hart, A.; Cann, P. Edge loading in metal-on-metal hips: low clearance is a new risk factor. *Proc. Inst. Mech. Eng. H* **2012**, *226*, 217–226. [CrossRef]
89. Kingery, W.D. *Introduction to Ceramics*; John Wiley: Hoboken, NJ, USA, 2016; ISBN 047155460X.
90. Hsu, S.M.; Shen, M.C. Ceramic Wear Maps. *Wear* **1996**, *200*, 154–175. [CrossRef]
91. Cuckler, J.M.; Bearcroft, J.; Asgian, C.M. Femoral head technologies to reduce polyethylene wear in total hip arthroplasty. *Clin. Orthop. Relat. Res.* **1995**, *317*, 57–63.
92. Willman, G. Ceramics for total hip replacement - what a surgeon should know. *Orthopedics* **1998**, *21*, 173–177.
93. Boutin, P. [Alumina and its use in surgery of the hip. (Experimental study)]. *Press. Med.* **1971**, *79*, 639–640.
94. Boutin, P.; Blanquaert, D. A study of the mechanical properties of alumina-on-alumina total hip prosthesis. *Rev. Chir. Orthop. Reparatrice Appar. Mot.* **1981**, *67*, 279–287.
95. Hamadouche, M.; Sedel, L. Ceramics in orthopaedics. *J. Bone Jt. Surg. Br.* **2000**, *82*, 1095–1099. [CrossRef]
96. Piconi, C.; Maccauro, G.; Muratori, F.; Branch Del Prever, E. Alumina and zirconia ceramics in joint replacements. *JABB* **2003**, *1*, 19–32.
97. Affatato, S.; Ruggiero, A.; Merola, M. Advanced biomaterials in hip joint arthroplasty. A review on polymer and ceramics composites as alternative bearings. *Compos. Part B Eng.* **2015**, *83*, 276–283. [CrossRef]
98. Affatato, S.; Jaber, S.A.; Taddei, P. Ceramics for hip joint replacement. In *Biomaterials in Clinical Practice*; Zivic, F., Ed.; Springer: Berlin, Germany, 2017.
99. Affatato, S.; Traina, F.; Mazzega-Fabbro, C.; Sergo, V.; Viceconti, M. Is ceramic-on-ceramic squeaking phenomenon reproducible in vitro? A long-term simulator study under severe conditions. *J. Biomed Mater Res. B Appl. Biomater* **2009**, *91*, 264–271. [CrossRef]
100. Jacobs, B.C.A.; Greenwald, A.S.; Oxon, D.; Anderson, P.A.; Matthew, J.; Mihalko, W.M. *Squeaky Hips Make Media, Medical Noise*; American Academy of Orthopaedic Surgeons: Rosemont, IL, USA, 2008.
101. Wu, G.L.; Zhu, W.; Zhao, Y.; Ma, Q.; Weng, X.S. Hip squeaking after ceramic-on-ceramic total hip arthroplasty. *Chin. Med. J. (Engl.)* **2016**, *129*, 1861–1866. [CrossRef]
102. De Aza, A.H.; Chevalier, J.; Fantozzi, G.; Schehl, M.; Torrecillas, R. Crack growth resistance of alumina, zirconia and zirconia toughened alumina ceramics for joint prostheses. *Biomaterials* **2002**, *23*, 937–945. [CrossRef]
103. Rahaman, M.N.; Yao, A.; Bal, B.S.; Garino, J.P.; Ries, M.D. Ceramics for Prosthetic Hip and Knee Joint Replacement. *J. Am. Ceram. Soc.* **2007**, *90*, 1965–1988. [CrossRef]
104. Kelly, J.R.; Denry, I. Stabilized zirconia as a structural ceramic: An overview. *Dent. Mater.* **2008**, *24*, 289–298. [CrossRef]
105. VanValzah, J.R.; Eaton, H.E. Cooling rate effects on the tetragonal to monoclinic phase transformation in aged plasma-sprayed yttria partially stabilized zirconia. *Surf. Coat. Technol.* **1991**, *46*, 289–300. [CrossRef]
106. Platt, P.; Frankel, P.; Gass, M.; Howells, R.; Preuss, M. Finite element analysis of the tetragonal to monoclinic phase transformation during oxidation of zirconium alloys. *J. Nucl. Mater.* **2014**, *454*, 290–297. [CrossRef]
107. Maccauro, G.; Rossi Iommetti, P.; Raffaelli, L.; Manicone, P.F. Alumina and Zirconia Ceramic for Orthopaedic and Dental Devices. In *Biomaterials Applications for Nanomedicine*; Pignatello, R., Ed.; InTech: London, UK, 2011; Volume 3, p. 485, ISBN 9533076615.
108. Pitto, R.P.; Blanquaert, D.; Hohmann, D. Alternative bearing surfaces in total hip arthroplasty: Zirconia-alumina pairing. Contribution or caveat? *Acta Orthop. Belg.* **2002**, *68*, 242–250.
109. Affatato, S.; Testoni, M.; Cacciari, G.L.; Toni, A. Mixed oxides prosthetic ceramic ball heads. Part 2: effect of the ZrO2 fraction on the wear of ceramic on ceramic joints. *Biomaterials* **1999**, *20*, 971–975. [CrossRef]

110. Affatato, S.; Goldoni, M.; Testoni, M.; Toni, A. Mixed oxides prosthetic ceramic ball heads. Part 3: Effect of the ZrO2 fraction on the wear of ceramic on ceramic hip joint prostheses. A long-term in vitro wear study. *Biomaterials* **2001**, *22*, 717–723. [CrossRef]
111. Piconi, C.; Burger, W.; Richter, H.G.; Cittadini, A.; Maccauro, G.; Covacci, V.; Bruzzese, N.; Ricci, G.A.; Marmo, E. Y-TZP ceramics for artificial joint replacements. *Biomaterials* **1998**, *19*, 1489–1494. [CrossRef]
112. Chevalier, J. What future for zirconia as a biomaterial? *Biomaterials* **2006**, *27*, 535–543. [CrossRef]
113. Affatato, S.; Torrecillas, R.; Taddei, P.; Rocchi, M.; Fagnano, C.; Ciapetti, G.; Toni, A. Advanced nanocomposite materials for orthopaedic applications. I. A long-term in vitro wear study of zirconia-toughened alumina. *J. Biomed. Mater. Res. Part B Appl. Biomater.* **2006**, *78*, 76–82. [CrossRef]
114. Gadow, R.; Kern, F. Novel zirconia-alumina nanocomposites combining high strength and toughness. In *Advanced Engineering Materials*; John Wiley & Sons: Hoboken, NJ, USA, 2010; Volume 12, pp. 1220–1223.
115. Dickinson, A.; Browne, M.; Jeffers, J.; Taylor, A. Development of a Ceramic Acetabular Cup Design for Improved in vivo Stability and Integrity. In *BIOLOX Symposium*; Sprimger: Edinburgh, UK, 2009; Volume 13, p. 227.
116. Merkert, P. Next generation ceramic bearings. In *Bioceramics in Joint Arthroplasty*; Springer: Berlin, Germany, 2003; pp. 123–125.
117. Affatato, S.; Modena, E.; Toni, A.; Taddei, P. Retrieval analysis of three generations of Biolox®femoral heads: Spectroscopic and SEM characterisation. *J. Mech. Behav. Biomed. Mater.* **2012**, *13*, 118–128. [CrossRef]
118. Deville, S.; Chevalier, J.; Fantozzi, G.; Bartolomé, J.F.; Requena, J.; Moya, J.S.; Torrecillas, R.; Díaz, L.A. Low-temperature ageing of zirconia-toughened alumina ceramics and its implication in biomedical implants. *J. Eur. Ceram. Soc.* **2003**, *23*, 2975–2982. [CrossRef]
119. Gutknecht, D.; Chevalier, J.; Garnier, V.; Fantozzi, G. Key role of processing to avoid low temperature ageing in alumina zirconia composites for orthopaedic application. *J. Eur. Ceram. Soc.* **2007**, *27*, 1547–1552. [CrossRef]
120. Massin, P.; Achour, S. Wear products of total hip arthroplasty: The case of polyethylene Produits d ' usure des arthroplasties totales de hanche: le cas du polyéthylène. *Morphologie* **2017**, *101*, 1–8. [CrossRef]
121. Guy, R.; Nockolds, C.; Phillips, M.; Roques-Carmes, C. Implications of Polishing Techniques in Quantitative X-Ray Microanalysis. *J. Res. Natl. Inst. Stand. Technol.* **2002**, *107*, 639–662.
122. Butler, M.F.; Donald, A.M.; Ryan, A.J. Time resolved simultaneous small- and wide-angle x-ray scattering during polyethylene deformation-II. Cold drawing of linear polyethylene. *Polymer1* **1998**, *39*, 781–792. [CrossRef]
123. Lewis, G. Polyethylene wear in total hip and knee arthroplasties. *J. Biomed. Mater. Res.* **1997**, *38*, 55–75. [CrossRef]
124. Landolt, D.; Mischler, S.; Stemp, M. Electrochemical methods in tribocorrosion: A critical appraisal. *Electrochim. Acta* **2001**, *46*, 3913–3929. [CrossRef]
125. Hodgson, A.W.E.; Kurz, S.; Virtanen, S.; Fervel, V.; Olsson, C.-O.A.; Mischler, S. Passive and transpassive behaviour of CoCrMo in simulated biological solutions. *Electrochim. Acta* **2004**, *49*, 2167–2178. [CrossRef]
126. Suñer, S.; Tipper, J.L.; Emami, N. Biological effects of wear particles generated in total joint replacements: trends and future prospects. *Tribol. Mater. Surfaces Interfaces* **2012**, *6*, 39–52. [CrossRef]
127. *StanDIN 50320 Wear; Terms, Systematic Analysis of Wear Processes, Classification of Wear Phenomenadards*; Beuth-Verlag: Berlin, Germany, 1979.
128. Chevalier, J.; Taddei, P.; Gremillard, L.; Deville, S.; Fantozzi, G.; Bartolomé, J.F.; Pecharroman, C.; Moya, J.S.; Diaz, L.A.; Torrecillas, R.; Affatato, S. Reliability assessment in advanced nanocomposite materials for orthopaedic applications. *J. Mech. Behav. Biomed. Mater.* **2011**, *4*, 303–314. [CrossRef]
129. Garino, J.P. Ceramic component fracture: trends and recommendations with modern components based on improved reporting methods. In *Bioceramics and Alternative Bearings in Joint Arthroplasty: Proceedings*; D'Antonio, J.A., Dietrich, M., Eds.; Steinkopff: Heidelberg, Germany, 2005; p. 218, ISBN 3798515409.
130. Weisse, B.; Affolter, C.; Stutz, A.; Terrasi, G.P.; Köbel, S.; Weber, W. Influence of contaminants in the stem—ball interface on the static fracture load of ceramic hip joint ball heads. *Proc. Inst. Mech. Eng. Part H J. Eng. Med.* **2008**, *222*, 829–835. [CrossRef]
131. Rehmer, A.; Bishop, N.E.; Morlock, M.M. Influence of assembly procedure and material combination on the strength of the taper connection at the head-neck junction of modular hip endoprostheses. *Clin. Biomech. (Bristol, Avon)* **2012**, *27*, 77–83. [CrossRef]

132. Nevelos, J.E.; Ingham, E.; Doyle, C.; Nevelos, A.B.; Fisher, J. Wear of HIPed and non-HIPed alumina-alumina hip joints under standard and severe simulator testing conditions. *Biomaterials* **2001**, *22*, 2191–2197. [CrossRef]
133. Dorlot, J.-M.; Christel, P.; Meunier, A. Wear analysis of retrieved alumina heads and sockets of hip prostheses. *J. Biomed. Mater. Res.* **1989**, *23*, 299–310. [CrossRef]
134. Mittelmeier, H.; Heisel, J. Sixteen-years' Experience With Ceramic Hip Prostheses. *Clin. Orthop. Relat. Res.* **1992**, *282*, 64–72. [CrossRef]
135. Brandt, J.-M.; Vecherya, A.; Guenther, L.E.; Koval, S.F.; Petrak, M.J.; Bohm, E.R.; Wyss, U.P. Wear testing of crosslinked polyethylene: Wear rate variability and microbial contamination. *J. Mech. Behav. Biomed. Mater.* **2014**, *34*, 208–216. [CrossRef]
136. Grupp, T.M.; Holderied, M.; Mulliez, M.A.; Streller, R.; Jäger, M.; Blömer, W.; Utzschneider, S. Biotribology of a vitamin E-stabilized polyethylene for hip arthroplasty—Influence of artificial ageing and third-body particles on wear. *Acta Biomater.* **2014**, *10*, 3068–3078. [CrossRef]
137. Moro, T.; Takatori, Y.; Kyomoto, M.; Ishihara, K.; Kawaguchi, H.; Hashimoto, M.; Tanaka, T.; Oshima, H.; Tanaka, S. Wear resistance of the biocompatible phospholipid polymer-grafted highly cross-linked polyethylene liner against larger femoral head. *J. Orthop. Res.* **2015**, *33*, 1103–1110. [CrossRef]
138. Zietz, C.; Fabry, C.; Baum, F.; Bader, R.; Kluess, D. The Divergence of Wear Propagation and Stress at Steep Acetabular Cup Positions Using Ceramic Heads and Sequentially Cross-Linked Polyethylene Liners. *J. Arthroplast.* **2015**, *30*, 1458–1463. [CrossRef]
139. Gremillard, L.; Martin, L.; Zych, L.; Crosnier, E.; Chevalier, J.; Charbouillot, A.; Sainsot, P.; Espinouse, J.; Aurelle, J.-L. Combining ageing and wear to assess the durability of zirconia-based ceramic heads for total hip arthroplasty. *Acta Biomater.* **2013**, *9*, 7545–7555. [CrossRef]
140. Reinders, J.; Sonntag, R.; Heisel, C.; Reiner, T.; Vot, L.; Kretzer, J.P. Wear performance of ceramic-on-metal hip bearings. *PLoS ONE* **2013**, *8*, e73252. [CrossRef]
141. Williams, S.; Al-Hajjar, M.; Isaac, G.H.; Fisher, J. Comparison of ceramic-on-metal and metal-on-metal hip prostheses under adverse conditions. *J. Biomed. Mater. Res. Part B Appl. Biomater.* **2013**, *101B*, 770–775. [CrossRef]
142. Halma, J.J.; Señaris, J.; Delfosse, D.; Lerf, R.; Oberbach, T.; van Gaalen, S.M.; de Gast, A. Edge loading does not increase wear rates of ceramic-on-ceramic and metal-on-polyethylene articulations. *J. Biomed. Mater. Res. Part B Appl. Biomater.* **2014**, *102*, 1627–1638. [CrossRef]
143. Al-Hajjar, M.; Jennings, L.M.; Begand, S.; Oberbach, T.; Delfosse, D.; Fisher, J. Wear of novel ceramic-on-ceramic bearings under adverse and clinically relevant hip simulator conditions. *J. Biomed. Mater. Res. Part B Appl. Biomater.* **2013**, *101*, 1456–1462. [CrossRef]
144. Al-Hajjar, M.; Carbone, S.; Jennings, L.M.; Begand, S.; Oberbach, T.; Delfosse, D.; Fisher, J. Wear of composite ceramics in mixed-material combinations in total hip replacement under adverse edge loading conditions. *J. Biomed. Mater. Res. Part B Appl. Biomater.* **2017**, *105*, 1361–1368. [CrossRef]
145. Al-Hajjar, M.; Fisher, J.; Tipper, J.L.; Williams, S.; Jennings, L.M. Wear of 36-mm BIOLOX ® delta ceramic-on-ceramic bearing in total hip replacements under edge loading conditions. *Proc. Inst. Mech. Eng. Part H J. Eng. Med.* **2013**, *227*, 535–542. [CrossRef]
146. Chan, F.W.; Bobyn, J.D.; Medley, J.B.; Krygier, J.J.; Tanzer, M. The Otto Aufranc Award. Wear and lubrication of metal-on-metal hip implants. *Clin. Orthop. Relat. Res.* **1999**, 10–24. [CrossRef]
147. RIPO Annual Report 2016. 2018. Available online: https://www.riotinto.com/documents/RT_2016_Annual_report.pdf (accessed on 1 February 2019).
148. Mayor, S. Registry data show increase in joint replacement surgery. *BMJ* **2017**, *358*, 1. [CrossRef]
149. Kurtz, S.; Ong, K.L.; Schmier, J.; Mowat, F.; Saleh, K.; Dybvik, E.; Kärrholm, J.; Garellick, G.; Havelin, L.I.; Furnes, O.; Malchau, H.; Lau, E. Future clinical and economic impact of revision total hip and knee arthroplasty. *J. Bone Joint Surg. Am.* **2007**, *89*, 144–151. [CrossRef]
150. Kurtz, S.; Ong, K.; Lau, E.; Mowat, F.; Halpern, M. Projections of primary and revision hip and knee arthroplasty in the United States from 2005 to 2030. *J. Bone Jt. Surg Am* **2007**, *89*, 780–785. [CrossRef]
151. Rajeshshyam, R.; Chockalingam, K.; Gayathri, V.; Prakash, T. Reduction of metallosis in hip implant using thin film coating. In *AIP Conference Proceedings*; AIP Publishing LLC: Melville, NY, USA, 2018; Volume 1943, p. 020090.

152. Bijukumar, D.R.; Segu, A.; Souza, J.C.M.; Li, X.; Barba, M.; Mercuri, L.G.; Jacobs, J.J.; Mathew, M.T. Systemic and local toxicity of metal debris released from hip prostheses: A review of experimental approaches. *Nanomed. Nanotechnol. Biol. Med.* **2018**, *14*, 951–963. [CrossRef]
153. Neuwirth, A.L.; Ashley, B.S.; Hardaker, W.M.; Sheth, N.P. Metal-on-Metal Hip Implants: Progress and Problems. In *Biomedical Applications of Metals*; Springer International Publishing: Cham, Switzerland, 2018; pp. 73–93.
154. Abdel Jaber, S.; Affatato, S. *An overview of In Vitro Mechanical and Structural Characterization of Hip Prosthesis Components*; Springer: Berlin, Germany, 2017; ISBN 9783319680255.
155. Lee, J.-M. The Current Concepts of Total Hip Arthroplasty. *Hip Pelvis* **2016**, *28*, 191–200. [CrossRef]

15

Development of a Novel in Silico Model to Investigate the Influence of Radial Clearance on the Acetabular Cup Contact Pressure in Hip Implants

Saverio Affatato [1,*], Massimiliano Merola [1] and Alessandro Ruggiero [2]

1 Laboratorio di Tecnologia Medica, IRCCS—Istituto Ortopedico Rizzoli, 40136 Bologna, Italy; massimiliano.merola@ior.it
2 Department of Industrial Engineering, University of Salerno, 84084 Salerno, Italy; ruggiero@unisa.it
* Correspondence: affatato@tecno.ior.it

Abstract: A hip joint replacement is considered one of the most successful orthopedic surgical procedures although it involves challenges that must be overcome. The patient group undergoing total hip arthroplasty now includes younger and more active patients who require a broad range of motion and a longer service lifetime of the implant. The current replacement joint results are not fully satisfactory for these patients' demands. As particle release is one of the main issues, pre-clinical experimental wear testing of total hip replacement components is an invaluable tool for evaluating new implant designs and materials. The aim of the study was to investigate the cup tensional state by varying the clearance between head and cup. For doing this we use a novel hard-on-soft finite element model with kinematic and dynamic conditions calculated from a musculoskeletal multibody model during the gait. Four different usual radial clearances were considered, ranging from 0 to 0.5 mm. The results showed that radial clearance plays a key role in acetabular cup stress-strain during the gait, showing from the 0 value to the highest, 0.5, a difference of 44% and 35% in terms of maximum pressure and deformation, respectively. Moreover, the presented model could be usefully exploited for complete elastohydrodynamic synovial lubrication modelling of the joint, with the aim of moving towards an increasingly realistic total hip arthroplasty in silico wear assessment accounting for differences in radial clearances.

Keywords: finite element analysis; total hip arthroplasty; UHMWPE; musculoskeletal multibody model; tribology

---

1. Introduction

Total hip replacement (THR) is the most successful application of biomaterials in the short term in order to alleviate pain, restore joint architecture, and increase functional mobility in diseased traumatized joints [1]. A major limiting factor to the service life of THRs remains the wear of the polyethylene acetabular cup. Preclinical endurance testing has become a standard procedure to predict the mechanical performance of new devices during implant development. Wear tests are performed on materials and designs used in prosthetic implants [1–3] to obtain quality control and acquire further knowledge on the tribological behavior in joint prostheses. To gain realistic results, a wear test should replicate the in vivo working conditions of the artificial implants [4]. However, it is well known that wear tests have a long duration and are expensive [1,5,6]. The simulation is run for several million cycles; assuming that one million cycles correspond to one year in vivo [7–9]. The running-in period encompasses approximately the first half a million cycles [10]; therefore, the steady-state wear is assessed by measuring the wear when the running-in period is over. Wear is measured either gravimetrically, measuring the weight loss of the component, or through a direct analysis of the volume that has been removed, optically or by coordinate-measuring [4,11–13].

Although in vitro wear evaluation of new medical devices is standardized [14], wear tests are not flexible enough. The prediction of wear in hip replacements has been a subject of intense study in recent years [15]. In silico investigation, where algorithms could be developed to model a biomedical process, is a logical extension of controlled in vitro experimentation. It is the natural result of the explosive increase in computing power available to scientists; thus, numerical models could be used to predict results of a wear test with less time and cost. Obviously, the in silico analysis integrates but does not replace the experimental tools.

Finite element analysis (FEA) has been widely used in many areas of biomechanics and biomechanical engineering to study parameters and boundary conditions, which are not accessible experimentally [15,16]. The numerical modeling tool of FEA has been widely applied to analyze the behavior of articular cartilage, joints, and bone structures under compressive and tensile stresses [17–21]. It was also used to improve the design of hip joint prostheses and to minimize experimental tests [22]. Structural applications include the design and development of joint prostheses and fracture fixation devices [23]. To make computational wear simulation meaningful, better wear models are needed, and those can only be built on experimental data that call for systematic experiments in which the relationships between the wear and the material properties, movements, lubrication, and loading are investigated.

FEA is a useful way to investigate the effects of changing parameters such as load, velocity, contact geometry, material properties, etc. This technique was introduced to orthopedic biomechanics in 1972 to evaluate stresses in a human bone [24]. Since then, it has been utilized with increasing frequency in the biomedical engineering context. FEA uses algorithms in which a domain is realized by a number of sub-domains referred to as elements [25,26]. The behavior of each element is readily defined and understood by numerical equations, which allow the study of complex behaviors of the entire body.

Many researchers use FEA to investigate the mechanical and tribological behavior of the most widespread hip implants. Maxian et al. [27] developed an adaptive re-meshing model to study the wear evolution on a long-term regime (20 years of follow up). He found that sliding distance was mainly responsible for the volumetric wear more than polyethylene thickness. Hu and collaborators [28] developed, in 2001, a fully thermo-mechanical coupled finite element model of a total hip prosthesis. The model simulating the wear test in a hip simulator was used to evaluate the transient contact stresses and to predict the rise of temperature due to the friction for different applied loads, sliding speeds, and frictional coefficients. Gao and co-workers [15] developed a wear model, on metal-on-metal hip replacements, which considered lubrication for the first time via a transient elastohydrodynamic lubrication regime. Sfantos et al. [29], on the other hand, performed a parametric study of the wear in total hip arthroplasty by using a boundary elements method.

The aim of this study was to develop a flexible finite element model, starting from the dynamic data retrieved by means of a multibody musculoskeletal model of the lower limb. In particular, in a previous work Ruggiero et al. [30] used this multibody model to estimate the loads and kinematic forces acting on the hip joint during walking and modelling with these inputs the deformation of an acetabular cup. Our study reported here focused on the influence that the radial clearance, namely the difference between the inner radius of the cup (R_c) and the radius of the femoral head (R_h)—see Figure 1—has on the pressure and deformation of the acetabular cup in a hard-on-soft bearing.

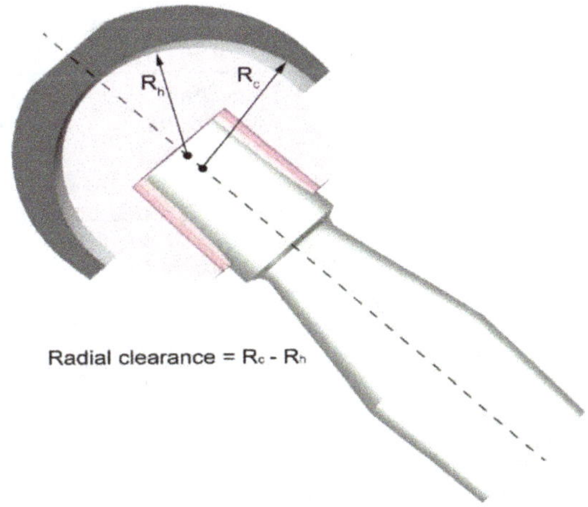

Figure 1. Schematization of the radial clearance between the inner surface of the acetabular cup (grey component in the picture) and the outer surface of the femoral head (pink component in the picture).

2. Materials and Methods

2.1. Finite Element Analysis (FEA) Model

Workbench Ansys® Software (v. 18.1, ANSYS Inc., Canonsburg, PA, USA) was used for the realization of the finite elements model. The model considered the hard-on-soft bearing configuration, typical of the most widespread hip implants [31]. To solve the contact problem, the solution algorithm must establish a relationship between the interacting surfaces, preventing the interpenetration. The software enforces contact compatibility through a penalty-based formulation that in this study is the augmented Lagrange, with a program-controlled penetration tolerance. With this formulation, a direct proportionality between the applied force and the penetration, where the coefficient is a contact stiffness, is established. Furthermore, the force is augmented by an extra term, making this method less sensitive to the magnitude of the contact stiffness. An asymmetric behavior was chosen for the contact, where the target body was the head and the contact body the cup, as all the resulting data belong to the contact side.

The simulations were performed comparing the effect of different clearances ranging from zero to 0.5 mm, namely 0, 0.05, 0.25 and 0.5 mm. The comparisons were in terms of magnitude and distribution of the contact pressure and of the deformation at the interface. As the sliding surfaces play a key role in the tribological performance of hip implants, the presence of the frictional force was considered. The coefficient of friction was obtained from experimental activities [32,33], considering a dry contact, and corresponded to 0.13. Even though the surface roughness could influence the friction and wear of a joint [34,35], the ease of computation and the very fine roughness—typical of actual hip replacements—led to a discharge of this aspect in the study. Contact area, pressure, and deformation were computed as a function of the angular displacements and dynamic loading calculated through a musculoskeletal model. Force components and orientations will be defined with respect to a pelvic reference frame that coincides with the true anatomic superior, anterior, and lateral directions.

Ultra-high-molecular-weight polyethylene (UHMWPE) type GUR 1050, was chosen for the acetabular cup whereas an infinitely rigid body was chosen as the femoral head, which is commonly realized in metal or ceramic. This choice is justified by the assumption that the site of wear interest is almost exclusively the soft body of the joint. Table 1 presents the main parameters of the acetabular cup material [36]. The presence of the pelvic bone has been neglected, since it has little influence on contact pressure [37]. The femoral head had a diameter of 28 mm, whereas the acetabular cup had a thickness of 5 mm. The cup was oriented with an anterior–posterior angle of 45°, and an inclination angle of 0°, these angles derived directly from the musculoskeletal model, from which forces and displacements were obtained. Therefore, it was not necessary to impose further inclination in the model.

Table 1. UHMWPE GUR 1050 properties.

Density	Young's Modulus	Poisson's Ratio	Bulk Modulus	Shear Modulus	Tensile Yield Strength	Tensile Ultimate Strength
(kg m^{-3})	(MPa)	(-)	(MPa)	(MPa)	(MPa)	(MPa)
930	690	0.46	1640	241	21	40

The finite element model is shown in Figure 2. A convergence study was performed to determine the optimum mesh aspect; contact pressure and cup deformation were used as performance metrics. For the cup the tetra patch conforming and tetra patch independent, the hex dominant quadrilateral/triangular and all quadrilateral, multizone hexagonal were compared; for the head, quadrilateral and triangular elements were compared. Regarding the head, quadratic elements were selected, for the cup a multizone hexagonal/prismatic hexagonal dominant meshing was chosen. The meshing of the entire model generated a total of 2012 elements and 3283 nodes, having 383 contact elements (Conta174 for the cup and Targe170 for the head). Elements of the mesh, having a minimum edge length of 53.7 mm, presented an average quality of 0.759 ± 0.152 and an average aspect ratio of 2.144.

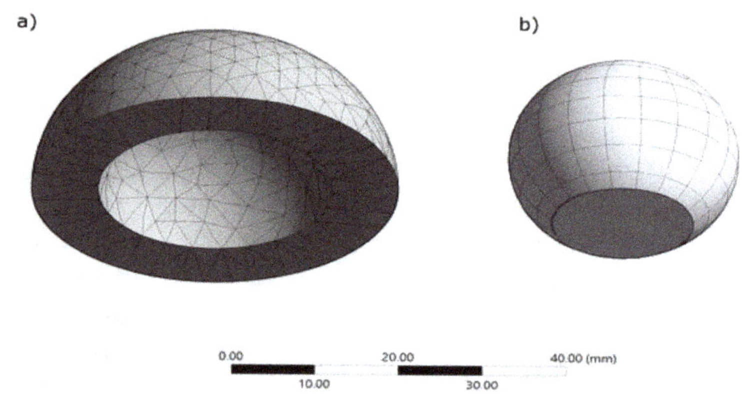

Figure 2. Meshing on (**a**) the acetabular cup and the (**b**) femoral head.

The input data obtained by the multibody system are in a local coordinates system, which follows the movements of the femoral head. As the software requires a global coordinates system, a conversion was required by using the rotational matrix. The three rotations around the axes are the Flexion/Extension (*Z* axes), Abduction/Adduction (*X* axes) and Inward/Outward (*Y* axes) (see Figure 3).

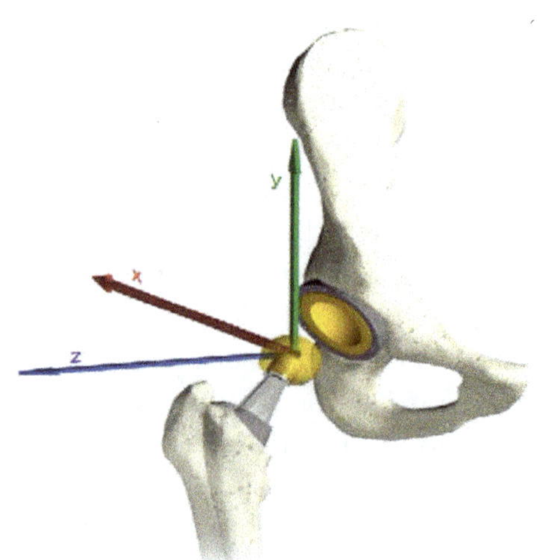

Figure 3. The three force directions.

2.2. Gait Cycles and Loads

In this study, we used musculoskeletal modeling software, to estimate loads acting on the hip joint during level walking. AnyBody Modelling System^{TM} (AnyBody Technology A/S, Aalborg, Denmark) is a musculoskeletal modeling and simulation software. It combines the principles of the inverse dynamics with different algorithms to define the muscle recruitment and analyze the loads acting on different joints of the human body [38]. To calculate the joint forces, the kinematic data and ground reaction force must be known and used as inputs. These data are collected using special motion capture tools in the gait analysis laboratories [39], which measure a subject gait by means of cameras that monitor markers on the person's skin.

In inverse dynamics, the motion and the external loads on the body are known, and the aim is finding internal forces. Since not enough equilibrium equations are available to solve the problem, the evaluation of the muscle forces is made possible by the so-called redundancy problem. The working method of the AnyBody Modelling System is amply defined in [38], stating that there is the need to use an algorithm to find the activation of the muscles to reproduce the function of the central nervous system. The resolution of the multibody problem is already described in a previous work [30].

3. Results

The force components and rotations, obtained from the multibody analysis, are shown in Figure 4, plotted along the gait cycle percentage.

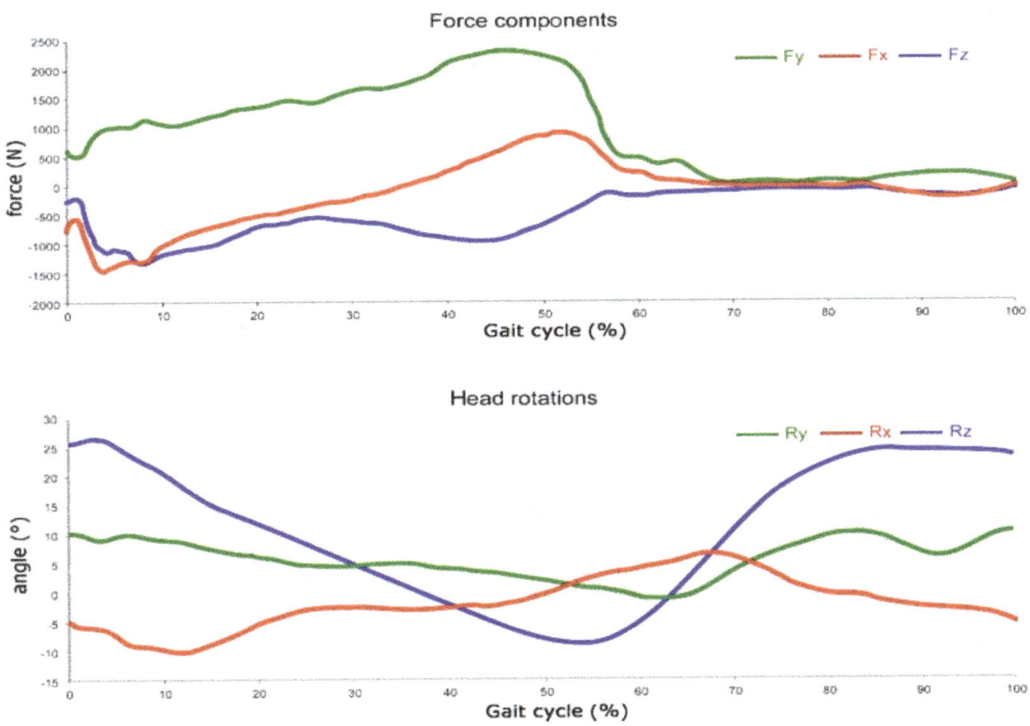

Figure 4. Forces and rotations obtained from multibody.

In Figure 5, pressure distribution, on the sliding surface of the acetabular cup during different steps are shown. Along with the cycle progressing, it is possible to observe the distributions of pressure and its magnitude. The rotation of the head (suppressed in the images for a better understanding) varies with the position of the highest value of pressure. When the pressure reaches its maximum values along the cycle, its major magnitude is in the edge zone of the cup.

In Figures 6 and 7 are the comparisons of the radial clearance on the pressure and the deformation, expressed in terms of the maximum value found on the inner surface of the cup in each timeframe.

From these images it is possible to highlight the divergences due to the clearance and the two peaks along the cycle. The presence of the two moments of high pressure and deformation already found in the previous analysis is clear.

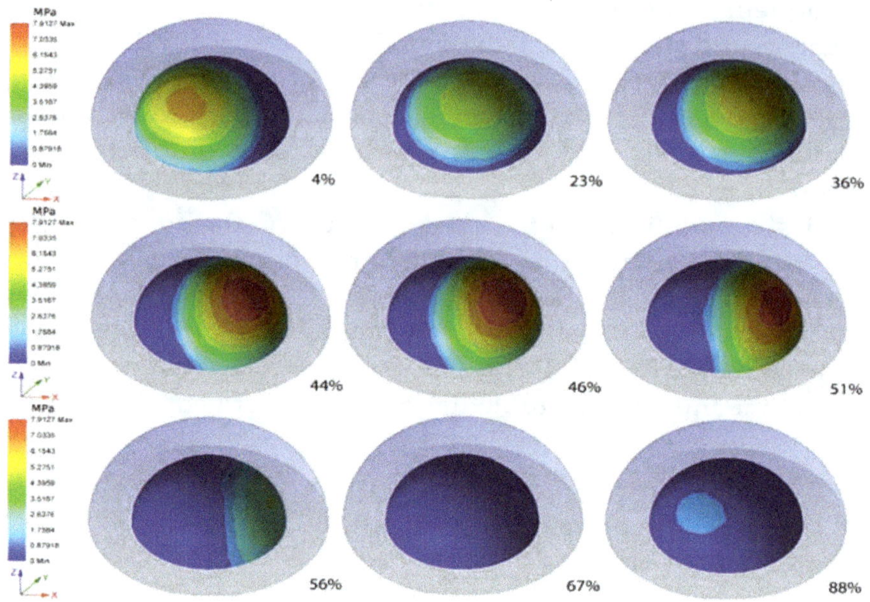

Figure 5. Pressure of the cup in several steps, as expresses in term of gait cycle percentage below each image.

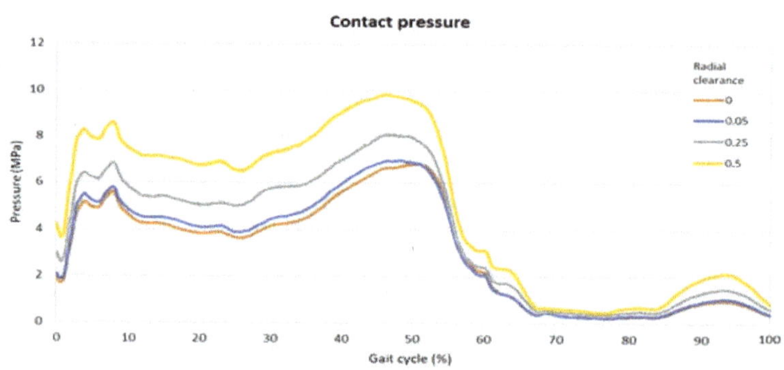

Figure 6. Maximum values of the pressure on the contact surface for different radial clearances.

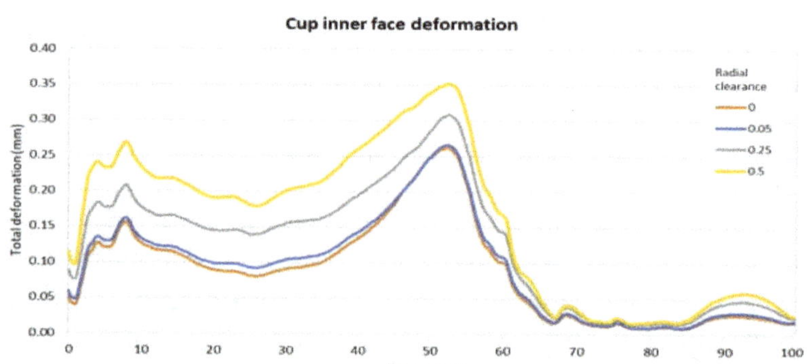

Figure 7. Maximum values of the deformation on the inner surface of the acetabular cup for different radial clearances.

Table 2 presents the highest values along the gait cycle found for pressure and deformation, comparing the radial clearances. These values were all located around the middle of the gait cycle, i.e., nearly 50%.

Table 2. Maximum values along the gait cycle of the pressure and deformation on the inner face of the cup.

Radial clearance	0	0.05	0.25	0.5
Maximum pressure (MPa)	6.82	7.00	8.12	9.84
Maximum deformation (mm)	0.26	0.27	0.31	0.35

4. Discussion

The increasing number of tribology studies to analyze polyethylene wear in total hip arthroplasty confirms the need for improved understanding and new solutions to avoid the failure of an implant due to polyethylene wear. Wear tests are performed on biomedical materials to solve or reduce failures or malfunctions due to material loss. It is well known that pre-clinical validation is considered as an extension in the risk analysis task, and wear tests in prosthetic hip implants are necessary in order to acquire quality control and further knowledge about the tribological processes in joint prostheses [7]. The "gold standard" accepted preclinical method to evaluate the wear performance of a hip implant design in the laboratory is performed using a joint simulator that simulates the physiological loadings and movements of the patients; these machines give important outcomes about the expected behavior of a hip implant in clinical use [7,30]. FEA methodology has been used for many years as a numerical technique to solve engineering problems related to stress and strain analysis of static or dynamic loaded contacts. The technique incorporates the principles of Newtonian mechanics to model and animate the realistic behavior of such contacts [40,41]. In addition, experimental studies are currently used, but they are quite expensive and time-consuming. In addition, these studies can analyze only limited configurations and load conditions. Some authors [42–45] used different protocols than those recommended by the ISO standard for hip and knee joint simulation [14,46,47] considering highly demanding activities such as stair climbing, chair sitting, squats, etc. Unfortunately, all these experimental approaches are time-consuming and very expensive. For these reasons, the use of computational modeling is expanding also in this orthopedic field, but unfortunately, few published papers present validated wear models to use.

The aim of this study was to investigate the influence of the radial clearance on the pressure and deformation of an acetabular cup made of UHMWPE. The investigation based its input data on a musculoskeletal multibody model, solved for a walking cycle. The results showed the behavior of the inner face of the cup, which is subjected to a dynamic pressure, changing magnitude and orientation along the gait cycle. In detail, the side zones of the cup are subjected to an elevated pressure during the first and last touching moments of the feet on the ground, when there is the impact and the release. These instants are known as heel strike and toe off, and their occurrence corresponds to an elevated bending in flexion.

The values of pressure find their agreement with previous studies, like the one performed by Liu et al. [16], where the maximum pressure corresponded to 8 MPa. The study on wear performed by Mattei et al. [48] showed a contact pressure of 8.2 MPa in correspondence with the maximum load. In the work of Matsoukas et al. [49] the highest values were almost 8 MPa and 12 MPa for the von Mises pressure and the contact pressure, respectively. These values were found in correspondence with the second peak of the stance phase, plus the pressure distribution concentrates in the edge zone of the cup. Maxian et al. [50] found a similar distribution of pressure reaching a maximum value of 9 MPa. The small differences that we found can be attributed to the dynamic loading retrieved from the musculoskeletal model, which differ from the standardized loads used in the literature. It is believed that before improving and making a more complex algorithm to find wear in silico, taking also into account realistic lubrication models, there is a need to apply more flexible and reliable loads as used in this study.

The comparison across the different radial clearance values highlighted that the there is a sensible divergence in term of pressure and deformation. From the 0 value of radial clearance to the highest, 0.5, there is a difference of 44% and 35% in terms of maximum pressure and deformation, respectively. This increment can be attributed to the modification of the contact distribution. In fact, when two convex–concave bodies pressing against each other are in perfect compliance the load is distributed across a wider area than if the same two bodies differ in dimension. Having a highly conformal contact means a wide area where forces are distributed and therefore a smaller pressure amplitude. As a consequence of a less intense pressure, the maximum values of the deformation are also smaller.

There is a very small variation between the two close cases of no clearance and 0.05 mm. In detail, the difference of these conditions is limited to the 3% of the maximum pressure and 4% of the maximum deformation. This variation is so little that it can be discarded in a first approximation, but even such a small difference can be relevant when lubrication comes into play. Lubrication in fact is dependent on different factors such as the viscosity of the lubricant, the finishing of the surfaces, and the shape of them. Research has demonstrated that lubricated hip joints could be modelled as a ball-in-socket or ball-on-plane equivalent configuration in boundary, mixed or hydrodynamic/elastohydrodynamic lubrication regimes. In this configuration, small radial clearances may benefit from lubrication phenomena by increasing minimum film thickness. Moreover, the greater entraining velocity in correspondence with low clearances could favor the hydrodynamic lubricating fluid film with a consequential positive effects on wear [24,51–54].

Obviously, our study has a number of limitations. The first limitation is due to the fact that our model was not validated experimentally on an in vitro simulation but it was validated only by comparison with international literature. It is stressed, however, that our model is in agreement with other in silico models. The second limitation is that our model was developed for a diameter of 28 mm, further studies are necessary to find out if there are differences with other dimensions. The model considered a single orientation of the cup, which is believed to be valid as stated by other studies [22], but limits its application to the specific case. Different cup inclination angles can influence the contact zone, as reported in the work of Hua et al. [55]: By increasing the cup inclination "the microseparation distances required to generate edge loading decreased". Other factors, such as additional effects of contact mechanics, or mechanics associated with three-body wear, temperature, and lubrication were not incorporated in this model and remain to be modelled.

5. Conclusions

The proposed finite element model allowed us to investigate the tribo-mechanical behavior of a hip implant subjected to dynamic loads derived from a multibody musculoskeletal model. The study focused on the differences found in pressure and deformation, in terms of distribution and amplitude, by varying the radial clearance in the range of 0–0.5 mm. The results highlighted the following main findings:

- along the walking cycle, the heel strike and the toe off are the instants of highest pressure, against these points the maximum pressure is located on the lateral side of the cup;
- radial clearance plays a substantial role on pressure and deformation magnitude across the gait cycle: the higher the clearance, the higher the pressure. Nevertheless, reducing the clearance to the smallest possible value is believed to affect the bearing lubrication;
- since radial clearance plays a key role in the lubricating phenomena, the proposed finite element model will be useful to exploit in the complete lubrication modelling of the joint toward a more and more realistic assessment of the in silico wear, accounting also for different radial clearances.

Author Contributions: S.A. and A.R. conceived and designed the investigation; S.A. developed the scientific framework; A.R. performed the multibody dynamical analysis; A.R. and M.M. developed the FEM model; S.A. and

M.M. selected the interest cases and analyzed the calculated data; S.A. and A.R. discussed the results; S.A., M.M. and A.R. wrote the paper.

Acknowledgments: The authors thank Simone Di Stasio for his key contribution to finite element modelling and Luigi Lena (Rizzoli Orthopaedic Institute) for his valuable help with the pictures.

References

1. Affatato, S.; Freccero, N.; Taddei, P. The biomaterials challenge: A comparison of polyethylene wear using a hip joint simulator. *J. Mech. Behav. Biomed. Mater.* **2016**, *53*, 40–48. [CrossRef] [PubMed]
2. Affatato, S.; Bersaglia, G.; Emiliani, D.; Foltran, I.; Taddei, P.; Reggiani, M.; Ferrieri, P.; Toni, A. The performance of gamma- and EtO-sterilised UHMWPE acetabular cups tested under severe simulator conditions. Part 2: Wear particle characteristics with isolation protocols. *Biomaterials* **2003**, *24*, 4045–4055. [CrossRef]
3. Affatato, S.; Bersaglia, G.; Rocchi, M.; Taddei, P.; Fagnano, C.; Toni, A. Wear behaviour of cross-linked polyethylene assessed in vitro under severe conditions. *Biomaterials* **2005**, *26*, 3259–3267. [CrossRef] [PubMed]
4. Grillini, L.; Affatato, S. How to measure wear following total hip arthroplasty. *Hip Int.* **2013**, *23*, 233–242. [CrossRef] [PubMed]
5. Affatato, S.; Zavalloni, M.; Spinelli, M.; Costa, L.; Bracco, P.; Viceconti, M. Long-term in-vitro wear performance of an innovative thermo-compressed cross-linked polyethylene. *Tribol. Int.* **2010**, *43*, 22–28. [CrossRef]
6. Affatato, S.; Testoni, M.; Cacciari, G.L.; Toni, A. Mixed oxides prosthetic ceramic ball heads. Part 2: Effect of the ZrO_2 fraction on the wear of ceramic on ceramic joints. *Biomaterials* **1999**, *20*, 971–975. [CrossRef]
7. Affatato, S.; Spinelli, M.; Zavalloni, M.; Mazzega-Fabbro, C.; Viceconti, M. Tribology and total hip joint replacement: Current concepts in mechanical simulation. *Med. Eng. Phys.* **2008**, *30*, 1305–1317. [CrossRef] [PubMed]
8. Dumbleton, J.H. *Tribology of Natural and Artificial Joints*; Elsevier: New York, NY, USA, 1981.
9. Petersen, D.; Link, R.; Wang, A.; Polineni, V.; Essner, A.; Sokol, M.; Sun, D.; Stark, C.; Dumbleton, J. The Significance of Nonlinear Motion in the Wear Screening of Orthopaedic Implant Materials. *J. Test. Eval.* **1997**, *25*, 239. [CrossRef]
10. Affatato, S.; Bersaglia, G.; Foltran, I.; Emiliani, D.; Traina, F.; Toni, A. The influence of implant position on the wear of alumina-on-alumina studied in a hip simulator. *Wear* **2004**, *256*, 400–405. [CrossRef]
11. Zanini, F.; Carmignato, S.; Savio, E.; Affatato, S. Uncertainty determination for X-ray computed tomography wear assessment of polyethylene hip joint prostheses. *Precis. Eng.* **2018**, *52*, 477–483. [CrossRef]
12. Affatato, S.; Valigi, M.C.; Logozzo, S. Wear distribution detection of knee joint prostheses by means of 3D optical scanners. *Materials (Basel)* **2017**, *10*, 364. [CrossRef] [PubMed]
13. Affatato, S.; Zanini, F.; Carmignato, S. Quantification of wear and deformation in different configurations of polyethylene acetabular cups using micro X-ray computed tomography. *Materials (Basel)* **2017**, *10*, 259. [CrossRef] [PubMed]
14. *ISO DIS 14242–1–Implants for Surgery–Wear of Total Hip-Joint Prostheses–Part 1: Loading and Displacement Paramenters for Wear–Testing Machines and Corresponding Environmental Conditions for Test*; International Organization for Standardization: Geneva, Switzerland, 2012.
15. Gao, L.; Dowson, D.; Hewson, R.W. Predictive wear modeling of the articulating metal-on-metal hip replacements. *J. Biomed. Mater. Res. Part B Appl. Biomater.* **2017**, *105B*, 497–506. [CrossRef] [PubMed]
16. Liu, F.; Fisher, J.; Jin, Z. Computational modelling of polyethylene wear and creep in total hip joint replacements: Effect of the bearing clearance and diameter. *Proc. Inst. Mech. Eng. Part J J. Eng. Tribol.* **2012**, *226*, 552–563. [CrossRef]
17. Suh, J.-K.; Bai, S. Finite Element Formulation of Biphasic Poroviscoelastic Model for Articular Cartilage. *J. Biomech. Eng.* **1998**, *120*, 195. [CrossRef] [PubMed]

18. Töyräs, J.; Saarakkala, S.; Laasanen, M.S.; Töyräs, J.; Korhonen, R.K.; Rieppo, J.; Saarakkala, S.; Nieminen, M.T.; Hirvonen, J.; Jurvelin, J.S. Biomechanical properties of knee articular cartilage. *Biorheology* **2003**, *40*, 133–140.
19. Li, G.; Gil, J.; Kanamori, A.; Woo, S.L.-Y. A Validated Three-Dimensional Computational Model of a Human Knee Joint. *J. Biomech. Eng.* **1999**, *121*, 657. [CrossRef] [PubMed]
20. Amirouche, F.; Solitro, G.; Broviak, S.; Goldstein, W.; Gonzalez, M.; Barmada, R. Primary cup stability in THA with augmentation of acetabular defect. A comparison of healthy and osteoporotic bone. *Orthop. Traumatol. Surg. Res.* **2015**, *101*, 667–673. [CrossRef] [PubMed]
21. Ghosh, R. Assessment of failure of cemented polyethylene acetabular component due to bone remodeling: A finite element study. *J. Orthop.* **2016**, *13*, 140–147. [CrossRef] [PubMed]
22. Uddin, M.S.; Zhang, L.C. Predicting the wear of hard-on-hard hip joint prostheses. *Wear* **2013**, *301*, 192–200. [CrossRef]
23. Huiskes, R.; Chao, E.Y.S.; Crippen, T.E. Parametric analyses of pin-bone stresses in external fracture fixation devices. *J. Orthop. Res.* **1985**, *3*, 341–349. [CrossRef] [PubMed]
24. Smith, S.; Dowson, D.; Goldsmith, A. The effect of diametral clearance, motion and loading cycles upon lubrication of metal-on-metal total hip replacements. *Proc. Inst. Mech. Eng. Part C* **2001**, *215*, 1–5. [CrossRef]
25. Felippa, C.A. Introduction to Finite Element Methods. 2004. Available online: https://www.colorado.edu/engineering/Aerospace/CAS/courses.d/IFEM.d/IFEM.Ch00.d/IFEM.Ch00.pdf (accessed on 19 July 2018).
26. Herrera, A.; Ibarz, E.; Cegoñino, J.; Lobo-escolar, A.; Puértolas, S.; López, E.; Gracia, L.; Herrera, A.; Lobo-escolar, A.; Mateo, J. Applications of finite element simulation in orthopedic and trauma surgery. *World J. Othop.* **2012**, *3*, 25–41. [CrossRef] [PubMed]
27. Maxian, T.A.; Brown, T.D.; Pedersen, D.R.; Callaghan, J.J. Adaptiive finite element modeling of long-term polyethylene wear in total hip arthroplasty. *J. Orthop. Res.* **1996**, *14*, 668–675. [CrossRef] [PubMed]
28. Hu, C.; Liau, J.; Lung, C.; Huang, C.; Cheng, C. A two-dimensional finite element model for frictional heating analysis of total hip prosthesis. *Mater. Sci. Eng. C* **2001**, *17*, 11–18. [CrossRef]
29. Sfantos, G.K.; Aliabadi, M.H.Ã. Total hip arthroplasty wear simulation using the boundary element method. *J. Biomech.* **2007**, *40*, 378–389. [CrossRef] [PubMed]
30. Ruggiero, A.; Merola, M.; Affatato, S. Finite element simulations of hard-on-soft hip joint prosthesis accounting for dynamic loads calculated from a Musculoskeletal model during walking. *Materials (Basel)* **2018**, *11*, 574. [CrossRef] [PubMed]
31. Affatato, S.; Ruggiero, A.; Merola, M. Advanced biomaterials in hip joint arthroplasty. A review on polymer and ceramics composites as alternative bearings. *Compos. Part B Eng.* **2015**, *83*, 276–283. [CrossRef]
32. Ruggiero, A.; D'Amato, R.; Gómez, E.; Merola, M. Experimental comparison on tribological pairs UHMWPE/TIAL6V4 alloy, UHMWPE/AISI316L austenitic stainless and UHMWPE/AL_2O_3 ceramic, under dry and lubricated conditions. *Tribol. Int.* **2016**, *96*, 349–360. [CrossRef]
33. Ruggiero, A.; D'Amato, R.; Gómez, E. Experimental analysis of tribological behavior of UHMWPE against AISI420C and against TiAl6V4 alloy under dry and lubricated conditions. *Tribol. Int.* **2015**, *92*, 154–161. [CrossRef]
34. Affatato, S.; Ruggiero, A.; De Mattia, J.S.; Taddei, P. Does metal transfer affect the tribological behaviour of femoral heads? Roughness and phase transformation analyses on retrieved zirconia and Biolox® Delta composites. *Compos. Part B Eng.* **2016**, *92*, 290–298. [CrossRef]
35. Affatato, S.; Ruggiero, A.; Merola, M.; Logozzo, S. Does metal transfer differ on retrieved Biolox® Delta composites femoral heads? Surface investigation on three Biolox® generations from a biotribological point of view. *Compos. Part B Eng.* **2017**, *113*, 164–173. [CrossRef]
36. Laurian, T.; Tudor, A. Some Aspects Regarding the Influence of the Clearance on the Pressure Distribution in Total Hip Joint Prostheses. In Proceeding of the National Tribology Conference RotTrib03, Annals, Galati, Romania, 24–26 September 2003.
37. Barreto, S.; Folgado, J.; Fernandes, P.R.; Monteiro, J. The Influence of the Pelvic Bone on the Computational Results of the Acetabular Component of a Total Hip Prosthesis. *J. Biomech. Eng.* **2010**, *132*, 54503. [CrossRef] [PubMed]
38. Damsgaard, M.; Rasmussen, J.; Christensen, S.T.; Surma, E.; de Zee, M. Analysis of musculoskeletal systems in the AnyBody Modeling System. *Simul. Model. Pract. Theory* **2006**, *14*, 1100–1111. [CrossRef]

39. Vaughan, C.; Davis, B.L.; O'Connor, J.C. Dynamics of Human Gait. Available online: https://isbweb.org/data/ (accessed on 6 April 2018).
40. Prati, E.; Freddi, A.; Ranieri, L.; Toni, A. Comparative fatigue damage analysis of hip-joint prostheses. *J Biomech.* **1982**, *15*, 808. [CrossRef]
41. Huiskes, R.; Chao, E.Y.S. A survey of finite element analysis in orthopaedic biomechanics: The first decade. *J. Biomech.* **1983**, *16*, 385–409. [CrossRef]
42. Abdel-Jaber, S.; Belvedere, C.; Leardini, Al.; Affatato, S.; Abdel Jaber, S.; Belvedere, C.; Leardini, Al.; Affatato, S. Wear simulation of total knee prostheses using load and kinematics waveforms from stair climbing. *J. Biomech.* **2015**, *48*, 3830–3836. [CrossRef] [PubMed]
43. Abdel-Jaber, S.; Belvedere, C.; De Mattia, J.S.; Leardini, A.; Affatato, S. A new protocol for wear testing of total knee prostheses from real joint kinematic data: Towards a scenario of realistic simulations of daily living activities. *J. Biomech.* **2016**, *49*, 2925–2931. [CrossRef] [PubMed]
44. Battaglia, S.; Belvedere, C.; Jaber, S.A.; Affatato, S.; D'Angeli, V.; Leardini, A. A new protocol from real joint motion data for wear simulation in total knee arthroplasty: Stair climbing. *Med. Eng. Phys.* **2014**, *36*, 1605–1610. [CrossRef] [PubMed]
45. Affatato, S. Towards wear testing of high demanding.pdf. *J Brazilian Soc. Mech. Sci. Eng.* **2018**, *40*, 260–266. [CrossRef]
46. *ISO-14243–2–Implants for Surgery–Wear of Total Knee-Joint Prostheses–Part 2: Methods of Measurement*; International Organization for Standardization: Geneva, Switzerland, 2000.
47. *ISO DIS 14243–3–Implants for Surgery–Wear of Total Knee Joint Prostheses–Part 1: Loading and Displacement Paramenters for Wear-Testing Machines with Displacement Control and Corresponding Environmental Conditions for Test*; International Organization for Standardization: Geneva, Switzerland, 2004.
48. Mattei, L.; Di Puccio, F.; Ciulli, E. A comparative study of wear laws for soft-on-hard hip implants using a mathematical wear model. *Tribol. Int.* **2013**, *63*, 66–77. [CrossRef]
49. Matsoukas, G.; Willing, R.; Kim, I.Y. Total Hip Wear Assessment: A Comparison Between Computational and In Vitro Wear Assessment Techniques Using ISO 14242 Loading and Kinematics. *J. Biomech. Eng.* **2009**, *131*, 41011. [CrossRef] [PubMed]
50. Maxian, T.A.; Brown, T.D.; Pedersen, D.R.; Callaghan, J.J. A sliding-distance-coupled finite element formulation for polyethylene wear in total hip arthroplasty. *J. Biomech.* **1996**, *29*, 687–692. [CrossRef]
51. Jin, Z.M.; Dowson, D. A full numerical analysis of hydrodynamic lubrication in artificial hip joint replacements constructed from hard materials. *Proc. Inst. Mech. Eng. Part C J. Mech. Eng. Sci.* **1999**, *213*, 355–370. [CrossRef]
52. Jalali-Vahid, D.; Jagatia, M.; Jin, Z.M.; Dowson, D. Prediction of lubricating film thickness in UHMWPE hip joint replacements. *J. Biomech.* **2001**, *34*, 261–266. [CrossRef]
53. Ruggiero, A.; Gòmez, E.; D'Amato, R. Approximate analytical model for the squeeze-film lubrication of the human ankle joint with synovial fluid filtrated by articular cartilage. *Tribol. Lett.* **2011**, *41*, 337–343. [CrossRef]
54. Ruggiero, A.; Gómez, E.; D'Amato, R. Approximate closed-form solution of the synovial fluid film force in the human ankle joint with non-Newtonian lubricant. *Tribol. Int.* **2013**, *57*, 156–161. [CrossRef]
55. Hua, X.; Li, J.; Wang, L.; Jin, Z.; Wilcox, R.; Fisher, J. Contact mechanics of modular metal-on-polyethylene total hip replacement under adverse edge loading conditions. *J. Biomech.* **2014**, *47*, 3303–3309. [CrossRef] [PubMed]

Permissions

All chapters in this book were first published by MDPI; hereby published with permission under the Creative Commons Attribution License or equivalent. Every chapter published in this book has been scrutinized by our experts. Their significance has been extensively debated. The topics covered herein carry significant findings which will fuel the growth of the discipline. They may even be implemented as practical applications or may be referred to as a beginning point for another development.

The contributors of this book come from diverse backgrounds, making this book a truly international effort. This book will bring forth new frontiers with its revolutionizing research information and detailed analysis of the nascent developments around the world.

We would like to thank all the contributing authors for lending their expertise to make the book truly unique. They have played a crucial role in the development of this book. Without their invaluable contributions this book wouldn't have been possible. They have made vital efforts to compile up to date information on the varied aspects of this subject to make this book a valuable addition to the collection of many professionals and students.

This book was conceptualized with the vision of imparting up-to-date information and advanced data in this field. To ensure the same, a matchless editorial board was set up. Every individual on the board went through rigorous rounds of assessment to prove their worth. After which they invested a large part of their time researching and compiling the most relevant data for our readers.

The editorial board has been involved in producing this book since its inception. They have spent rigorous hours researching and exploring the diverse topics which have resulted in the successful publishing of this book. They have passed on their knowledge of decades through this book. To expedite this challenging task, the publisher supported the team at every step. A small team of assistant editors was also appointed to further simplify the editing procedure and attain best results for the readers.

Apart from the editorial board, the designing team has also invested a significant amount of their time in understanding the subject and creating the most relevant covers. They scrutinized every image to scout for the most suitable representation of the subject and create an appropriate cover for the book.

The publishing team has been an ardent support to the editorial, designing and production team. Their endless efforts to recruit the best for this project, has resulted in the accomplishment of this book. They are a veteran in the field of academics and their pool of knowledge is as vast as their experience in printing. Their expertise and guidance has proved useful at every step. Their uncompromising quality standards have made this book an exceptional effort. Their encouragement from time to time has been an inspiration for everyone.

The publisher and the editorial board hope that this book will prove to be a valuable piece of knowledge for researchers, students, practitioners and scholars across the globe.

List of Contributors

Kazuhiro Imai, Xiao Zhou and Xiaoxuan Liu
Department of Life Sciences, Graduate School of Arts and Sciences, The University of Tokyo, Tokyo 153-8902, Japan

Marcus Jäger and Florian Dittrich
Department of Orthopaedics and Trauma Surgery, University of Duisburg-Essen, Hufelandstrasse 55, D-45147 Essen, Germany

Herbert P. Jennissen
Department of Orthopaedics and Trauma Surgery, University of Duisburg-Essen, Hufelandstrasse 55, D-45147 Essen, Germany
Institute of Physiological Chemistry, University Hospital, University of Duisburg Essen, Hufelandstrasse 55, D-45147 Essen, Germany

Alfons Fischer
Institute of Metal Engineering, University of Duisburg-Essen, Campus Duisburg, Lotharstraße 1, D-47057 Duisburg, Germany

Hedda Luise Köhling
Institute of Medical Microbiology, University of Duisburg-Essen, Virchowstr. 179, D-45147 Essen, Germany

Chris Steffi, Zhilong Shi, Chee Hoe Kong and Wilson Wang
Department of Orthopaedic Surgery, Yong Loo Lin School of Medicine, National University of Singapore, NUHS Tower Block, Level 11, 1E Kent Ridge Road, Singapore 119228, Singapore

Alice Acciaioli, Giacomo Lionello and Massimiliano Baleani
IRCCS—Istituto Ortopedico Rizzoli, Laboratorio di Tecnologia Medica, 40136 Bologna, Italy

Wei Xu, Ming Li, Shaomin Lv and Chengcheng Liu
Institute for Advanced Materials and Technology, University of Science and Technology Beijing, Beijing 100083, China

Cuie Wen
School of Engineering, RMIT University, 3083 Melbourne, Australia

Xin Lu and Xuanhui Qu
Institute for Advanced Materials and Technology, University of Science and Technology Beijing, Beijing 100083, China
Beijing Key Laboratory for Advanced Powder Metallurgy and Particulate Materials, University of Science and Technology Beijing, Beijing 100083, China
Beijing Laboratory of Metallic Materials and Processing for Modern Transportation, University of Science and Technology Beijing, Beijing 100083, China

Żaneta Anna Mierzejewska
Faculty of Mechanical Engineering, Bialystok University of Technology, Wiejska 45c Street, 15-351 Białystok, Poland

Sami Abdel Jaber
Medical Technology Laboratory, IRCCS—Rizzoli Orthopaedic Institute, Via di Barbiano, 1/10, 40136 Bologna, Italy

Pierangiola Bracco
Chemistry Department and Nanostructured Interfaces and Surfaces (NIS) Centre, University of Turin, Via Giuria 7, 10125 Turin, Italy

Yong-Gon Koh
Joint Reconstruction Center, Department of Orthopaedic Surgery, Yonsei Sarang Hospital, 10 Hyoryeong-ro, Seocho-gu, Seoul 06698, Korea
Department of Mechanical Engineering, Yonsei University, 50 Yonsei-ro, Seodaemun-gu, Seoul 03722, Korea

Hyoung-Taek Hong and Kyoung-Tak Kang
Department of Mechanical Engineering, Yonsei University, 50 Yonsei-ro, Seodaemun-gu, Seoul 03722, Korea

Muhammad Jamshaid Zafar, Dongbin Zhu and Zhengyan Zhang
School of Mechanical Engineering, Hebei University of Technology, Tianjin 300130, China

Blanca Teresa Perez-Maceda, María Encarnación López-Fernández and Rosa María Lozano
Cell-Biomaterial Recognition Lab., Department of Cellular and Molecular Biology, Centro de Investigaciones Biológicas (CIB-CSIC), Ramiro de Maeztu 9, 28040 Madrid, Spain

Iván Díaz, María Lorenza Escudero and María Cristina García-Alonso
Department of Surface Engineering, Corrosion and Durability, Centro Nacional de Investigaciones Metalúrgicas (CENIM-CSIC), Avda. Gregorio del Amo 8, 28040 Madrid, Spain

Aaron Kavanaugh and Fabrizio Billi
Department of Orthopaedic Surgery, David Geffen School of Medicine, University of California Los Angeles, Orthopaedic Hospital Research Center, 615 Charles E. Young Dr. South, Room 450A, Los Angeles, CA 90095, USA

Rafał Zieliński and Marcin Kozakiewicz
Department of Maxillofacial Surgery, Medical University of Lodz, 1st Haller Plac, 90-647 Lodz, Poland

Jacek Świniarski
Department of Strength of Materials and Structures, Technical University of Lodz, Stefanowskiego 1/15, 90-924 Lodz, Poland

Saverio Affatato
Medical Technology Laboratory, IRCCS–Rizzoli Orthopaedic Institute, Via di Barbiano, 1/10, 40136 Bologna, Italy

Massimiliano Merola
Department of Industrial Engineering, University of Salerno, 84084 Fisciano, Italy
Medical Technology Laboratory, IRCCS–Rizzoli Orthopaedic Institute, Via di Barbiano, 1/10, 40136 Bologna, Italy

Alessandro Ruggiero
Department of Industrial Engineering, University of Salerno, Via Giovanni Paolo II, nr. 132, 84084 Fisciano, Italy

Index

www.ingramcontent.com/pod-product-compliance
Lightning Source LLC
LaVergne TN
LVHW081014210926
848485LV00004B/859